D1595617

Miraculous Plagues

Miraculous Plagues

*An Epidemiology of Early
New England Narrative*

CRISTOBAL SILVA

OXFORD
UNIVERSITY PRESS

OXFORD
UNIVERSITY PRESS

Oxford University Press

Oxford University Press, Inc., publishes works that further
Oxford University's objective of excellence
in research, scholarship, and education.

Oxford New York

Auckland   Cape Town   Dar es Salaam   Hong Kong   Karachi
Kuala Lumpur   Madrid   Melbourne   Mexico City   Nairobi
New Delhi   Shanghai   Taipei   Toronto

With offices in

Argentina   Austria   Brazil   Chile   Czech Republic   France   Greece
Guatemala   Hungary   Italy   Japan   Poland   Portugal   Singapore
South Korea   Switzerland   Thailand   Turkey   Ukraine   Vietnam

Published by Oxford University Press, Inc.
198 Madison Avenue, New York, New York 10016

www.oup.com

Oxford is a registered trademark of Oxford University Press

Library of Congress Cataloging-in-Publication Data
Silva, Cristobal.
Miraculous plagues : an epidemiology of early New England narrative / Cristobal Silva.
p.   cm.
Includes bibliographical references and index.
ISBN 978-0-19-974347-6
1. Epidemics—New England—History—17th century—Sources. 2. Epidemics—Social aspects—
New England—History—17th century—Sources. 3. Epidemiology—New England—History—
17th century—Sources. 4. New England—History—Colonial period, ca. 1600–1775—Sources.
5. Great Britain—Colonies—America—History—17th century—Sources. 6. Epidemics—
New England—Historiography. 7. Epidemics in literature. 8. Narration (Rhetoric)—
Social aspects—New England—History—17th century. I. Title.
RA650.5.S57   2011
614.4'974—dc22   2010039733

1 3 5 7 9 8 6 4 2

Printed in the United States of America
on acid-free paper

For my Parents

CONTENTS

ACKNOWLEDGMENTS

The process of writing *Miraculous Plagues* has fundamentally changed my understanding of what books are, and of how they come into being. There were, as I had always imagined, many hours spent working in solitude, but none of that work would have produced this book had it not been for the many acts of friendship, generosity, and encouragement that helped shepherd it into print.

I thank Cyrus Patell, who first helped to refine the vague set of ideas that developed into my dissertation at NYU. His guidance gave me the confidence that this was a project worth pursuing, and led me to recognize the various paths that eventually culminated in *Miraculous Plagues*; his advice and pointed questions have continued to shape my work long after leaving graduate school. Thank you to Phil Harper, whose early enthusiasm encouraged me to keep thinking through the relation between seventeenth- and twentieth-century epidemiology; I am in his debt for teaching me to be a careful reader. Ross Posnock took an immediate interest in the project, and continues to be a strong advocate on my behalf. I thank him for his encouragement, for his questions, and for his advice, which have stayed with me during the revision process. Nancy Ruttenburg's personal and intellectual generosity are difficult to quantify, except to say that they helped me to see this project through, and to navigate my early years in the profession. Also from my time at NYU, I would like to thank Elizabeth McHenry, Virginia Jackson, Tim Reiss, Bryan Waterman, Richard Sieburth, Pam Schirmeister, as well as Karen Kupperman, who were all instrumental in my training, and had strong influences on this book.

One of the joys of graduate school lies in the many collaborations and friendships that one forms during a period of intense coursework, teaching, and research; the many conversations that I had at NYU continue to resonate years after the fact. I thank Natalie Friedman, Elizabeth Bradley, and Anne

Green, who were all there at the inception of the project, and helped to focus it in important ways. Likewise, I thank Raphael Allison, Tania Friedel, Will Kenton, David Tully, and Mike Kelly, who were there late in the dissertation process, and helped put an end to it. A special thank you to Robert Gunn, who, as much as anyone else, has seen this book through its various forms; his feedback has always been helpful, and I value his and Jonna Perrillo's friendship as one of the great gifts of being in this profession.

I would like to thank a number of scholars who were generous and patient enough to take an early interest in my work: Priscilla Wald's encouragement and support came at a critical stage of this project, and her work has been instrumental in its development. Likewise, Elizabeth Dillon's guidance has helped me to look beyond the immediate limits that I had set for the book, and to consider its broader historical, geographic, and political implications. Dennis Moore welcomed me into the Society of Early Americanists while I was still a graduate student, and his continued generosity in the SEA and at Florida State has been inspiring. David Shields challenged me to think more widely about the boundaries of the field, and his insights continue to pay dividends. I thank him and the readers at *Early American Literature* for their valuable comments on early drafts of Chapter 1, an excerpt of which was previously published as "Miraculous Plagues: Epidemiology on New England's Colonial Landscape," *EAL* 43, no. 2 (2008): 249–75. Tita Chico's friendship and advice have been invaluable; she has been generous with her time, and has helped me to think through a number of important intellectual and professional questions; her comments early in the revision process helped me to understand what the book would eventually look like. I thank Tita as well as Bob Markley for inviting me to join *The Eighteenth Century: Theory and Interpretation* in 2005—a position that has influenced my own work immeasurably. Over the years, many others have given advice, read material, and talked through key issues with me. For those conversations, I am grateful to Ralph Bauer, Jeffrey Richards, Frank Shuffelton, Tom Krise, Sean Goudie, Sarah Rivett, Matt Cohen, Jeffrey Glover, and Eirik Steinhoff.

From my time at Texas Tech, I would like to thank Jen Shelton, Madonne Miner, Jennifer Snead, Megan Nelson, and Doug Crowell, who all provided feedback on revisions. Likewise, Bryce Conrad, John Samson, Bruce Clarke, Yuan Shu, Michael Borshuk, Julie Couch, Min-Joo Kim, Amy Koerber, and my Chair, Sam Dragga, were all supportive of this work, and taught me how to be a colleague. I thank Jenni Frangos and Michael Holko, who made the transition from New York to West Texas at the same time as Elizabeth and I did; my work with Jenni began with the exchange of dissertation chapters, and has continued since then. Our collaborations on the transatlantic eighteenth century allowed me to bring much of this material into the classroom, where it developed in new and unexpected ways. I am grateful to her for her intellectual generosity, for her patience, and for her continued friendship.

Ralph Berry, my Chair at Florida State, has been unfailingly supportive, and I greatly appreciate his candor, as well as his professional and intellectual advice; his engagement with this project played a critical role as the process neared its completion. I thank both he and Kathi Yancey, my Interim Chair, for their leadership during my time at FSU. I thank Robin Goodman (and Mona), Barry Faulk, Andrew Epstein, Helen Burke, Jim O'Rourke, Elizabeth Spiller, Tim Parrish, Dan Vitkus, Elaine Treharne, Candace Ward, Meegan Kennedy, Leigh Edwards, Paul Outka, David Ikard, Robert Patterson, and Joe Gabriel, who created a vibrant intellectual community, and provided helpful feedback during my years in Tallahassee. I would also like to thank the many graduate students, including Lindsey Phillips, Nick Young, Kelly Wisecup, and Ayanna Jackson, who had the patience to indulge my interest in colonial American, Caribbean, and African epidemiology over the years. While I hope that they found those many seminar hours and countless readings to be productive, the questions they asked helped me to refine and clarify my arguments.

Thank you to Robert Olen Butler, whose sponsorship of the FSU English Department's visiting editors series was instrumental in placing the manuscript at Oxford University Press. I appreciate the critical eye that Oxford's anonymous readers brought to the manuscript; their questions and comments clarified a number of important issues, and had a significant impact on the final form of this book. I am grateful to my editor, Shannon McLachlan, for her enthusiastic support, and to Brendan O'Neill for his patience and careful attention. I have been fortunate to receive funding from various sources over the life of this project: while I was writing the dissertation, the NYU Graduate School of Arts and Sciences supported me with the Shortell-Holzer dissertation fellowship; in 2005, the National Humanities Center offered a Summer Institute stipend; FSU's First-Year Assistant Professor grant, and its generous junior leave program gave me the time to finish the initial draft of the manuscript. I am grateful to Columbia University for funding my parental leave that, in the midst of turbulent life changes, allowed me to complete the revisions to this book. In particular, I would like to thank my Chair Jean Howard, for welcoming me to Columbia, and for making the transition so seamless.

I would like to thank the various librarians and staff members who helped me to discover new materials, and without whom this project could never have been started, let alone completed. The New York Historical Society, the New York Academy of Medicine Library, the Fales Library and Special

Collections at NYU, the New York Public Library, and the Rare Book and Manuscript Library at Columbia were all important sources when I began investigating the trajectories of early epidemiology. Though I began my research in the pre-digital era, it was transformed by access to electronic materials. I have been fortunate to work at institutions that subscribe to databases like *Early English Books Online, Eighteenth Century Collections Online, Early American Imprints (Evans)*, and *Early American Newspapers*. Though these collections aren't an end in and of themselves, they are remarkable resources for scholars trying to understand the variety of printed material that circulated in the seventeenth and eighteenth centuries.

Finally, this book would never have been possible without the extensive support of my family. John T. and Sylvia Ronan opened their doors to me and supported this project in ways that are too numerous to count. John Ronan introduced me to many new ideas when I was just beginning as a graduate student, and he helped me to negotiate my early years in the profession. Joel and Diane Freed welcomed me into their home when I was far from mine, and I thank Joel for the useful lens that his reading brought to this project. I can always rely on my siblings Lucanor, Leonardo, and Cordelia to keep me grounded in the present when my thoughts turn too much to the seventeenth and eighteenth centuries; the past four years would not have been possible without their generosity. *Miraculous Plagues* is dedicated to my parents, Anne and Julio Silva, who taught me to see the world, and then to look at it again; though my mother did not live to see it, she inspired this book, and is in every page. Last, I thank Elizabeth, who has lived through the project from beginning to end, and has followed its circuitous path across the country. Her patience has been remarkable, and without her continued faith, love, and support, the book would have been abandoned long ago. Vera and Roxanne have been around just long enough to be perplexed by what it is that I do, and yet they have made me look forward to doing it every day since they were born. In a bid of solidarity as my work was nearing completion, Vera rarely left home without a sheaf of papers tucked under her arm, so that she, too, could finish her book.

—Cristobal Silva
February, 2011

Miraculous Plagues

Introduction

The doctors believe they can find the secret of the fever in the
victims' dead bodies. They cut, saw, extract, weigh, measure. The
dead are carved into smaller and smaller bits and the butchered
parts studied but they do not speak. What I know of the fever I've
learned from the words of those I've treated, from stories of the
living that are ignored by the good doctors. When lancet and fleam
bleed the victims, they offer up stories like prayers.

—John Edgar Wideman, *Fever*[1]

When I first settled on the subtitle of *Miraculous Plagues* during the initial
stages of the project, *An Epidemiology of Early New England Narrative* was
whimsical, rather than analytic, and meant to intrigue readers, rather than
illuminate them. Although it brought together the primary terms that would
be central to my research, I had only vague notions of how those terms fit together at the time; I certainly did not foresee *what* an epidemiology of narrative would look like, nor did I have much more than an intuitive grasp of how
such a study would eventually unfold. Despite the fact that "literature and
medicine" was an active, well-defined field of study, and biological histories
published in the prior thirty years had provided increasingly complex accounts of the effects of epidemics on indigenous peoples in the Americas
during the colonial era, neither the disciplinary and nationalist paradigms
that had long driven the study of literature, nor the statistical and mathematical tools of modern epidemiology suggested obvious ways to produce a coherent model for the kind of interdisciplinary work that I planned to
undertake.[2] And while my primary goal was to bring the analytical methods of
literary criticism and epidemiology to bear on one another, the fact that I was
trained in a literature department rather than in a medical school made it

almost inevitable that my work would look a certain way. Indeed, as I began to trace the intertwined histories of colonial New England's epidemiological, theological, and legal discourses, this study became increasingly recognizable as literary criticism: close reading as well as formal and thematic analysis framed my methodological approach to the field, and informed the major historiographic concerns that guided my research into colonial epidemics. This being the case, it was clear that I had to address three questions from the outset: first, what exactly does "epidemiology" mean in the context of literary criticism? Second, what is the relation between epidemiology and early New England narrative? And finally, what is an "epidemiology of narrative"?

In plain terms, epidemiology is the branch of medical science that investigates patterns of infection, immunity, and epidemic so that public health professionals may locate, organize, treat symptoms of, and finally disrupt the progress of disease in a community. Where an epidemic is defined by an unexpectedly high incidence of illness in a given population or region, epidemiologists search for behavioral differences between the sick and the healthy in order to identify possible disease vectors and transmission routes; they map their data onto spatial and temporal axes to visualize health and illness as functions of behavior, which, depending on the disease in question, might range from washing hands to tobacco use to sexual practices to food consumption.[3] For example, a sudden outbreak of e. coli would prompt epidemiologists to investigate the eating habits of those who fell ill, and to monitor processing, storage, and shipping techniques at appropriate nodes in the food services industry until they could pinpoint both the source of the bacteria, and its geographic trajectory over time. While epidemiological maps are shaped by specialized statistical and observational techniques, they are, in the sense that I present them here, representations of disease that encode bodies, health, illness, social habits, geographic spaces, communities, and borders into coherent narratives that reveal the progress of epidemics over time in provisionally bounded spaces.[4] Given this framework, I approach epidemiology as a literary critic would a narrative genre: specifically, epidemiology formalizes a set of vocabularies and grammars that articulate why epidemics act as they do, and why certain people get sick while others do not. Thus, the task of this book is to imagine a method of formal and thematic analysis that untangles the generic conventions of epidemiological texts, and demonstrates how regional and generational patterns of illness reposition our understanding of the relation between immunology and ideology in the formation of communal identity.

That said, epidemiology has a very specific historical context, and only emerged as a coherent field in the late nineteenth and early twentieth centuries. As I will describe shortly, my appropriation of epidemiology into the colonial era (a period when neither the word nor the concept existed) does great violence to the term, so I would like to justify the move by outlining what I see as epidemiology's discursive power to redefine spaces and behaviors in the modern era. I begin, therefore, with a brief outline of John Snow's prototypical study of London's 1854 cholera epidemic. Snow's study is perhaps the first to be recognized as epidemiological in the modern sense of the word, and my interest lies in how his analysis of cholera maps bodies and behaviors in relation to public health. Snow kept a detailed record of individual cholera cases during the epidemic, and while this was hardly an innovation in itself, his conceptual breakthrough came as a result of literally plotting those cases on a map to produce a visual record of the epidemic.[5] Unlike later twentieth-century epidemiologies, this map said very little about the temporal progress of the disease. Instead, it aggregated cases, and in doing so provided a visual representation of the concentration of cholera victims relative to one another, and to urban landmarks. Snow's map indicated to him that infections clustered around—or radiated outward from—the Broad Street water pump, which he had suspected to be a possible source of infection. He verified his conjecture by disabling the water pump, and noting that the incidence of cholera decreased almost immediately. Epidemiologically speaking, Snow had identified a specific behavior (in this case, drinking water from the Broad Street pump) and pathologized it by drawing a detailed map and pinpointing the geographic source of illness. The map thus redefined this behavior as a local phenomenon, and gave it new meaning because of its effects on bodies. Although Snow did not discover the pathogen that caused cholera (the definitive link to the *vibrio cholerae* bacillus would not be made for another three decades), his inference about the source of the disease highlights the power of epidemiology to reinscribe otherwise unremarkable behaviors as dangerous, and to extrapolate this danger to the community at large.[6]

Snow's groundbreaking observation was essential for identifying the source of infection in this specific instance, and it also transformed the management of urban infectious diseases, and had an even greater transformative impact on reshaping cityscapes by making water treatment and urban planning matters of public health. Indeed, the implications of Snow's map are far deeper than the spatial distribution of illness that it rendered. In the act of redefining urban spaces and quotidian behaviors, Snow demonstrated that cholera was *not* an inevitable fact of life in large nineteenth-century cities, but that it was a disease with a clear chain of transmission that could be disrupted with relative ease: clean water, better drainage, and effective sanitation measures quickly made cholera a disease of the past in cities like London.

Ideologically speaking, this reconfiguration of urban environments and behaviors effectively normalized health and all of its attendant privileges as London's natural state—a radical shift for a city where virulent diseases had long been endemic. And if, as Snow's study suggests, drinking clean water is just such a privilege, then every new cholera outbreak in the twenty-first century reminds us that it has become a privilege of modern industrialized societies, while communities that suffer such epidemics are regularly defined by their susceptibilities to illness, and by their essential belatedness (e.g., their status as "developing" rather than modern societies—a not too subtle echo of stadialist theories of colonialism). Aside from clean drinking water, other such privileges include mobility, education, and access to capital—each of which is naturalized as a metonym for good health. On the flipside of this equation, epidemiology all too often encodes illness as disenfranchisement or alienation from these same privileges: the ill are fixed in place—in locations like the developing world, or inner cities, that, in the case of HIV/AIDS, are coded as unhealthy[7]; they are ill because they have limited access to capital (this includes medicine and health insurance), or to education about healthful practices (such as nutrition or safe sex). Thus, the study of epidemiology that I undertake here is not simply a biological history of epidemics in a given region or era, but a broader inquiry into the shaping influence that epidemiology has on landscapes and cultural practices.

This approach to critiquing epidemiology owes a debt to Priscilla Wald and Cindy Patton, who have both conducted important analyses of the subject— Wald, with an eye toward theorizing the nation in terms of what she calls "imagined immunities," and Patton, to underscore the power of epidemiology to reconfigure spaces and behaviors.[8] Significantly, Patton and Wald are both clear about the ethical dimensions that accompany any work touching on public health policy: each makes a conscious commitment to rethinking the moral and political stakes of public health on a global scale, and each displays a conviction that these types of analyses are necessary to draw attention to— if not overturn—the "legacies of colonialism and modernization" that have exacerbated health-care inequalities around the world, even as Western medicine has become increasingly effective at identifying and treating a wide spectrum of illnesses.[9] Although my own work is rooted in the seventeenth and eighteenth centuries rather than the twentieth or twenty-first, it is guided by an abiding interest in modern epidemiology and public health. As such, I share Patton's and Wald's commitments and convictions in ways that I hope will become clear as I expand on their critical engagements with epidemiology to address the genre's effect on narrative and colonial practices in New England.

Patton's analysis focuses on Western responses to the global HIV/AIDS pandemic. She begins by highlighting the conceptual difference between *tropical medicine* and *epidemiology*, which she describes as two representational frameworks for understanding contagion. Whereas tropical medicine evolved in concert with colonial history, its legacy lies in the West's continuing representation of the developing world as pathological—as the site and source of innumerable diseases (ranging from malaria to HIV/AIDS and Ebola) that threaten the American or European who ventures there.[10] Patton argues that in contrast to tropical medicine, epidemiology is interested in the movement of pathogens first, and in the bodies they infect, second. She claims that when epidemiology marks those bodies that are the "most likely to harbor and transport infection," it creates, in the process, a "space-time" for epidemic disease, which is to say a map that structures the spaces where bodies and pathogens come into contact with one another, giving them extension, duration, and boundary.[11] This transformation, which we might characterize as historical and geographic (or spatial and temporal), makes the trajectory of epidemics visible by turning ill-defined blank spaces into legible landscapes that are imprinted with their own historical experience of disease. And if the epidemiologist reads these maps to trace the history of an epidemic, the literary critic reads that history as a function of epidemiology's narrative conventions. For example, epidemiological maps reflect—or even structure—the economic and geographic assumptions that give shape to the world in which we live: mountains, oceans, and deserts all naturalize the history of disease, and circumscribe place according to the geological boundaries that hinder or facilitate the progress of epidemics. Likewise, epidemiology's appropriation of economic frameworks highlights the relationship between trade and movement that mirrors the evolution of epidemics.

Wald is equally interested in epidemiology's discursive power, though her work leans more self-consciously on the tools of literary criticism than Patton's does, as it engages the politics of community and nation. Focusing on what she calls the *outbreak narrative*—a formulaic genre that systematizes "individuals, groups, populations, locales (regional and global), behaviors and lifestyles"—Wald argues that immunities and susceptibilities to disease imprint communal bonds on (or in) the bodies of citizens, while outbreak narratives make those bonds visible.[12] By conjuring the immunological foundation of community, Wald temporarily destabilizes political and territorial models of nationhood, and produces a useful matrix through which to naturalize and reimagine national affiliations. Indeed, this biological framework allows Wald to evoke a powerful set of tropes to critique the politics of nationhood. The primary one of these—"imagined immunities"—is a deliberate nod to Benedict Anderson's work on "Imagined Communities," and draws attention to the way that the outbreak narrative "articulates community on a national scale."[13] Wald pivots elegantly from the link Anderson makes between shared reading practices and the acts of imagination that form community, to the immunological bonds that structure imaginative communities in her account. This shift occurs along two axes: an individual imagines him or herself as part of a community defined by shared immunities and susceptibilities to disease, while professional and lay epidemiologies formalize these immunological bonds, multiplying individual acts of imagination to transform social groups into a "mystically connected biological entity"—for example, the nation (signs of which can range from the vaccination certificates that children must produce before entering public school in the United States to the face-masks that often appear in public when infectious diseases such as H1N1 break out).[14] What is most powerful about this model of imagined immunities is that when epidemiology historicizes and circulates narratives about the progress of disease—whether this be on the news, on the Internet, in print, in movies, or by word of mouth—it renders specific immunities visible, and signifies these as essential preconditions to (or markers of) citizenship. In other words, epidemiology draws attention to the actions and behaviors that determine the progress of an epidemic over time so that these behaviors are themselves appropriated into models of citizenship.

While focusing on imagined immunities appears to work against the grain of political and territorial modes of nationhood, epidemiology quickly recuperates and naturalizes those modes as it imprints them with immunological significance. Thus, specific preventative behaviors can be recognized for their political significance even as they are a function of public health. The links between politics and epidemiology are perhaps most visible when a community or nation appears to be under attack from foreign invaders (real or imagined), at which point nationalist discourses marshal epidemiological practices in the form of quarantines and xenophobia to reassert sovereignty over borders and cultural identity, and to demonstrate the fundamental health of the body politic; conversely, one might talk about this relation in mutually constitutive terms, and posit that in such instances, epidemiology marshals nationalist discourses to figure public health as a function of citizenship. For Wald, this move describes the nation as an immunological ecosystem "configured in cultural and political as well as biological terms," though biology here is taken to mean something other than simple "kinship."[15] Wald's ecosystem trope underscores the interrelation of the political and the biological, but it also points to the fragility of these acts of imagination, which simultaneously require the very real threat of pathogens to harness nationalist impulses, alongside a willful suspension of disbelief to maintain the illusion that epidemiology is a totalizing narrative that can fully account for the trajectories of foreign pathogens, and restore the nation to its underlying natural state of health. In addressing this mechanism, the literary critic reveals the ways that epidemiology repeatedly draws on the national imaginary to invoke the cultural and ideological ties that define immunological ecosystems.

The histories of smallpox, yellow fever, cholera, HIV/AIDS, SARS, and H1N1 all trace important geopolitical shifts, as well as evolutions in the technologies of travel, from the seventeenth to the early twenty-first centuries. But even as these political, economic, and geographic trajectories underscore the porousness of national borders, time and again giving proof that epidemics behave transnationally, both Patton and Wald demonstrate that pathogens reify the very nationalist impulses they undermine. Herein lies the ideological power of epidemiology to reshape social as well as geographic spaces: epidemiology represents political, economic, and territorial borders contiguously with a nation's health, and the health of its citizens; it structures colonial landscapes, and formalizes the rules through which bodies, behaviors, and movements become legible alongside their respective immunities and susceptibilities to disease. As epidemiological narratives circulate in both professional and popular contexts, the national imagination aligns itself with normative images of healthfulness, and further represents the security of its borders as a matter of public health policy. Indeed, by delimiting physical boundaries between healthy and sick spaces, and by developing public health practices to monitor pathological behaviors, epidemiology helps to consolidate civic duties and territorial borders as impermeable buffers against epidemic in the minds of citizens. Significantly, these effects turn epidemiology's gaze outward, to project pathogens as foreign bodies while representing community (or nation) as the fundamentally healthy site that protects its citizens, and needs, in turn, their protection. Such strategies afford critics the opportunity to inquire into the role that illness and health play in transforming landscapes, and into the very nature of boundary and identity—whether these are considered from individual, national, territorial, or even disciplinary vantage points.

Wald and Patton push us to think of the ways that epidemiology structures spaces, behaviors, and communities, and to consider the very real political and health consequences of this structuring. Their work challenges literary critics to theorize the genre's formal trajectories as these impact on political and medical discourses in moments of immunological stress, and to read epidemiological texts with an eye to unpacking the representational practices that encode specific ideological assumptions about what it means to be healthy or sick, and how medical treatments are distributed. Of course, literary criticism is not in the business of developing treatments or testing their effectiveness in the field—and for good reason. Yet, the vibrancy of narrative medicine programs, and the broad scholarly interest in fields such as literature and medicine suggest an ever-increasing acknowledgment that strong attention to the rules, the forms, and the language of narrative does have its place in the practice of medicine and public health. So to answer the question of what literary criticism has to do with epidemiology, I would argue that the critic's role is to analyze the formal and thematic properties of professional and lay epidemiologies, and to demonstrate how these discourses are bound up in the cultural assumptions of the communities that produce them—how, for example, their representational practices regulate access to medicine, and define the boundaries of citizenship.

The second question that I raised at the outset of this introduction—about the relation of seventeenth-century texts to epidemiology—is a bit more complicated for historiographic reasons, given the fact that epidemiology only came into being as a medical science in the latter half of the nineteenth century, and matured during the twentieth. When I refer to epidemiology in the context of colonial New England, I mean those texts—including journals, diaries, exploration narratives, political tracts, medical pamphlets, correspondence, newspapers, and poems—which, regardless of their medical or scientific pretensions, aim to represent the etiologies of illness, and to explain why epidemics act as they do. This is a broad definition, and as will appear at various times in *Miraculous Plagues*, these etiologies are quite far afield from anything we would expect out of traditional models of epidemiology. But the point, once again, is to think in terms of generic properties rather than specific tools or techniques—I am not looking to find early methodological precursors to modern epidemiology, but to identify formal narrative analogues that shape political and cultural spaces. Indeed, to pretend that the first generations of New England settlers thought "epidemiologically" in a way that would be recognizable to twenty-first-century medical professionals and public health advocates flirts with anachronism, if it assumes an understanding of modern immunological and statistical processes on their part. This is certainly not a claim that I make in this book.

I want to emphasize that *Miraculous Plagues* is not epidemiological in the familiar sense of the word: I do not employ statistical methods in my research. I do not study specific population distributions, nor do I calculate the rates of incidence and prevalence of historical epidemics. What I do, however, is look at the narratives behind such epidemiological methods—behind both professional and popular strategies—to better understand how those methods make the notion of community formation transparent as a function of illness and health. The disciplinary intervention that I propose does not deny the power of epidemiological discourse to form effective public health policy, but it does affirm its power to shape literary, economic, and geopolitical networks, and it recognizes that those networks play an important role in determining how medical knowledge is disseminated, as well as where and for whom medical treatment programs are deployed. And though my use of the term "epidemiology" in the context of the seventeenth century is anachronistic at face value, my purpose in appropriating the term for Early American studies is to defamiliarize epidemiological analysis from its modern medical and statistical operations in order to read it *as* narrative. The stakes of such a move are obviously high. For example, I risk losing sight of seventeenth- and eighteenth-century medical knowledge and practices—knowledge of how (or even whether) the subjects of my study conceived of the biological mechanisms at work in illness, and of how these mechanisms were to be treated; but those concerns tend to be the subject of traditional biological histories of the New World, which have covered the ground rather well, and thus they are a secondary interest of mine in this book. On the other hand, my interest in seventeenth-century conceptions of illness, contagion, and treatment lies in their parallel evolution to theological, juridical, and political discourses.

As a case in point I offer this book's title—*Miraculous Plagues*—which was inspired by John Winthrop's justification for the Puritan migration to New England. In calling the epidemics that decimated Native American populations along the eastern seaboard of New England between 1616 and 1619 a "miraculous plague," Winthrop helped set the stage for the rhetoric of infection that dominated seventeenth-century historiography of the Antinomian controversy, helped shape new theological practices like the halfway covenant and the jeremiad in response to the unexpected cyclical epidemic patterns that afflicted Anglo-American communities at midcentury, and affected the reception and evolution of inoculation in early-eighteenth-century Boston. Each of these events forms its own node in New England Puritan studies, but an epidemiological approach reveals how those nodes are connected narratively by immunology as much as by ideology or theology; they behave epidemiologically insofar as they imagine specific relationships between sick and well populations, and form coherent narratives for describing those relationships. And even if modern audiences do not immediately recognize texts associated with these events as "medical" or "epidemiological," they imagine spaces according to detailed behavioral models, and therefore share a basic investment in the practice of epidemiology.

Instead of importing statistical tools into the seventeenth century to describe rates of infection and mortality, or to chronicle the biological effects of specific epidemics, *Miraculous Plagues* is concerned with uncovering the narrative impact of epidemiology on New England's colonial landscape—with seeing how epidemiology gave shape to that landscape. At first glance, this might seem like a minor semantic difference, but a study of epidemics would highlight the historical effects of disease on specific populations, while a study of epidemiology is concerned with how those effects are narrated as a means of politicizing behaviors, and reconceptualizing community. The goal here is thus not to add one more biological history of the New World to an already considerable list, or to trace evolving technologies of observation and treatment. Instead, it is to consider the relation between how and what epidemiologies observe, and how they circulate within medical, economic, and political circles. In this respect, *An Epidemiology of Early New England Narrative* does not describe literature or narrative as a sickness, but embodies a philosophy of analysis that calls for a spatial, temporal, and formal rearticulation of critical research—a task for which epidemiology is ideally suited because its primary investment lies in rethinking the relationship between body and place.

What is gained through this work is a deeper insight into how the formal and thematic properties of epidemiology shaped the ideological and historiographic legacies of colonial New England, and how, in turn, new approaches to those legacies help us to think about public health practices today. For example, the first generation of colonists in New England relied on epidemiology to create legal justifications for their appropriations of Native American lands. My reading of the texts that relate specifically to the 1616–19 epidemics suggests that epidemiology provided colonists with the vocabulary to transform the landscape from undefined to "wilderness" to "property." It is this transformative act that I refer to as epidemiological mapping—the legible imprint of epidemics on open spaces. What I want to emphasize is that this nature of epidemiological mapping is not specific to seventeenth-century colonial New England, but is a generic property of epidemiology that reconfigures twenty-first-century spaces as well. The payoff of this approach is that it argues for a productive concept of anachronism that positions health and epidemiological rhetoric as integral to theology and political thought in Puritan New England. This is a self-consciously transhistorical and transdisciplinary vision of anachronism that provides for a fruitful analysis of the colonial era precisely because it defamiliarizes narrative histories that segregate medicine, theology, and law into their own specialized modern disciplines, and it transforms our relation to the materials of literary history. At its best, the violence that I commit against the term by analyzing the generic conventions and narrative modes of seventeenth-century epidemiological texts reshapes our relationship to contemporary epidemiology, and opens modern discourses to similar cultural criticism. It simultaneously allows literary critics and cultural theorists to understand early American historical processes through a contemporary biomedical lens, and clarifies the narrative and ideological effects of epidemiology on contemporary landscapes. Again, I conceive of these effects on two planes: for those Early Americanist critics who wish to explore new frameworks for the evolution of the field, and for those cultural critics who wish to develop tools for understanding the relation between contemporary contagion and ideology.

The third and perhaps most fraught question that I am committed to answering in this introduction asks what is an epidemiology of narrative? To be clear, my use of the term "epidemiology" is meant as something more than a metaphor to describe traditional genealogical history. Indeed, what I intend my subtitle to suggest is that epidemiology functions not just as the subject of this book, but as a method of literary and historiographic analysis—as a set of analytical practices that inquire into the spatial and temporal trajectories of epidemics, and map the dynamic interplay of disease, migration, immunology, and colonialism in narrative terms. In this vein, an epidemiology of narrative describes an analytical framework that charts a genealogy of New England's literary history according to the temporal and geographic specificity of epidemical outbreaks—a specificity that relates to shifting migration patterns and immunological conditions over time as much as it does to factionalism, political intrigue, and religious orthodoxy. The net effect of this analysis is to consider literary history within a deeply local—and embodied—historical experience of illness. For example, I argue that it matters how epidemics appear and recede; who gets sick and when; and how treatment options are debated in public. It also matters how these facts are understood by local communities, and described in their epidemiological texts. Finally, it matters that as local as these experiences were in seventeenth-century New England, they nevertheless remained dependent on relations to the broader Atlantic World. The ongoing circulation of pathogens between Europe, Africa, the Caribbean, and North and South America altered longstanding immunological patterns, and ultimately forced a reassessment of the epidemiologies that had previously formalized what local communities understood about their place in the world.

The genealogy that I describe in this book troubles traditional monolithic accounts of New World epidemics, such as the so-called virgin soil hypothesis that represents the transfer of pathogens as relatively monolithic and unidirectional; this hypothesis suggests that Native Americans had no prior exposure to Old World diseases, and were therefore "virgin soil" to the pathogens that wreaked havoc among them. Although the immunological mechanism it relies on is correct, I follow David Jones's critique of virgin soil, which, because it stands as a totalizing narrative, tends to foreclose deeper analyses into the dynamics of colonial immunology.[16] To this end, rather than conceiving of epidemics as independent, discrete events, I consider them within a continuous immunological history. It is therefore no coincidence that the hundred-year period that I have chosen to work with is bookended by two major outbreaks: the 1616–19 Native American epidemics, and the 1721 smallpox epidemic that infected half the inhabitants of Boston. The first question that arises when thinking of these epidemics in relation to one another is how do we account for the dramatic shift in which pathogens attacked Native bodies in the earlier epidemics, and European (or what I come to call "Anglo-American") bodies later on in the century? This question is especially important in the context of the virgin soil hypothesis, which is predicated on a stark immunological distinction between Native American and European populations during the early colonial era, but which nevertheless gets projected forward as a timeless (if not essential) account of racial immunology. In addressing this century-long epidemiological shift, *Miraculous Plagues* inquires into the immunological dynamics that produced it, and traces the formal, thematic, and generic conventions of epidemiology that evolved to account for these new patterns of illness. Thus, an "epidemiology of narrative" deciphers these radically different immunological experiences by tracing the links between New England's narrative conventions, and its shifting epidemiological patterns over the course of the seventeenth century, when illnesses seemed to turn inward on Anglo-American communities.

The practice of charting the history of New England's epidemics alongside a genealogy of its narrative conventions and theological traditions puts pressure on otherwise static analytical models of colonial history by considering the temporal as well as spatial axes along which illness and immunity operate. This approach to epidemics and epidemiology gives rise to what I call New England's *immunological syntax*—a term that points to the interplay between language and biology, and which I use, in this context, to highlight the function of epidemiological history as a system that orders and gives meaning to immunological and demographic mechanisms as these impact narrative and generic conventions. Thus, immunological syntax describes the specific immunities and susceptibilities of a population (or region) at a given moment, it describes how (and why) those conditions change over time, and, most importantly for this study, it accounts for the formal properties of epidemiological texts in terms of how communities understand their own role in the behaviors of epidemics. From a critical perspective, immunological syntax does two things: first, it compels a historiographic investigation into specific epidemiological mechanisms operating in seventeenth-century New England. That is, it seeks to understand the immunological and demographic conditions that shaped the history of colonial epidemics. An inquiry along this track resembles traditional historical and epidemiological analysis—from the focus on behavioral differences between sick and well populations, to the mapping of observational data along spatial and temporal axes in order to identify specific patterns in epidemic outbreaks, and to understand how and why epidemics function as they do.

Second, and more germane to the field of literary studies, immunological syntax offers a detailed set of reading practices for moving beyond representations of illness as metaphor or allegory, and theorizing the translation of epidemic events into narrative and generic terms according to a region's demographic and immunological histories. From this perspective, immunological syntax helps critics decipher the relation between epidemiology and the communal narratives that account for experiences of illness—whether these narratives are primarily medical, juridical, political, or even fictional. Immunological syntax is a useful term for historians and literary critics because it helps to formalize the relationship between epidemic outbreaks and the behaviors of citizens as a means of defining the shifting physical and cultural boundaries that a given community might establish for itself over time. While corporeal representations of the body politic make illness a potent metaphor for cultural and political upheaval (and certainly, these metaphors predate the Puritan migration to New England), the purpose of thinking about immunological syntax is to move away from metaphor, or to consider how metaphors and representations shift over time as a reflection of biological processes. This call to account for the temporal dynamics at play in epidemiological history considers individual epidemics as interrelated components in a dynamic immunological trajectory rather than as discrete or isolated events. For example, the early justification narratives that I discuss in Chapter 1 offer a snapshot of New England's epidemiological history at a fixed point in time, but as the book progresses, its attention to immunological syntax constructs an increasingly complex picture of how colonial epidemics functioned over a period ranging from the early seventeenth to the early eighteenth centuries, and of how succeeding generations of settlers accounted for this complexity in their narratives. Beyond this, I argue that attention to the generic conventions of epidemiological narratives gives scholars insights into the politics of community, as familiarity with immunological histories shifted over time. By paying attention to the epidemiological assumptions that account for these shifts, we better understand the thematic and formal structure of New England's literary history. Thus, *An Epidemiology of Early New England Narrative* creates a framework for literary critics and medical historians alike to visualize how the analytical practices of both fields reshape one another.

Given this theoretical framework, I would now add a final question to the prior three: Namely, what does an epidemiology of narrative tell us about early America and Early American studies? On the one hand, it reminds us that colonialism was deeply invested in local and regional experiences, and that these experiences were embedded in the materiality of human bodies. That said, my characterization of local experiences is complicated by the fact that this localism should always be envisioned within a transatlantic network of narratives, bodies, and pathogens. By this, I mean that the history of colonial epidemics is never distinct from the transatlantic movements that transported pathogens from one location to the next, producing epidemic outbreaks in some places, while quickly petering out in others; indeed, the trajectory of local epidemics is fundamentally tied to the relation between specific locations and the rest of the Atlantic World. To this end, it would have been equally productive to pursue a self-consciously transatlantic or hemispheric epidemiological analysis, or an epidemiology of the Atlantic slave trade centered on the exchange of pathogens and of Western and African medical narratives in the Caribbean basin. But the circulation of pathogens throughout the Atlantic world only tells half of the story, while human bodies (or immune systems) fill in the blanks. Local population densities, demographics, and proximity to other cities, towns, and colonies all have a determinant effect on the shape and outcome of epidemics, and this is especially true in an era when virulent diseases like smallpox, measles, and yellow fever circulated far and wide. And yet, despite—or perhaps because of—this circulation, the local experience of illness in a dense English city like London was much different from experiences in a Caribbean colony like late-eighteenth-century St. Domingo, or in a physically and geographically isolated New England town like seventeenth-century Boston. Though New England settlers could not explain the reasons for this difference biologically, their epidemiologies nevertheless sought to account for them in terms that we recognize today as political, juridical, and theological.

Where early justification narratives were grounded on reports of Native American susceptibility and European immunity to disease, the immunological distinctions that settlers observed between themselves and Native Americans were crucial to how they understood their place in the New World. But New England's immunological history was far more complex than these justification narratives would indicate, and English anxieties about the threat of infectious disease became increasingly acute as the years progressed and ep-idemics turned inward on them. Specifically, these anxieties were a direct consequence of New England's physical isolation from Europe, so I want to argue for a patient elaboration of the way that regionalism (or localism) mediates transatlantic networks through the material experience of bodies. At times, these experiences are visible—as in the case of widespread epi-demic eruption and war, or when organized around other forms of colonial violence, such as in the Atlantic slave trade. But at other times, these experi-ences seem to be guided, as Cotton Mather wrote about Boston's history of smallpox, by a "peculiar agency of the invisible world."[17] The theological valence of Mather's phrase is clear, but there is a deeper, immunological dy-namic at work that, even if Mather couldn't account for it, nevertheless becomes visible to us in the twenty-first century, as we read it through the appropriate epidemiological lens.

Chapter 1 of *Miraculous Plagues* focuses on the epidemics that struck the eastern seaboard of present-day New England between 1616 and 1619, killing up to 95 percent of the indigenous population living there at the time. In 1629, John Winthrop identified those epidemics as a "miraculous plague" sent by God to "vacate" New England prior to (and as an invitation for) the Puritan migration.[18] Winthrop's is but one of many texts that blend medical, legal, and theological discourses to help justify the colonial project in New England by reorganizing the civil-law rhetoric of property rights around im-munity and susceptibility to disease. Although such representations are not biological in the modern sense of the word, they are epidemiological in that they create a framework for understanding a set of behavioral and cultural mechanisms for infection. Indeed, the phrase "miraculous plagues" points to a cosmology wherein medical and theological rhetorics are deeply intertwined. These New England epidemiologies map immunological distinctions between Native American and English bodies by relying on Christian/heathen and civ-ilized/savage tropes, and transform the landscape in the process. While Chris-tianity is what purportedly maintains the health of English colonists, the Native American body is represented as immunologically inferior, and this inferiority becomes legible as a failure to improve the land. Where epidemics depopulated wide swaths of New England, epidemiological rhetoric subse-quently contextualized this emptiness as a vacant wilderness free to be appro-priated by English Christians. Thus, colonial epidemiology seizes on ideological and cultural difference to articulate strategies for appropriating the American landscape into an historical European colonial framework.

The balance of this chapter investigates the circulation of epidemiolog-ical rhetoric as a means of appropriating and consolidating power during

English/Native American encounters in New England by focusing specifically on what I call the *counter-epidemiologies* attributed to Native Americans like Tisquantum of Patuxet. These counter-epidemiologies offer alternative readings of how and why epidemics spread as they did in the wake of colonial encounters, invariably implicating European explorers and settlers in their appearance. And yet, as is frequently the case with Native American narratives from this era, these counter-epidemiologies are ventriloquized through English voices, and printed in English texts. My analysis traces the relation between colonial epidemiologies and counter-epidemiologies, and highlights the parallel political and economic function of each. Ultimately, it demonstrates that counter-epidemiologies are, in fact, part of a complex colonial apparatus that negotiates the relations between English settlers and Native Americans during the first twenty years of New England colonial history.

Chapter 2 departs from the remainder of the book insofar as it focuses on a figural, rather than literal, epidemic by way of arguing that the social manifestations of diseases (their etiologies, diagnoses, and prognostications) are a driving force behind their treatment. Where epidemiology seeks to categorize and modify behaviors in order to treat disease, its ideological nature manifests itself in the regulation of public spaces, and in the abstraction of social behaviors as epidemical—a policing model of public health. I argue that because early justification narratives had been so successful in shaping colonial discourses during the decade that framed the initial migration to New England, John Winthrop and the Massachusetts Bay ministerial elite deployed epidemiological rhetoric as a strategic maneuver to contain Antinomianism, and to protect the colony from what Thomas Weld called this "great and sore affliction" in his preface to John Winthrop's history of the controversy.[19] In much the same way as earlier providential readings of physical epidemics assumed a stable communal core under attack from contagious disease, so too could a Puritan "Orthodoxy" constitute and represent itself as the focal point of a healthy colony by representing Antinomians as the source of infection. My work here is neither dependent on, nor claims the existence of a religious Orthodoxy in Massachusetts Bay, so much as it reveals the context and strategies through which a political faction manifests itself as a coherent and orthodox voice by silencing dissent. In positioning Antinomianism as a dangerous and contagious behavior, the ministerial elite in Boston represented itself as the source of healthy religious doctrine over and against the monstrosities of Antinomianism. In this manner, I argue that what came to be known as the "Orthodox" rhetoric of the controversy—including the prosecution of male Antinomians for sedition, and of Anne Hutchinson for various (at times unnamed) crimes—successfully represented social transgression as pathological behavior, and in so doing, stabilized and reified the boundaries of proper, "healthful" conduct.

But where Puritans like Winthrop figured Antinomianism as a physical danger to the community, Anne Hutchinson—who came to be its central figure at the end of the crisis—complicates the relation between subversion and contagion. Her subversiveness was not easily contained by her theological belief. Had it been, she would have been prosecuted for sedition like her brother-in-law John Wheelwright (who had been preaching the same ideas publicly), and disposed of just as swiftly by the ministerial elite. Instead, Hutchinson's extended civil and church trials implied that the danger she represented to the community manifested itself in her ability to transgress social as well as religious boundaries, and to disseminate her ideas in unsupervised and unregulated pathways. This transgression was most violently figured in gendered rather than religious terms, and was expressed as an anxiety about the fact that her "helpfulness" in times of childbirth could be exploited to the detriment of the community.[20] Because this kind of work appeared to be a ready conduit for the dissemination of Antinomian ideas, the language of the controversy quickly represented womanhood in America as a pathological category to be policed for the greater health of the community. By the time that Winthrop's *A Short Story of the Rise, reign, and ruine of the Antinomians, Familists & Libertines, that infected the Churches of New-England* was published in 1644, Hutchinson had variously been called "the breeder and nourisher of all these distempers," an "American Jesebel," a "Husband [rather] than a Wife," as well as a "Magistrate [rather] than a Subject," and, most tellingly, she was accused of having "stept out of [her] place."[21] The Antinomian controversy reveals that epidemiological rhetoric is not only helpful in identifying the sources of contagion, but, read alongside Cindy Patton's model, it performatively reinvents "the meaning of quotidian acts by placing them within a model of transmissibility"—it reinvents acts like midwifery and nursing as behavior that places the community at risk.[22] Although the Antinomian controversy was not a physical epidemic, its presence in *Miraculous Plagues* models a shift in which my reading of epidemiology reflects a conscious interest in narrative, rather than disease.

This type of analysis comes into better focus in Chapter 3, where I examine the ongoing history of midcentury epidemics in New England. Whereas the first generation of Puritan settlers read Native American susceptibility to illness as a sign justifying their colonial project, the cyclical recurrence of epidemics later in the century undermined those readings when Anglo-Americans succumbed to such illnesses on a large scale. This shifting epidemical pattern is due in large part to a concept known as *herd immunity*, which depends on

changing ratios between immune and susceptible populations in a given location.[23] Unlike England, where smallpox was a fact of day-to-day existence in
large, densely populated cities, New England communities did not have the
critical population base to support a disease like smallpox endemically.[24] And
because smallpox was not endemic in New England during the seventeenth
century, there were large periodic swings in the ratio of susceptible to immune
subjects, thereby radically altering the pattern of epidemics, and causing an
attendant shift in the Puritan framework for understanding the place of English bodies in America. The narrative strategies used to explain these shifts
(which included the evolution of the New England jeremiad and the halfway
covenant) figured epidemics as national punishments. While it is in keeping
with traditional providential readings of historical events, this figure assumes
that communities are built as stable corporate entities: like human bodies
that suffer illnesses, communal bodies can be afflicted by epidemics when
their "behaviors" became pathological. But as providential signs of God's
wrath, epidemics also take their meaning alongside any number of other national traumas like earthquakes, floods, droughts, Indian wars, and heresy,
insofar as these events are essentially substitutable for one another. In this
context, the providential representation of epidemics as national afflictions is
thematic: its importance lies in the legibility of disease as a sign of wrath,
rather than in the spatial or temporal dynamics that mark the nature of infection and immunity. Thematic readings therefore import epidemics into static
frameworks, and shape nationalist discourses by offering communal coherence as the ontological ground upon which epidemics signify.

   In opposition to this, I claim that the illusion of cultural homogeneity in
Puritan New England reflects shifting and emerging disease patterns in the
seventeenth century, rather than any essential nature of Puritan culture.
Therefore, by examining the relation between immunology and demographics,
my intention is to account for the shifting dynamics of epidemics in New England's history, to stand apart from ontological assumptions about culture and
homogeneity, and to reappropriate the temporal axis of epidemiology into the
field of Early American studies. To this end, historians of New England Puritanism have quite rightly recognized the thematic nature that describes the
interpretation of disease in the seventeenth century; however, they have too
often continued to participate in this thematic discourse, and this has led to
the elision of epidemics and epidemiology from criticism. To counteract such
thematic readings, I offer immunological syntax as a strategy for moving
beyond thematic representations of epidemics—which nevertheless tend to
be ahistorical—and modeling the spatial as well as temporal narrative organizing principles of epidemiology. The intergenerational scales that reveal the

demographic and immunological significance of cyclical smallpox epidemics require a dynamic conception of history that obviates thematic readings, and reveals the ideological frames of reference that such readings employ to conceptualize the place of disease in New England. An assertion of this temporal relation reappropriates epidemics as a central object of study, and helps to explain both the biological evolution of citizenship in America, as well as the attendant evolution of proto-national narratives.

Chapter 4 of *Miraculous Plagues* jumps to Boston's 1721 inoculation controversy, and pays close attention to the relation between epidemics and formal narrative concerns. Thus, my focus is not so much the technology of smallpox inoculation, as it is the controversy that the issue of inoculation engendered in Boston. Taking Perry Miller's dismissive characterization of the controversy as a "tiff about style" as my point of departure, I examine the key figures used to represent inoculation in order to understand the manner in which style and form are implicated in the self-imaginings of community.[25] The fact that the controversy played itself out as a pamphlet and newspaper war—with James Franklin's *New England Courant* most widely known as a mouthpiece for anti-inoculation views—provides a model for the interplay between Benedict Anderson's work on *imagined communities*, and Priscilla Wald's subsequent analysis of *imagined immunities*.[26] These self-imaginings appropriate their public voice in anti-inoculation narratives such as William Douglass's satirical plan to eradicate Indians with a bounty-system of inoculation—where inoculators would be paid a certain fee if Indians died soon after inoculation, and would receive a larger one if inoculees successfully spread the infection to other Native Americans. Although meant facetiously, this plan recuperates the long history of Native American susceptibility to Old World disease into the rhetoric of eighteenth-century Boston's public health policies, and its circulation in print offers a coherent model for the community to coalesce around its shared fear of two potential threats. Furthermore, it explicitly places Native American susceptibility to smallpox in a model where style and satire—as understood by Miller and Douglass, respectively—have a transparent relation to economics and colonialism. Neither Miller nor Douglass could fully conceive of the way in which Native American susceptibility to diseases had always been a fundamental building block of New England's economic and medical discourse, but the terms of Douglass's plan reflect the axis along which public health operated in early Boston, and how its application was shaped by the ideology of eighteenth-century economic markets in America.

This economic and colonial framework is drawn even more starkly in Cotton Mather's public advocacy of inoculation. One of the most intriguing aspects of the controversy is the mode of transmission through which Mather came to learn about the procedure. In a 1716 letter to John Woodward of the Royal Society, Mather recounts that his slave Onesimus told him about inoculation, and explained that it conferred a lifelong immunity to smallpox.[27] To supplement his narrative, Onesimus revealed an inoculation scar to Mather, which, coupled with later testimonials from the Royal Society, appeared to confirm the case once and for all. But if Mather took Onesimus's story at face value, he seemed to recognize that others would not so easily be convinced. When he made Onesimus's testimony public, Mather shaped the narrative, and tried to supplement it with formal and stylistic clues to support its factual nature. In successive iterations, Onesimus's voice becomes increasingly ungrammatical, to the point that Douglass would call it "blundering and Negroish."[28] Conversely, pro-inoculators called attention to these manufactured stylistic features as evidence that the slaves who spoke of the procedure were so naïve that they could not possibly mislead Bostonians. While this formal manipulation is part of an attempt to popularize inoculation in New England, it effectively distracts attention from the narrative's African source, and toward Mather's style of argument. What is lost in the process is the relation between slavery and the migration of narrative: Onesimus's story ought to draw attention to the African source of Western medical practices, and to the way that African narratives infiltrate Western ones, and are appropriated by them.

Whether one reads epidemics thematically to untangle formal epistemological questions, or to explore the modes of circulation in public markets, *Miraculous Plagues* seeks to make the narrative modes of epidemiology visible. My primary method is to examine the intersection between medical and communal narratives in order to understand how conceptions of health, of immunity, and of infection shape—and are shaped by—early colonial discourses in New England. In so doing, a direct consequence of my work has been to reexamine key moments in the history of Early American studies, and to model this history as part of the same nation-building rhetoric that it has sought to analyze. My work does not seek to revive outdated questions about the status of cultural coherence and homogeneity in Puritan New England, or about American exceptionalism, but it suggests a way to conceive of how these questions came to hold such sway over the field since its inception, and why they came to be asked in the first place. My reading of epidemiological mechanisms is an intervention into the history of American literary studies, and positions that history as a critical response to the same dynamic at work in colonial New England; whether in the context of cultural homogeneity or exceptionalism, epidemiological rhetoric positions these discourses in a dynamic framework that encompasses legal, economic, and theological, as well as medical, practices. The complexity of this dynamic underlies migratory patterns and immunological mechanisms, but is undermined by the relative ease with which thematic and allegorical readings of epidemics suggest themselves. At their base, questions about homogeneity and exceptionalism are representational in nature, and each reveals ontological assumptions about the way that America and American citizenship can be articulated, as well as the way that health is conceptualized in American culture.

I repeat an earlier assertion that epidemiology is of great use to the Western world; my analysis is not meant as a critique of modern treatments in and of themselves. But the late twentieth and early twenty-first-centuries have taught us that epidemiology is neither infallible nor all-seeing, and it would be a grave mistake to credit it with the same omniscience that the early Puritans ascribed to their God. The way that we conceptualize disease, the way that we treat it, and the way that we talk about it, is deeply inflected by the way that we think of self and of nation. I am therefore interested in the function of epidemiology as narrative; I draw few distinctions between illness and treatment, or between transmission and immunity because each of these is part and parcel of a larger discourse. When I first embarked on this project, I suggested (again, with more irony than insight) that at its most ambitious, it was meant to be a diagnostic endeavor: I wanted to expose the epidemiological roots of New England—and American—literature, and to understand the place of epidemics in the production of national history and national myths. If I can now articulate what I meant by an epidemiology of narrative more clearly, it is an analytical framework that inquires into the positioning of discursive practices in order to conceptualize the historical and ideological forces that shape communal narratives. Traditional epidemiology takes the histories of epidemics and of population movements as a point of departure for inquiries into the dynamics of illness. I take them as a starting point for inquiries into the dynamics of ideology and culture in America.

1

New England Epidemiology

But they did not understand that the Jes Grew epidemic was
unlike physical plagues. Actually Jes Grew was an anti-plague. . . .
Terrible plagues were due to the wrath of God; but Jes Grew is the
delight of the Gods.
So Jes Grew is seeking its words. Its text. For what good is a liturgy
without a text?

—Ishmael Reed, *Mumbo Jumbo*[1]

I

During his 1605 voyage down the coast of present-day New England, Samuel de
Champlain made note of the numerous people and cultivated fields that he
encountered along the way: at the mouth of the Saco River in what is now southern Maine, he described the corn "which [the Almouchiquois] raise in gardens,"
as well as the "many squashes, and pumpkins, and tobacco, which they likewise
cultivate," and in Boston Harbor, he noted that "all along the shore there is a
great deal of land cleared up and planted with Indian corn."[2] A decade later,
John Smith wrote about the same region in idyllic terms, observing that "the
Countrie of the Massachusets . . . is the Paradise of all those parts: for, here are
many Iles all planted with corne; groves, mulberries, salvage gardens, and good
harbors. . . . The Sea Coast as you passe, shewes you all along large corne fields,
and great troupes of well proportioned people."[3] These images of bountiful
gardens and a populated paradise presented potential settlers and investors
with visions of an inviting, Edenic landscape that could support European
planters with minimal effort. And yet these very same images stand in stark
contrast to those that would be painted by the first generation of English settlers

in Plymouth and Massachusetts Bay. Within a decade of Smith's visit, men like William Bradford and Edward Winslow described an increasingly transformed landscape as they sought to establish their own rights to appropriate land, and to live alongside the Native Americans. Indeed, efforts to settle New England permanently produced a class of narratives whose primary goal was to justify migration, rather than to describe new territory. A typical justification narrative—Robert Cushman's *Reasons and Considerations touching the lawfulness of removing out of England into the parts of America* (1622)—went so far as to base its argument on a description of New England as a "vast and empty chaos."[4]

Ironically, although Cushman's characterization differs from de Champlain's and Smith's, it would prove to be just as inviting to English settlers, whose concerns by then focused as much on widespread anxieties about the inherent dangers of migrating to the New World and potential hostility from Native Americans, as they did on how fertile the land was. To address this second set of concerns, justification narratives (which took varied forms, including pamphlets, sermons, journals, and correspondence) borrowed tropes and generic conventions from earlier European explorers to represent the region as hospitable to the English, healthy for their constitutions, and free for them to appropriate.[5] Furthermore, these texts shared a common detail described in a 1619 letter from Thomas Dermer to Samuel Purchas, which highlights an astonishing transformation that would prove to shape the physical and ideological landscapes of New England for generations to come. Addressing a catastrophic collapse in the Native American population during the intervening half-decade since Smith's visit, Dermer wrote, "I passed alongst the coast where I found some antient Plantations, not long since populous now utterly void; in other places a remnant remaines, but not free of sicknesse. Their disease the Plague, for wee might perceive the sores of some that had escaped, who described the spots of such that usually die."[6]

Historians have long since acknowledged it unlikely that the (bubonic) plague actually made its way from Europe to New England in the early seventeenth century, but Dermer's more general reference to "sicknesse" points to the root cause of this depopulation: a series of epidemics that struck the eastern seaboard of New England between 1616 and 1619, killing up to 95 percent of the Native Americans who were living there at the time.[7] These epidemics were so widespread and so devastating that no explorer or settler could fail to notice their effects. In *New Englands Trials* (1622), which chronicled his return voyage to the region, Smith reported that "God had laid this country open for us, and slaine the most part of the inhabitants by cruell warres and a mortall disease; for where I had seene 100 or 200 people [in 1614], there is scarce ten to be found. From Pembrocks bay to Harrintons bay there is not 20; from thence to Cape An, some 30; from Taulbuts bay to the River Charles, about 40."[8] Others such as Bradford would go on to describe the "late great mortality" in graphic detail, noting that it killed so many Native Americans, that they were not "able to bury one another, [and] their bones and skulls were found in many places lying still above the ground where their houses and dwellings had been, a very sad spectacle to behold."[9]

As accounts of these New England epidemics proliferated, they became increasingly elaborate in scope. Rather than simply describing the effects and consequences of disease as Smith and Dermer had apparently done, writers theorized the root causes of the epidemics, and constructed etiologies in order to locate their meaning within seventeenth-century medical and theological cosmologies—though one can't help but notice how often the theological overshadows (and even stands in for) the medical; because the physical impact of epidemics was so readily apparent, English colonists understandably attached special providential significance to them, and used them to frame their encounters with the New World. For this very reason, it is difficult to tell the story of European conquests in North America adequately, without paying close attention to the history of epidemics. And while this history has been described by scholars such as Alfred Crosby, David Jones, Noble David Cook, William McNeill, and Francis Jennings, the physical and environmental effects of disease only tell half the story. Epidemics certainly facilitated settlement in New England, but as important as these effects were, the seventeenth-century colonial justification narratives that described diseases rendered them legible to English audiences by providing settlers with the language through which to understand and legitimate their migration. In this chapter, I investigate those texts that chronicle early-seventeenth-century colonial epidemics with the aim of repositioning familiar histories of New England by recognizing the centrality of epidemiological discourses to justification narratives—and, therefore, to the migration itself. In doing so, I will reveal the process that translates epidemic events into narrative terms according to differences of susceptibility between populations, and explore how this translation played a foundational role in shaping New England's landscape for colonialist ends.

An illustrative place to begin this analysis is Thomas Morton's *New English Canaan* (1637), which describes the effects of epidemics on Native American populations in apocalyptic terms—a striking contrast to Smith's earlier vision of Massachusetts as a "Paradise." The Natives, Morton writes, suffered:

> Such a mortall stroake, that they died on heapes, as they lay in their houses and the living that were able to shift for themselves would runne away, & let them dy, and let there Carkases ly above the ground

without buriall. For in a place where many inhabited, there hath been but one left a live, to tell what became of the rest, the livinge being (as it seems) not able to bury the dead, they were left for Crowes, Kites, and vermin to pray upon. And the bones and skulls upon the severall places of their habitations, made such a spectacle after my comming into those partes, that as I travailed in that Forrest, nere the Massachussets, it seemed to mee a new found Golgotha.[10]

Morton's combative relationship with New England's Pilgrim and Puritan communities only highlights the breadth of this scene's narrative impact on English writers, as he echoes Bradford's observations, and displays his own mastery of the narrative conventions of providential rhetoric. But instead of focusing on the more obvious colonialist and Old Testament figure of plague that would represent Native Americans as the enemies of God's Chosen People (a representation one might expect from traditional Protestant reform theology), Morton shifts our attention to the region itself, imagining the landscape as a "new found Golgotha"—the site of Christ's crucifixion—less a sign of divine punishment against a cursed people, than it is a proleptic vision of New England's future. Morton reflects on this transformation even more directly in succeeding paragraphs by describing the effects of the "plague" on the region as having made it "so much the more fitt for the English Nation to inhabit in, and erect in it Temples to the glory of God."[11] Although perhaps only a fantasy conjured by the images that early settlers encountered, Morton's narrative draws attention to a colonial ideology that framed the settlement of New England as a divinely ordained mission, and that understood the epidemics to play a crucial role in that mission. Looking forward rather than backward at history, the figure of Golgotha reinscribes the scene of untold Native American deaths as the primal origin of Christianity in the New World. Although not literally a paradise, it consecrates the English migration on the site of Christ's sacrifice.[12]

By midcentury, Edward Johnson would reflect on the epidemics of 1616–19 in his *Wonder-Working Providence* (1654), and underscore the connection between migration and providence even more directly, identifying Christ as the prime agent behind the epidemics, and, by extension, behind the migration to New England:

Their Disease being a sore Consumption, sweeping away whole Families, but chiefly yong Men and Children, the very seeds of increase, their *Powwowes*, which are their Doctors, working partly by Charmes, and partly by Medicine, were much amazed to see their *Wigwams* lie

full of dead Corpes . . . howling and much lamentation was heard
among the living, who being possest with great feare, oftimes left
their dead unburied. . . . But by this meanes *Christ* (whose great and
glorious workes the Earth throughout are altogether for the benefit
of his Churches and chosen) not onely made roome for his people to
plant; but also tamed the hard and cruell hearts of these barbarous
Indians, insomuch that halfe a handfull of his people landing not long
after in *Plimoth*-Plantation, found little resistance.[13]

Johnson's reading of epidemics is certainly more conventional than Morton's,
but the convention itself bears investigating in the context of New England's
colonial history. How, for example, do epidemics signify in early colonial histories? What narrative purpose do epidemics serve in relation to the establish-
ment of colonies? A partial answer to these questions was obvious to Johnson:
epidemics shaped the meaning of the English migration, as well as its success,
they simplified the endeavor by physically clearing the land of Native Americans prior to the arrival of the English at Plymouth, and they stood as providential evidence that Christ had endorsed the migration wholeheartedly.

Although these are rather generic early-modern interpretations of disease
that one would expect to read on either side of the Atlantic, Johnson's narrative is significant because it fuses the local history of epidemics with agricultural tropes in order to reimagine the New England landscape in English
hands. For example, his claim that the "consumption" destroyed "the very
seeds of increase" represents epidemics as agricultural (rather than strictly
immunological) events acting on the land through their actions on Native
Americans, whose dead bodies he reads as metonymic symbols of failed crops.
As with Morton's description, these deaths have a meaningful impact on
Johnson's reading of the New England landscape, implying that Native Americans are unsuited to life in the region, and that the English are, by extension,
constitutionally fit for it. Not surprisingly, Johnson expands on the agricultural trope in the second half of the excerpt, drawing English settlers into the
equation as examples of fertile plantations in the New World, although it is
worth noting that the English remain agents—not crops—in this representation. Explaining that the epidemics have created enough "roome . . . to plant"
for the colonists, Johnson situates English and Native American communities
at opposite ends of an agricultural spectrum. While both play important roles
in New England's history, the divinely ordained epidemics essentially clear the
land so that a fertile model of European agriculture replaces the older, sterile
growth, and provides the English with an opportunity to supplant the Native
Americans even as they plant themselves in Plymouth.

The parallel relation that Johnson creates between Native Americans and English settlers operates as part of a well-developed colonial discourse, and highlights the importance of agricultural tropes in early-seventeenth-century narratives (as seen in de Champlain's and Smith's earlier accounts that portrayed the region as a garden-filled paradise). Jorge Cañizares-Esguerra argues that narratives like Johnson's function in what he calls the "epic" tradition of the Spanish colonial *reconquista* that was appropriated by English writers in the seventeenth century. For Cañizares-Esguerra, New England historians have too long "exaggerate[d] the cultural differences between Anglo-Protestant and Catholic-Iberian discourses of colonial expansion in the New World," and have consequently ignored the influences and intersections between those discourses.[14] One of the intersections that Cañizares-Esguerra traces, and that is particularly salient to Johnson's representation of epidemics, is the "gardening" trope (what I have referred to above as "agricultural"), which, he suggests, was "as central to Puritan pietism as . . . to Catholic mysticism." Cañizares-Esguerra argues that in losing sight of this specific language, historians have overdetermined the "mercantilist meanings of the term 'plantation'" in New England, and his aim is to resituate Anglo-Protestant narratives within the wider Atlantic context.[15] In this vein, his elaboration of the gardening trope focuses our attention onto the landscape itself as a central figure in colonial rhetoric, and provides a useful lens through which to trace justifications for English migrations to the New World. In turning to Johnson's use of agricultural tropes, we can achieve two things: first, we recognize how closely epidemics and landscape are bound to one another in seventeenth-century New England justification narratives, and second, we rediscover the ways in which those narratives are centered on long-standing rhetorical traditions that shaped emerging legal theory. Therefore, I'd like to complicate Cañizares-Esguerra's claim that many of these narratives were based not on "legal" but on "epic" arguments by suggesting that Johnson's agricultural tropes operate in dual modes. Certainly, the narrative refers back to a Spanish epic tradition, as Cañizares-Esguerra has demonstrated, but these tropes overlay an emerging juridical discourse that specifically emphasizes the natural world in order to accommodate English colonial experiences.[16] Rather than the either/or model that Cañizares-Esguerra's reading of the "legal" and the "epic" implies, I would argue that earlier epic traditions provide English writers with the language through which to naturalize the juridical discourse that was so important to the colonial project in New England.

As a case in point, Johnson's observation that New England epidemics created "roome" for English settlers to plant themselves in the New World is meant to soothe anxieties about the legitimacy of England's colonial endeavor, and to gloss over any difficulties that settlers may have faced during the migration.[17] In doing so, the term "roome" mediates between agricultural and mercantilist forms as it calls attention to the colonizing doctrine of *vacuum domicilium*, which was used by settlers and legal theorists alike to rationalize the appropriation of North American land. This doctrine held that unimproved wilderness belonged to no one in particular, and was therefore available to those who were willing to enclose and improve it. Terms such as "desert," "wilderness," "chaos," "void," and "waste" (and, in Johnson's case, "roome . . . to plant") were the building blocks of justification narratives because they helped to construct a legal basis for the colonists' ongoing presence in America; if the land could be declared "vacant," then it was free to all, and settling it was not to be considered a form of theft. The foundation of *vacuum domicilium* rested, in turn, on the twin concepts of natural and civil law, which held that God had granted the world to humankind in common, and that this gift ensured a "natural right" by which all humans shared equally in the earth's spontaneous produce. But as populations increased, making it impossible for the earth to support them "naturally," human beings were compelled to work the land in order to raise crops, improve yields, and survive. Legal theorists and theologians posited that God rewarded this labor by providing humans with a "civil right" that defined the fruits of an individual's work as his own; not only did cultivating an apple orchard transform the fruit into property, but so too did the labor of clearing, enclosing, plowing, and fertilizing vacant wilderness turn it into private property. The upshot of these theories as far as the English colonists in New England were concerned is that their civil right to property always superseded the natural right of Native Americans who lived in vacant lands.[18] Ultimately, the agricultural and juridical valence of the tropes that Johnson uses to situate epidemics within civil and natural law implies that it is the settlers' Christian duty to appropriate and improve these lands, and to transform them, in Cañizares-Esguerra's words, from "the 'wilderness' into blossoming spiritual 'plantations.'"[19] For Johnson, the groundwork for this transformation had already been performed by Christ in clearing land for the settlers.

Johnson's agricultural trope signals that *vacuum domicilium* would be the controlling legal framework for this segment of his history of New England, but he was by no means the first English writer to identify a link between epidemics and property rights in the seventeenth century. Insofar as Johnson mediates between the Spanish epic tradition of colonial history and the English colonists' desire to provide legal justifications for the settlement of New England, we can return to those earlier narratives to uncover the rhetorical and ideological work they do in their observations about epidemics. Even

Dermer, who had previously described New England as "utterly void" of in-habitants, used a term ("void") that is instantly recognizable for its parallels with the rhetoric of civil and natural law. To illustrate this point further, John White's *The Planters Plea* (1630)—an advertisement to attract settlers to New England—echoes Dermer's language, and elaborates the link between land use and epidemics:

> The Land affords void ground enough to receive more people then [*sic*] this State can spare, and that not onely wood-grounds, and others, which are unfit for present use: but, in many places, much cleared ground for tillage, and large marshes for hay and feeding of cattle, which comes to passe by the desolation hapning through a three yeeres Plague, about twelve or sixteene yeeres past, which swept away most of the Inhabitants all along the Sea-coast, and in some places utterly consumed man, woman, & child, so that there is no person left to lay claime to the soyle which they possessed.[20]

Drawing attention to the agricultural potential of "cleared ground," White's use of terms like "void," "claime," and "possessed" signals an implicit argument about land rights. But whereas Dermer's reference had only touched on the issue obliquely, White frames his observations about illness in New England with these civil law concepts: here, epidemics consume Native Americans and create a "void" landscape that consequently leads to English possession of land. If White does not ascribe divine agency to this "three yeeres Plague" directly, he is nevertheless sure to point out that it lies at the root of present English land rights, as none are "left to lay claime to the soyle." In other words, White uses the evidence of Native American susceptibility to argue that plagues are the catalyst for the settlement of New England, and then implies that English land rights are contingent on New England's epidemiological history.[21]

One of the striking features of White's narrative is the fact that it repre-sents these epidemics in an abstract—or disembodied—state, as if Native Americans are peripheral to the effects of disease; yes, they were "swept away" by illness, but this detail is significant to White only insofar as he filters it through civil-law rhetoric, and projects it onto the landscape. This level of abstraction may be due, in part, to the fact that unlike Bradford and Morton, White had not been in America to witness these events, but regardless of the reason, Native American bones are conspicuously absent from his text—an absence that marks land, rather than body, as the site on which disease regis-ters in his argument. This formula represents land and body as apparently interchangeable, and is further evident in Cushman's *The Sin and Danger of*

Self-Love, a 1621 sermon that internalizes its epidemiological rhetoric, and draws an insistent link between bodies, land, and disease. Cushman's text makes a passing reference to the epidemics of 1616–19, reminding the Plymouth settlers that Native Americans had been "very much wasted of late, by reason of a great mortalitie that fell amongst them three yeares since, which together with their own civill dissensions and blouddie warres, hath so wasted them, as I thinke the twentith person is scarce left alive."[22]

I am particularly interested in Cushman's use of the word "wasted," which, like Dermer's reference to "void," resonates unmistakably with the rhetoric of civil and natural law. More emphatically, Cushman's repetition of the term locates the Native American body at the nexus of epidemics and civil law, and therefore as the site of colonial expansion. Native Americans were certainly "wasted" by epidemics (as any number of explorers and settlers reported back to England), but Cushman's words should also be read for their relation to landscape, because they imply that Native American deaths transformed the land into a "waste," free for appropriation by the English. In playing off of the dual meaning of "waste," Cushman equates the effects of epidemics on Native American bodies with those on the landscape; his representation essentially creates a metonymy between land and body, where the apparent immunological weakness of one becomes a ready means of establishing the legal status of the other. Indeed, this metonymy is far from accidental, as Cushman was clearly aware of its dual valence when he argued that it was legal for Europeans to appropriate land that lay "idle and waste" in his *Reasons and Considerations*.[23] As with the metonymy Johnson would use when describing Native American bodies as failed crops, White and Cushman both rely on a rhetorical figure that forms the cornerstone of justification narratives because it paves the way for colonists to treat Native Americans and land as a coherent joint entity under the law.

If Johnson, White, and Cushman all fuse legal, theological, and epidemiological rhetoric in the service of colonizing New England, John Winthrop would capitalize on this rhetoric less than a year before crossing the Atlantic, when he wrote his *Generall Considerations for the Plantation in New England, with an Answer to Several Objections* (1629) as a justification of the intended Puritan migration to Massachusetts Bay. Winthrop addresses civil and natural law more explicitly than the narratives examined thus far, in part because he is so clear about his purpose. Responding to the charge that English settlers had no right to "take that land, which is and hath been of long time possessed of others the sons of Adam," he relies on the discourse of civil and natural law to argue that Native Americans had no a priori property rights in New England, because "this savage people ruleth over many lands without title or property; for they inclose no ground, neither have cattell to maintayne it."[24] In contrast to Johnson's and White's more elliptic narratives, Winthrop implies that failure to cultivate land is an essential component of the Native American's constitution.[25] It is worth noting that in doing so, his defense engages in a rhetorical sleight-of-hand: where his paraphrase of the objection to migration represents Native Americans as "sons of Adam"—and therefore as co-inheritors of the earth alongside Christians—Winthrop's response points in a different direction. With its Latin root *silvaticus*, the term "savage" literally locates Native Americans in a state of wilderness; savages both live *in* the wilderness, and their presence (like the absence of cattle, enclosure, or cultivation) reflects the legal status of land *as* wilderness.[26] Similarly to Cushman, Winthrop's reliance on "savage" as a rhetorical marker produces a metonymy that merges land and body, and in so doing, implies that Native Americans are inherently subject to natural law.

Of course Winthrop's argument leans toward theoretical abstraction rather than the practical concerns of day-to-day settler life. It is one thing to represent a sovereign agent as a rhetorical figure in a text written for an English audience, and quite another to make the same point in situ. And despite the fact that justification narratives like Winthrop's *Generall Considerations* relied on the rhetorical presence of the Native American ("savage") for their arguments, English settlers nevertheless felt that Native Americans posed an ongoing physical threat to the New England colonies, and a legal threat to their land claims.[27] This concern produced a double bind in which colonists deployed the figure of Native Americans ("savages") in justification narratives so that they could recognize vacant lands and establish land claims, while simultaneously working to remove them physically from the landscape in order to protect English settlements—either via conversion and assimilation, or through violence. Perhaps not unexpectedly, given the rhetorical parallel between his and Cushman's text, Winthrop locates the solution to this double bind in the epidemics of 1616–19. Epidemics fit elegantly within the rhetorical framework of the justification narrative, but Winthrop also represents them as having literally removed Native Americans from the New England landscape, thereby easing the colonists' endeavors in the process. Indeed, Winthrop supplements his civil-law argument with the observation that "God hath consumed the natives with a miraculous plague, whereby the greater part of the country is left voide of inhabitants."[28]

Echoing Dermer's and White's double use of the word "void," Winthrop's attention to plague at this juncture of his argument asserts the connection between epidemics and civil law.[29] In doing so, he effects the transition from a relatively abstract theoretical argument to one that relies on the local specificity of New England's history. By the time Winthrop wrote this justification in 1629, the epidemics were well known in England, so these observations about Native American susceptibility to disease permit him to argue that the migration would be made much easier by their effects, and that civil law has an intrinsic application in New England: by apparently clearing the land of Native Americans, epidemics produced a recognizable wilderness, and they retroactively authorized the civil-law rhetoric that established English rights to appropriate vacant lands in the first place. Just as significantly, the "miraculous" nature of this plague reasserts the providential character of the New England migration, and reinforces God's central role in maintaining civil and natural law; it yokes epidemics to theology and civil law, and gives colonists the means through which to read the New England landscape as vacant, but also through which to posit their own physical superiority on this landscape. Winthrop would repeat this language in a 1634 letter to Sir Simonds D'Ewes, only this time making the relation between epidemic and property rights explicit by encoding "title" as a function of immunological susceptibility to disease: "For the natives in these parts, Gods hand hath so pursued them, as for 300 miles space, the greatest parte of them are swept awaye by the small poxe, which still continues among them: So has God hathe hereby cleered our title to this place."[30]

Whereas the Old Testament Mosaic representations of plague relied on disease to help free God's Chosen People from their Egyptian captors, the underlying metonymy in Winthrop's argument implies that the miraculous plague was a divine force acting directly on the Promised Land itself, creating a void in New England, and opening the space of wilderness to migration and cultivation. By virtue of their own health, God's Chosen People were compelled to run toward the site of epidemics (i.e., the new Promised Land), rather than away from it (the biblical Egypt). Significantly, this inversion of the traditional Old Testament story highlights certain critical assumptions about the mechanics and etiologies of disease in New England. Johnson and Winthrop were well aware that the epidemics occurred prior to the great wave of migration to New England in the 1620s and 1630s, but the justification narrative form they use does not seem to allow for the possibility that the Europeans themselves were almost certainly the source of the Native American epidemics.[31] Instead, they superimpose epidemical events onto colonial narratives, and read the plagues as an invitation to settlement—a precursor to migration, rather than vice versa. This interpretation represents disease as a static force imposed on specific regions—independent of human interaction—thus freeing movement and migration from the important relationship to epidemics that modern theories of contagion would assign to them. Epidemics stay in place, consuming their Native American victims who remain fixed to the landscape, leaving "heapes" of bones in their wake, while healthy Englishmen are free to explore the country, make settlements, enclose, and appropriate land.[32] Under this vision of contagion, either English settlers did not recognize their own role in producing a wasteland in New England, or, perhaps more likely, they willfully ignored it. Justification narratives tied epidemics so closely to Native American bodies that both became geographic features of the landscape in the rhetoric of colonialism, and guaranteed the colonists a right to plant themselves in America so long as they remained healthy. Indeed, these actions and behaviors essentially preserved the English body as a model of health in the colonial environment.

In drawing the link between disease and place, Winthrop implies that epidemics strike land and body simultaneously, leaving legible effects on each. The upshot of this claim is that movement and migration are represented as a privilege of healthy, civilized bodies. Conversely, the land/body metonymy at the heart of justification narratives ensures that immunologically susceptible Native American "savages" become static figures in the wilderness. William Cronon characterizes this transformation in his analysis of nature, property, and colonialism, as one where the Native American becomes "as passive and 'natural' as the landscape" itself, essentially maintaining a narrative value in colonial discourses, even while succumbing to epidemics.[33] This transformation permits English colonists to read the effects of epidemic on the land through their effects on passive Native Americans bodies. And while this epidemiological discourse is specific to the early settlement of New England, such representations of passivity were not uncommon in seventeenth-century European colonial rhetoric. For example, Barbara Arneil argues that the Native American—considered either as "savage" or "natural man"—is a rhetorical figure who "belongs to no nation and has no political or ethical codes. . . . Rather he is [part of] an undifferentiated and ahistorical mass of non-European, non-civil savages."[34] By this "ahistorical mass," Arneil means, quite simply, that notions like *nation, property, politics, ethics,* and *history* are alien to the rhetorical figure of "Native American" constructed in European colonial narratives because these are, by definition, European legal, political, and theological concepts, and their use serves to elide individual and cultural differences between tribes by representing a homogeneous, monolithic population. Indeed, "savage" is also a colonial concept imposed on Native Americans as a means of preventing them from participating as agents in the order of history and law. It is a figure, in other words, that colonizes the Native American body by specifically excluding it from European civil law.

These exclusionary practices are formed by binding European literary traditions (including the epic conventions and "gardening" tropes investigated by Cañizares-Esguerra) with the rhetoric of seventeenth-century New England justification narratives to appropriate the "ahistorical mass" of Native Americans into the realm of European legal, political, and theological discourse, and to narrate historical fact by transforming disease into a normative occurrence in society. The term "appropriation" should, in this case, be heard in its full valence: Native Americans are appropriated into a historical discourse (through their representation as savages), and this representation is managed to the effect of appropriating land for the English settlers. Because concepts like *land, wilderness, nature,* and *natural law* themselves function in opposition to *property,* their projection onto America through justification narratives implies the subjection of Native Americans to English law. Indeed, as Eric Cheyfitz argues, "The use of *English* terms *property, possession,* and *ownership* to refer to the Algonquians' land usages in seventeenth-century New England risks collapsing the cultures and histories of these peoples into the English histories . . . which was precisely the prime mode of expropriation that the colonists used in their 'legal' dealings with the Indians."[35] Cheyfitz's discussion of land and property situates these English justifications within their proper rhetorical context—or what he calls a *Poetics of Imperialism.* That is, where Cheyfitz writes of the translation of empire ("*translatio imperii*"), he refers to the displacement of Native Americans "into the realm of the proper, into that place where the relation between *property* and *identity* is inviolable, not so these Americans could possess the proper but so that having been translated into it they could be dispossessed of it (of what, that is, they never possessed) and relegated to the territory of the figurative."[36] Likewise, my own use of "appropriation" is intended to echo Cheyfitz in both its literal and rhetorical functions. Even as the Native Americans succumb to disease, New England is simultaneously colonized—or appropriated—by Old World pathogens and by the colonial rhetoric that will create space for English settlers.

Arneil further summarizes the influence that colonial experiences had on evolving seventeenth-century theories of natural and civil rights, claiming that "Christianity and legal theory are fused and become, through natural law, the singular viewpoint for understanding the new world and its inhabitants."[37] I would only add that with the rhetoric of New England's justification narratives, epidemiological discourse mediates between Christianity and legal theory, naturalizing them—or binding them under natural law—via the action of pathogens on Native American bodies. Where disease clears the land of its inhabitants, justification narratives give shape to the wilderness by constructing a frame of reference through which the English settlers can read America as subject to civil and natural law—concepts that have already been projected onto Native Americans because of their immunological susceptibility to disease. Finally, the settlers redeploy their understanding of epidemics in the context of natural and civil rights, and create a framework to represent disease as a causal agent of—an invitation for—the migration, rather than vice versa. Early English justification narratives thus did not read epidemics as a response to European migration, but represented the migrations as a response to the epidemics—a fact intended to help underpin the legality of North American colonization. In their most obvious juridical and political manifestation, epidemics were used by King James as evidence for granting Plymouth Plantation's patent:

> Within these late years, there hath, by God's visitation, reigned a wonderful plague, together with many horrible slaughters and murders, committed amongst the savages and British people there heretofore inhabiting, in a manner to the utter destruction, devastation, and depopulation of that whole territory, so as there is not left, for many leagues together, in a manner, any that do claim or challenge any kind of interest therein . . . whereby we, in our judgment, are persuaded and satisfied, that the appointed time is come in which Almighty God, in his great goodness and bounty towards us, and our people, hath thought fit and determined, that those large and goodly territories, deserted as it were by their natural inhabitants, should be possessed and enjoyed by such of our subjects.[38]

James's reference to "horrible slaughters and murders" complicates the standard justification narrative by highlighting violence in addition to epidemic, though the patent remains ambiguous about the temporal source of that violence. Like the savages themselves, the "British people" have fallen victim to violence here, though the text brackets them off from the effects of illness. On the other hand, the reference to God's "wonderful plague" works on the same level as Winthrop's "miraculous plague" by representing disease as a divine tool in the service of England's appropriation of American lands—protecting the "interests" of the British. Epidemiological rhetoric is thus the narrative mechanism through which the secular and sacred worlds are held together and bound as one in justification narratives, and where religious and civil law underpin one another.

II

The New England epidemics of 1616–19 are as well known to modern historians as they were to seventeenth-century settlers, but most of the twentieth-century criticism on the subject aimed to identify the diseases in question, or to describe their physical and ecological impact on populations and on the environment; the historiographic project to date has largely been etiological and forensic, rather than interested in ideology or generic conventions.[39] My purpose here is not to repeat the work of those earlier critics, but to trace the relation between New England's epidemiological history and the evolution of its rhetorical practices, to consider the shaping effects of epidemiological narratives on the landscape into which the settlers were stepping, and to reflect on how these settlers' experiences of health and illness in America forged their communal narratives. Doing so reveals the underlying epidemiological nature of justification narratives, as well as the manner in which the history of epidemics influenced the settlement of New England for generations to come. The key to this analytical strategy lies in identifying those seventeenth-century justification narratives that described New England epidemics as *early epidemiologies*—texts that explain the appearance and modes of infection associated with disease, and that create a historical, as well as a geographic, frame of reference for mapping the progress of sickness in New England.[40] This is not to say that such narratives offer a biological or statistical conception for the spread of epidemics as one would expect from the familiar (i.e., modern) definition of epidemiology. On the contrary, it is clear that they do not. The goal, rather, is to recognize how epidemiology functions as *narrative*, to conceptualize the generic qualities of epidemiology itself, and to consider what the formal discursive structure of early epidemiology reveals about the joint operation of medicine, law, and theology in seventeenth-century New England.

Winthrop's, White's, and Johnson's texts all share a number of important epidemiological qualities relating to the frameworks they create for understanding the appearance and function of epidemics in early New England. In simplest terms, Winthrop identifies God as the source of epidemic, and "savagery" as its immunological trigger—although here again, the ideological complexity of his narrative is predicated on a circular argument in which savagery produces susceptibility to disease, but is also defined by it. Winthrop does not track individual cases of illness (he represents Native Americans as an unindividuated "savage" mass in the *Generall Considerations*), but his narrative reconfigures New England's landscape as a blank wasteland, and thus maps its epidemiological environment in spatial and juridical terms. Whereas a modern epidemiologist would chart the progress of disease as a set of data points in an attempt to identify and disrupt its causative agents, Winthrop sees through the effects of illness on Native American bodies in order to observe those effects directly on the land, thus marking its transformation into wilderness for the Christian settlers to appropriate, improve, and enclose. But if his epidemiological narrative is not what a twenty-first-century epidemiologist would recognize as medically or statistically significant, its implied emphasis on the underlying causes of illness (Native American savagery, violence toward Christians, laziness, etc.) is. These etiologies are significant because they represent illness and health as functions of savagery and civilization, and because they assign specific causes to illness, where being Christian (or not) and tilling land (or not) are behavioral qualities that can presumably protect people from (or make them susceptible to) disease in seventeenth-century New England. To understand these functions as behavioral acts is to understand the epidemiological nature of texts like Winthrop's. Indeed, contemporary epidemiologists note that their primary task is to compare the behaviors of people who get sick with those who do not in order to identify why epidemics erupt where and when they do. Thomas Timmreck describes the work as follows: the epidemiologist's job is to "ascertain, in a population, those groups with high rates of disease, disability, injury or death and those with low rates . . . [and to] discover what the well group is doing that the ill group is not doing or what the sick population is doing that is different from the well population."[41] By highlighting the behavioral claims that early epidemiologies make about the Native American victims of disease, we reveal the important generic links between seventeenth-century texts and their modern counterparts, and we can strip away the methodological apparatus of twentieth- and twenty-first-century medical practices to expose epidemiology's underlying narrative core.[42]

Although my aim is to stretch the boundaries of how contemporary critics think about epidemiology, I do not wish to suggest that any and all narratives that treat disease ought to be called epidemiological. After all, epidemiology does not merely describe symptoms and illnesses. Instead, one of its main functions is to track movement and behavior in order to develop a clear picture of how and why diseases spread as they do. For example, where Winthrop theorizes a causal link between epidemic and migration, and sees this as a useful end in and of itself, modern epidemiologists describe epidemics by calculating rates of incidence, prevalence, and distribution—each of which is to be mapped along spatial and temporal axes. It matters to an epidemiologist *where* and *when* someone gets sick because this information shapes public health policies; likewise for Winthrop. But even in view of modern epidemiological successes such as the treatment of polio and smallpox in the twentieth century, the statistical apparatus at the heart of these practices occurs within a highly inflected context that reduces patients to static points in a dataset even as they operate dynamically, as carriers of infection. As Wade Hampton Frost suggests, these contexts are deeply meaningful, because epidemiologists are concerned "not merely with describing the distribution of disease, but equally or more with fitting it into a consistent philosophy."[43] Frost recognizes that medical discourses operate within meaningful frameworks, and I would like to suggest that these frameworks are important objects of analysis in and of themselves. Such philosophies of medicine reveal how communities conceive of illness and health in relation to the world, and help to regulate the behavioral practices of their citizens— a consequence that has significant political implications beyond the treatment and management of illness. The stakes of analyzing the generic conventions of epidemiology (whether in the seventeenth century or the twenty-first) ought to be clear: even as epidemiologists work to identify and combat diseases, they are necessarily constrained by their models of health, of the human body, of community, and of behavior—whether this means advocating abstinence or safer-sex practices, regulating malaria through the use of DDT or mosquito nets, introducing disinfectants to the home, mandating vaccinations for school-age children, or, in the case of seventeenth-century settlers in New England, being Christian and cultivating the land. Because epidemiology translates the natural (i.e., biological) manifestations of disease to social and ideological spheres, the study of epidemiology's historical and cultural inflections—its *colonialist* philosophical model in seventeenth-century New England—reveals its epistemological roots and generic structures, and provides an important critique of the medical communities that produce them.[44]

In this broader generic context, it is hardly surprising that Winthrop and Johnson would seek to make sense of epidemics within familiar Puritan theology. Even if their narratives fail to read Native American illness as a biological consequence of European migration, they create a recognizable etiology and assign coherent meanings to illness. Indeed, the epidemics suggest to Winthrop and Johnson that Native Americans are unfit to live in New England, and this unfitness helps to ensure the legality of English land claims in North America. Although the symptoms of illness necessarily manifest themselves on individual bodies, the decimation of Native New England tribes between 1616 and 1619 registered with English colonists through the effect of epidemics on the land. Thus, the manner in which epidemics discriminated between Natives and Europeans during New England's early colonial history provided writers like Winthrop with the opportunity to conflate land and body metonymically, and to recontextualize their effects in terms of arguments about property rights.[45] And where modern medicine might understand the disproportionate mortality rates among Native Americans according to various environmental factors that include population distribution and immunological sensitivity to European pathogens, this discrepancy underpins the English settlers' sense of self in New England. In effect, this recontextualization means that key civil law concepts like cultivation and enclosure were not the only source of property rights in America—for these would always remain subject to Native Americans behaving "savagely"—but that property could be grounded in a broader immunity to disease. So long as diseases appeared to have different effects on Native Americans than they did on Europeans, the English would maintain their land-ownership rights, and read their migration to New England as a Christian project under the law.

Native American susceptibility to epidemics was crucial to the success of the English migrations, but it is difficult to overstate the impact that representations of European immunity had during the first years of settlement. After all, if settlers succumbed to the same epidemics that marked Native Americans as unfit to possess land, they could hardly argue for an inherent civil right to property in New England.[46] And although English mortality was universally high during the first year of any new settlement, the rhetoric colonists used to describe this mortality is quite different from that used in the case of Native American deaths. Cushman, for example, follows his remarks about Native American deaths in *The Sin and Danger of Self-Love* with the acknowledgment that "many of us were sicke, and many dyed." However, he cites neither plague nor God in this passage, and he certainly doesn't use the same metonymy that he had when referring to "wasted" Native American bodies. Instead, he ascribes this mortality to the climate, and to poor planning—to the "colde and wet, it being the depth of winter, and having no houses, nor shelter."[47] Even more tellingly, White talks about English settlers in the context of these early epidemics as well, but does so in order to highlight their fitness for life in North America by drawing attention to their remarkable immunity, which persisted in the face of regular contact with sick Native Americans. He writes that the plague did not "seiz[e] upon any other but the Natives, the *English* in the heate of the Sicknesse commercing with them without hurt or danger."[48]

Beyond his observation about English immunity to epidemics, however, White insists on the healthfulness of New England's environment for the settlers. He writes:

No Countrey yeelds a more propitious ayre for our temper, then *New-England*, as experience hath made manifest by all relations: manie of our people that have found themselves alway weake and sickly at home, have become strong, and healthy there: perhaps by the dry-nesse of the ayre and constant temper of it, which seldome varies suddenly from cold to heate, as it doth with us: So that Rheumes are very rare among our English there.[49]

This image contrasts with the portrait of dying Native Americans that White includes in the facing pages of his text, and further establishes the English colonists' immunological claims to property rights in New England. Likewise, narratives such as Francis Higginson's *New England's Plantation* (1630) also made note of the "great and grievous plague" that swept away the Native Americans, while emphasizing the salutary effects that New England's environment had on settlers.[50] Taking himself as the prime example of a man who had been "verie sickly" but gained "perfect health" in New England, Higginson claims that "there is hardly a more healthfull place to be found in the World that agreeth better with our English bodyes."[51] This fascination with the settlers' health held important political significance for English audiences in addition to the epidemiological justification for appropriating land in the face of Native American epidemics. For example, Jim Egan argues that English healthfulness helped soothe anxieties about the migration by demonstrating that "living in a different climate did nothing to compromise one's political identity."[52] In other words, while epidemics reconstituted the notion of property rights in America by focusing attention on the ability of English bodies to remain healthy—if not become stronger and healthier—this attention also helped to inaugurate a rhetoric for describing the body politic in which a mobile, healthy human body became the signifier of communal identity, ultimately endowing that body, Egan explains, with a "rhetorical authority . . . to which Locke would lay claim later in the century."[53] Such a political transformation points to the transatlantic implications of epidemiological rhetoric, broadening the scope of justification narratives to underscore the political importance of representing the English body in the New World as healthy. I want to emphasize that even as epidemics helped English writers to conclude that they were "better suited to the climate" than Native Americans, epidemiological rhetoric acts as the catalyst for fusing political, juridical, theological, and epic traditions into a colonial framework that would become fundamental to Locke's theories of property and government.[54]

To recapitulate, the apparent distinction between English and Native American responses to disease allows bodily difference to be transformed through epidemiological analysis into the lifestyle and behavioral triggers that are perceived to cause illness. And because the epidemics of 1616–19 seemed to discriminate between Native Americans and the English, the legibility that epidemiology imposes on bodies manifests itself in the fusion of theology and legal theory. The savage Native American body that had already been marked by absence—both the absence of God and the absence of labor— adds immunological susceptibility to the list, and this susceptibility frames his inability to improve the land, setting the scene for God's intervention. The advent of epidemics in New England presents the Native American as always already marked by a weak constitution, which then supplements the absence of his labor on the landscape as justification for displacement; lack of enclosure becomes the legible manifestation of God's intervention in the context of civil law. In other words, even as Native Americans succumb to disease, New England is already colonized—both by European pathogens and by the colonial rhetoric that will create space for English settlers.

Where epidemics are seen as clearing the land of its inhabitants, justification narratives give shape to the wilderness by constructing a frame of reference through which the English settlers can read America as subject to civil and natural law—concepts that have already been projected onto the Native Americans because of their immunological susceptibility to disease. Naturally, the converse is also true: the fullness inherent in the English settler (the fullness of God's presence and the fullness of labor) is reflected in his body's ability to withstand illness. The English settler's immunity marks him as the inheritor of these now recognizably vacant lands, while justification narratives naturalize that ownership. As the settlers redeploy their understanding of epidemics in the context of natural and civil rights, they represent disease as a causal agent of the migration rather than vice versa; justification narratives did not represent epidemics as a response to European migration, but the migrations, rather, were a response to these epidemics—a chronology that served to underpin the legality of New England colonialism. The deployment of epidemiology in the colonial context thus functions as a double erasure, at once ratifying European rights under civil law by dispossessing the Native Americans of their land in point of law, while disease physically removes them from it, rendering the region legible as an empty wilderness. If the untilled soil is not enough to confirm the settler's legal rights, then the epidemics certainly are. And yet the argument turns back on itself, becoming hopelessly tautological: the Native American is dispossessed of the land because it is dispossessed of him.

Even as Winthrop fixes Native American "savages" within European legal codes in order to justify the appropriation of land in America, epidemiology makes this appropriation signify meaningfully by projecting Native American bodies onto the newly historicized space of the New England landscape. In the terms that Arneil uses to describe the European colonization of the New World, the Native American body is supplanted by an ahistorical *savage* body, and colonized by the historicizing framework of civil and natural law as it succumbs to disease. Thus, as epidemics physically clear the land, epidemiology creates a discursive framework for appropriating Native Americans within European civil law, for legally dispossessing them of their property rights, and for reifying that law as a reflection of "natural" (or "divine") immunological processes. Dispossession and appropriation are ideologically significant because of the dual valence they prescribe for the Native American body—on the one hand, victim of pathogenic agents, and on the other, of the historicizing colonial forces of epidemiology. These historicizing impulses imply not only that European immunity sets the stage for epidemiology to rearticulate notions of land ownership in seventeenth-century New England, but also that it forms the basis for the eventual biological evolution of citizenship in America, where the properly American body is always a healthy one, and is one that always has God to thank for its health. From the first generation of settlers onward, the Anglo-American immune system guided the shaping of legal and political rights in New England. The New England settler's body—and later the American citizen's—is thus imagined from the outset with an attending fullness and coherence that excludes sickly others, and that is reified by a historiographic tradition that if more nuanced, nevertheless inherits its tropes from the same colonial tradition that it seeks to study or critique.

My continued interest in this critical discourse is geared specifically toward uncovering the close alignment of epidemiological, theological, and juridical rhetoric on the colonial landscape. As a case in point, a seemingly simple phrase like "miraculous plague" asks us to stop and reflect on how closely interwoven these discourses are in seventeenth-century thought, but as the remainder of this chapter—and this book—seeks to demonstrate, it would be a mistake to suggest that these colonialist implications are relics of a distant history. Indeed, these rhetorical operations are historiographically as well as historically significant, and they continue to shape the terms through which we understand regional and national histories, and through which we describe contemporary epidemics to this day. While seventeenth-century justification narratives constructed a metonymy between land and body that would ground arguments for migrating to the New World, the influence of this metonymy resonates in contemporary practices and tropes as its colonial legacy replicates itself rhetorically. Perhaps the most famous example in American

Studies is Henry Nash Smith's "virgin land," which anthropomorphizes the American landscape in a way that echoes earlier colonial rhetoric; the "vacant" wilderness described by New England settlers is appropriated by Smith, and given the characteristics of a "clean," "unsullied," or even "innocent" human body, and projected onto a national myth.[55]

While Smith's version of the metonym would itself be troped numerous times later in the century—notably in Francis Jennings's use of the phrase "widowed land" to highlight the violence of England's colonial legacy, it bears noting that these later tropes redirect the land/body metonymy as part of their critiques of colonialism, rather than escaping it entirely.[56] Jennings's phrase provides a much clearer echo of New England's epidemiological history than does Smith's, but clearer still is Alfred Crosby's popularization of the metonymy with his phrase "virgin soil epidemics" to characterize the devastating effects of European pathogens on Native Americans with "weaker" or "virgin" immune systems. Even as Crosby's explanation of colonial processes is steeped in the New World's history of epidemical eruptions, his concept of Native American susceptibility pivots on an ambiguity between the internalized weakness of human bodies and the legal status of colonial lands, both represented here as virginal and unsullied. As elegantly as the phrase encapsulates a complex immunological history of colonialism in the New World, it remains deeply invested in the rhetorical legacy of that colonial history. David Jones offers a compelling critique of this analytic paradigm, explaining that "virgin soil theory combines these older narratives, replacing a virgin, vacant land with a land filled with virgin, vulnerable people. . . . Virgin Indians were helpless before the thrust of European pathogens. Their bodies provided fertile soils for the growth of European seeds."[57] Jones's critique turns on recognizing the metonymic substitution of Native American bodies for land in the virgin soil model, and revealing that in addition to the very real effects of early colonial epidemics on Native populations, the phrase is part of an equally real legacy of colonial rhetoric that continues to be normalized even as it comes under the scrutiny of modern scholars.

As a counterweight to the static model of "virgin soils," I would like to think about the relation between early colonial epidemics and epidemiology in terms of *immunological syntax,* which is to say that the effects of the 1616–19 epidemics should be understood within the temporal and geographic contours of the colonial era, rather than as an ahistorical, monolithic (read universal) representation of Native American and European susceptibilities and immunities. Thus, where the justification narratives that framed New England's landscape in terms of natural and civil law provided an epidemiological snapshot at a fixed point in time, this snapshot reflects a local history that was contingent on a particular set of immunological disparities—in which first-generation settlers were most likely immune to an array of European pathogens that devastated Native American populations; thus, the genesis of a "virgin soils" model. On the other hand, an analysis that considers epidemiological history through the lens of immunological syntax does not downplay immunological disparities, but it does necessarily recognize their local and temporal specificity. The function of immunological syntax, in other words, is to render the narrative process of encoding immunities and susceptibilities within epidemiological rhetoric visible, and to push critics to consider how these encodings mapped New England as a coherent, legible colonial landscape. In the case of justification narratives, for example, these mappings are not so much a history of who fell ill and who did not (as in the virgin soils model), or of where and when epidemics erupted (as one would expect from modern epidemiological maps), as they represent a complete transformation of landscape into a legible historical space. Immunological syntax intends to disrupt monolithic biological models of colonial history in favor of a model that traces epidemics through their local impact in shaping colonial narratives.

The legacy of such a model can be seen in the work of Cindy Patton, whose analysis of the late-twentieth-century HIV/AIDS epidemic makes it clear that this colonialist apparatus continues to be central to the operation of epidemiology. Echoing Arneil's work on seventeenth-century legal and political theory, Patton describes the effect that epidemiology has on bodies with respect to the constitution of subjectivities and communities in colonial spaces, explaining that history, in this case, "means the possible destruction of natural history, the supplanting of the disease's history with a history of the healthy body."[58] The implication of Patton's critique is that epidemiology functions as a colonialist tool by disrupting local chronologies, and appropriating these within the philosophies and ideologies of Western medical practice. The history of the healthy seventeenth-century New England body is thus inevitably the history of the European colonial body—in both its narrative and physical manifestations. Epidemiology (as distinct from disease) becomes the event through which the history of migration can be measured and told as fact, and through which westward expansion can be justified; it becomes the inaugurating event of colonial history in New England in that it appropriates the ahistorical Native American into the realm of English religious, juridical, and medical discourse, figuring him as "savage," and figuring New England as a legible space with a history to narrate—a history that is, in fact, complicit with the teleological colonialist historiography which produced it. Where the logic of colonial rhetoric was always threatened by the presence of Native Americans in proximity to English plantations, epidemics and epidemiology succeed in confirming English rights to the land by erasing that presence.

The historical and temporal dimensions of Patton's and Arneil's arguments are significant because they provide insight into the operative practices of seventeenth-century colonial epidemiology, and into the ongoing impact of these practices on the historiographic record. For example, the "ahistorical mass" of savages that Arneil describes as fundamental to colonial rhetoric erases the differences between various Native American bodies, and abstracts these with a singular figure (the "savage") who stands as a symbol of a coherently legible whole. And yet, while this singular figure clearly belies the political and cultural complexity of Native American societies, it also masks their immunological heterogeneity in a determinist "virgin soil" narrative. Unlike the near universal mortality reported by Smith, Dermer, Cushman, and Winthrop, for example, New England's early epidemiological history was far more nuanced. While some tribes were decimated, others, such as the Narragansett centered around Rhode Island, appear to have escaped relatively unscathed, and accrued significant regional power during the period of colonization; right on the heels of his description of the unburied skulls and bones found in the region, Bradford writes that "the Narragansetts lived but on the other side of that great bay, and were a strong people and many in number, living compact together, and had not been at all touched with this wasting Plague."[59] In other words, the image of a "virgin population" or "virgin soil" vastly oversimplifies the effects of European pathogens on Native populations, whereas attention to the local dynamics of epidemics reveals the representational stakes of epidemiology in the colonial setting.

Thus, the ideological work done by rhetorical figures such as the "savage" or "natural man" in colonial justification narratives helps to elide individual and communal difference, and to represent New England's epidemiological history as a foregone conclusion—what seventeenth-century Calvinists might call predestination. But it remains incumbent on scholars to consider what this predestinarian epidemiological streak signifies, and to imagine the stakes of its historiographic persistence. For David Jones, when biological factors like immunity and susceptibility to disease are inscribed on the human body, or when, for example, "naturally weak" Native American immune systems are represented as the catch-all explanation for New England's epidemiological history, these are manifestations of an "immunological determinism" that pervades modern criticism.[60] Despite the nearly four centuries that separate Winthrop's *Generall Observations* from twentieth-century epidemiological histories, this determinism exists as a faint echo of seventeenth-century thought, where genetics have come to replace predestination as the prime causal agent of epidemics.

The concept of immunological determinism is not simply a vestige of colonial rhetoric that descends to us from seventeenth-century justification narratives. Indeed, it is deeply imbedded in the tools and methods of contemporary epidemiological practices that cannot so easily escape their discursive origins, especially as these are appropriated for historiographic ends. For example, Crosby's argument about the implicit differences between human immune systems would be formalized more insistently by epidemiological historians when increasingly sophisticated tools of genetic and statistical analysis became available to them, such as when Francis Black offers a hypothesis about the high death rates among Native Americans during the early colonial era by studying the relation between "New World population homogeneity [and] pathogen mutability."[61] Black begins by self-consciously distancing himself from Crosby's formulation, and suggesting that high Native American death rates were not due to inferior (or "virgin") immune systems, but were a function of genetic homogeneity in small populations. Extrapolating from the effect of measles on modern South American indigenous peoples, he notes that mortality rates tend to increase in relation to the genetic proximity of individuals who infect one another. Thus, for "a hut-mate, who would have had both mother and father in common, the [mortality] rate was 3.8 times higher" than cases contracted by strangers on village streets.[62] Black argues that small, genetically homogeneous population clusters—such as those traditionally expected to be found in indigenous tribal communities—tend to magnify the effects of epidemics because the immune systems of individual community members are themselves so genetically similar, that when one person becomes infected, he or she will more readily spread disease to other family members, who share similar susceptibilities.

While Black's hypothesis may well reflect a significant factor contributing to Native American mortality in the seventeenth century, three aspects of his study are worth noting: first, genetics and epidemiology come together in his argument to form a potent framework for visualizing communities according to their shared immunities. Black's notion of genetic homogeneity suggests a coherent model for conceiving of communal boundaries in which the science of genetics maps bodies onto specific locations. Here, racial, cultural, and national characteristics can be reduced to genetic traits—a genomic identity— and these traits can presumably predict the future viability of individuals as well as communities. By extension, "healthy" communities can ascribe their immunities to the internal, and inescapable fate of "good genes"; in other words, the survival or success of a given community can retroactively be understood as genetically predetermined (again a Calvinist might say predestined).[63] Second, Black's work becomes an unwitting argument for miscegenation as public health policy:

An implication [of the study] is that racial mixing is the best way to preserve the genetic traits of New World people, and the relative success of mixed race populations has been noted. If the theory is correct, mixing individuals would serve as well as mixing genes, but, either way, indigenous cultures are likely to be lost. For the people most affected, there is a choice, but it may be a bitter one.[64]

Aside from the assumption that "genetic traits" are the basic markers of a community's identity, and the apparent paradox that racial mixing is the best way to preserve the genetic traits of distinct populations, Black's analysis implies that indigenous cultures are immunologically and evolutionarily unfit for a modern world in which humans live in large cities, migrate, and interact regularly with others.[65] His argument moves very quickly from a hypothesis about the fates of indigenous populations in the sixteenth and seventeenth centuries, to an immunologically deterministic conclusion about modern communities and cultures. Black's argument echoes earlier justification narratives insofar as it essentially fixes indigenous populations to specific locations, technologies, and chronologies, while representing Western bodies as those whose power to migrate protects them from illness, and assures them their survival. Contrary to his assertion that the concept of immunological "inferiority" had no place in his theory, Black suggests that the fate of indigenous bodies in the modern world is always already inscribed in their genes, while the definition of a modern Western body is therefore naturalized as that which is healthy, and genetically preordained to survive infection in a technological age. His argument becomes one for the power of globalization to shape populations and communities biologically.

Because Black takes it as a given that indigenous cultures are likely to be "lost," the question of miscegenation suggests a deep ontological dilemma with regard to categories of community. This dilemma is more fully revealed in a third aspect of his study, which provides a technical explanation for the fact that mortality rates among siblings who infect each other tend to be higher than among strangers. This fact, Black argues, is due to the genetic similarity of siblings: when a first sibling becomes ill, his or her immune system destroys the weakest pathogens most easily, leaving the stronger microbes to survive longer, and eventually be passed on to others. Because their immune systems are so similar, siblings generally have similar immunities and susceptibilities;

the pathogens that survive longest in one sibling's immune system will be better adapted against the second, and will more likely be fatal to both than had they been strangers with entirely different immune systems.

The issue here—as with many biological histories—is that susceptibility is reduced and internalized as an essential biological weakness, and recorded as genetic homogeneity in a world that places a premium on heterogeneity and mobility. Over a period of five centuries, this reductive vision has been replicated at sites throughout the Americas until it formed a deterministic axiom that manifests itself, for Black, as a foregone conclusion that indigenous cultures will "be lost." And while this claim bears an uncanny resemblance to the early colonial epidemiologies promulgated in justification narratives, only substituting genetic homogeneity for Native American savagery—both leading to population extinction—Jones offers a word of caution that sheds light on how wide-ranging our understanding of epidemiology ought to be. He explains that the existence of near universal disparities between European and Native American susceptibility to disease "regardless of the underlying disease environment provides a powerful argument against the belief that each disparity reflected an inherent susceptibility of American Indian populations. Instead, the disparities in health status must actually reflect the disparities in wealth and power that have endured since colonization."[66] Indeed, Jones's warning offers an important admonition about the complexity that underlies local epidemical outbreaks, and about the power of epidemiology to naturalize political and economic disparities in the world. In the genealogy that I propose here, the antidote to such deterministic impulses lies in thinking about epidemiological history through a model of immunological syntax, that pushes us to consider the temporal and geographic specificity of epidemics, and to account for their translation into narrative terms.

III

One of the most striking ironies about the fact that justification narratives helped to erase Native American land rights in New England is that this erasure obscures what was an obvious presence of agriculture and labor prior to the arrival of English settlers—an observation certainly confirmed by de Champlain, Smith, and Dermer, among others, in the decade prior to the settlement of Plymouth. Because such observations were so widespread, it is worth noting that justification narratives often did not argue that Native Americans *never* cultivated the land, but relied instead on epidemiological rhetoric to discount or pass over the signs of agriculture by visualizing empty fields and "plaine ground" as wastelands that settlers could appropriate legiti-mately.[67] It quickly becomes evident from even a cursory reading of early colo-nial histories, that Morton's new-found Golgotha was not the vacant wasteland Winthrop had imagined in his *Generall Considerations,* so much as a land dotted with fields that were left empty in the wake of catastrophic events; the bones and skulls of the Natives that Bradford had described were those of people who were indeed practiced in the art of cultivation. And whereas Boston was once the site of plantations and "large corn-fields,"[68] William Wood notes:

Of the severall plantations in particular mount Walleston, a very fertile soyle, and a place very convenient for Farmers houses, there being great store of plaine ground, without trees. This place is called Massachusetts fields where [Chickatabot] the greatest Sagamore in the countrey lived, before the Plague, who caused it to be cleared for himselfe.[69]

Wood's description is notable both for his observation that lands had been cleared by the Massachusetts Indians, and because it offers further evidence that agriculture and disease are deeply interwoven in the early histories of New England. The empty fields signaled that the Massachusetts Indians did cultivate the land and did succumb to disease, and the fields thus stood as a reminder of the inherent contingency of English land claims until Chick-atabot, the sagamore who had seen his tribe reduced from 30,000 to 300 men fifteen years earlier, died in the smallpox epidemic of 1633.[70] With his death, and with the dramatic increase in the number of English settlers over the next ten years, the Native Americans' invisibility and the myth of their invisible labor made it all but inevitable that the English would maintain their expan-sionist narrative.

The fact that land was cleared and cultivated by Native Americans prior to the epidemics had a major—if unforeseen—impact on the development of English plantations. Wood's remark that Walleston had been a convenient place of "plaine ground" recognizes that the English could settle on older Na-tive American sites, and, by all accounts, this was not an uncommon practice. In his analysis of the ecological impact of European settlement in the New World, for example, William Cronon suggests that "more than 50 of the ear-liest settlements" in New England—including Plymouth—were planted in such fields, "thus saving their inhabitants much initial work in clearing trees."[71] Not simply a labor-saving strategy, settling plantations on old Native American fields had a significant ideological impact insofar as these new English plantations literally covered over—or erased—the signs of prior Na-tive American labor, and thus helped to naturalize the rhetoric of justification

narratives and colonial epidemiologies on the land. Similarly, early Pilgrim
accounts testify both to the presence of Native American agriculture, and to
the fact that Native Americans often taught the English how to tend their
crops in this new environment. Wood, who had described Native Americans
as "too lazy" to fertilize their fields properly, went on to praise them as:

> our first instructors for the planting of their Indian Corne, by teaching
> us to cull out the finest seede, to observe the fittest season, to keepe
> distance for holes, and fit measure for hills, to worme it, and weede it;
> to prune it, and dresse it as occasion shall require.[72]

Likewise, Bradford described the help offered by the Wampanoag Tisquantum, a man who had "stood them in great stead, showing them both the
manner how to set [their corn], and after how to dress and tend it."[73] This kind
of evidence that so clearly challenges the foundation of justification narratives also demonstrates a fundamental tension between the practical and theoretical concerns of New England's early colonists. Where epidemics and
epidemiological rhetoric mediated this tension by shaping the landscape for
colonialist ends, the evidence of Native American agriculture asks us to reconsider the various trajectories that epidemiology might have taken in colonial
New England had the need to establish land rights not been paramount.
Indeed, such alternate trajectories do exist, and we might call them *counter-
epidemiologies* to distinguish them from the early epidemiologies of Winthrop, Cushman, Johnson, and White, if only to ask what the relationship of
this genre to colonial ideology is.

By counter-epidemiology, I mean those narratives that treat the 1616–19
epidemics, but which seem to act counter to—or at cross-purposes with—justification narratives. These texts fall in two categories, both of which offer at
least an implicit acknowledgment that English settlers had a more nuanced
understanding of the genealogy of epidemics in the earliest years of New England's history than their justification narratives suggest. While I will explore
the narratives attributed to Native Americans at greater length below, I point
first to writers like Smith and Morton, who both acknowledge the presence of
Europeans among the Native Americans prior to the Pilgrim and Puritan migrations (a detail that is almost universally elided in justification narratives).
Immediately prior to his description of the "new found Golgotha," for example, Morton describes an encounter between several Frenchmen and the
Natives of Massachusetts Bay. Having been captured by the Natives, one of
the Frenchmen "rebuke[d] them for their bloudy deede, saying that God would
be angry with them for it, and that hee would in his displeasure destroy them,

but the Salvages (it seemes boasting of their strenght,) replyed an sayd, that they were so many, that God could not kill them."[74] Morton is clear about the epidemiological implications of this vignette, as he describes God's "mortall stroake" sent to punish the Natives. While this narrative outlines a causal and temporal relation between the arrival of Europeans and the eruption of epidemics, a similar story is reprised by Smith, who describes a lone European castaway who converted the Natives to Christianity, and warned them that God would "bring in strangers to possesse their land: but so long they mocked him and his God, that not long after such a sicknesse came, that of five or six hundred about the Massachusets there remained but thirty, on whom their neighbours fell and slew twenty eight: the two remaining fled the Country till the *English* came, then they returned and surrendred their Countrey and title to the *English*."[75] Once again, this narrative contextualizes illness in terms of property rights, making the cession of the Native Americans' "title" an explicit consequence of the epidemic, but it also suggests that the English were at least aware of alternate temporalities for epidemics.[76] Indeed, by implicating Europeans into the prehistory of these epidemics—even if only as rhetorical agents—counter-epidemiologies like this one point to a far more nuanced etiology than those represented in justification narratives. As Joyce Chaplin argues, colonial texts that asserted English superiority over Native American bodies and constitutions "had to ignore both European theories of infection . . . *and* Indian statements that they had been healthier before the arrival of the English, to which colonists were deaf. Their selective interpretations naturalized their emerging control over American territory."[77]

The more vexed set of counter-epidemiologies that I would like to investigate in depth are those attributed directly to Tisquantum, who is an interesting figure because of his own transatlantic history, having made the return trip to Europe at least once (if not more) before the Pilgrims settled at Plymouth. He was captured by Thomas Hunt (a ship's master under the Smith expedition) in 1614, and transported across the Atlantic to be sold into slavery in Spain. He escaped to England, where he eventually found his way to the Newfoundland fishery, and back to New England with Thomas Dermer in 1619, only to discover that his home in Patuxet (soon to be resettled and renamed Plymouth) had disappeared.[78] The thing that makes Tisquantum such a compelling figure is that his absence from New England coincided with the epidemics of 1616–19, and as the only survivor of his tribe, he would seem well-positioned to describe the impact of early colonial diseases on Native American populations. He learned to speak English during his absence, and was, along with Samoset, one of two Native Americans with whom the Pilgrims communicated directly when they settled at Plymouth. It is specifically in his role as an interpreter who could circulate between English and Native American communities that Tisquantum tested the boundaries of the epidemiological genre, destabilized those boundaries with his self-conscious counter-epidemiology, and offered insights into the genre's broader colonialist function.

Whereas the application of epidemiology is an important feature of early seventeenth-century English colonial rhetoric, I introduce the term "counter-epidemiology" because there is no reason to believe that Native American voices could not appropriate the genre for their own ends by describing how and why epidemics spread as they did. Indeed, one of the measures of epidemiology's discursive power to frame bodies and to shape spaces lies in the efficiency with which it can be cited and redeployed, and in the effectiveness that it maintains through such translations. But whether Tisquantum's counter-epidemiology replicated English etiologies or introduced alternate explanations for the spread of disease, a complicating factor is that like virtually all Native American narratives from the era, it survives in a mediated form, having gone through multiple iterations as it was retold by Winslow, Bradford, and Morton, among others. One of the central considerations to bear in mind while reading his story is what it means for English colonial writers to reproduce and recirculate this counter-epidemiology so obsessively—what the actual telling of the story signifies—and how it might naturalize the colonialist assumptions of the writers who produced them.

The first and most detailed iteration of Tisquantum's narrative was transcribed by Winslow, who wrote that:

> one notable, though wicked practice of this Tisquantum; who, to the end he might possess his countrymen with the greater fear of us, and so consequently of himself, told them we had the plague buried in our store-house; which, at our pleasure, we could send forth to what place or people we would, and destroy them therewith, though we stirred not from home. Being, upon the forenamed brabbles, sent for by the Governor to this place, where Hobbamock was and for some other of us, the ground being broke in the midst of the house, whereunder certain barrels of powder were buried, though unknown to him, Hobbamock asked him what it meant. To whom he readily answered, That was the place wherein the plague was buried, whereof he formerly told him and others. After this Hobbamock asked one of our people, whether such a thing were, and whether we had such command of it; who answered, No; but the God of the English had it in store, and could send it at his pleasure to the destruction of his and our enemies.[79]

Tisquantum's etiology is significant because he associates the settlers with the plague, saying that they have it in their possession, and can "send [it] forth" at their pleasure. This observation is not simply about who can deploy epidemics as a weapon because it offers direct evidence that for these Native Americans, there was a clear causal relation between the arrival of Europeans and plagues in New England. Presumably, the factor that makes Tisquantum's explanation believable to Hobbamock is that the association of Europeans with plagues was fairly widespread among Native American communities— even to the point that the conversation between Tisquantum and Hobbamock contradicts English temporalities of the epidemics, which claimed that diseases preceded the migration, and were therefore an invitation from God to embark upon it. Notably (although perhaps not surprisingly), even as Winslow transcribes this alternate vision of how the epidemics operate, the counternarrative itself implicitly acknowledges that the English were aware of alternate etiologies and temporalities, but it doesn't drive them to reassess their own epidemiological explanations. On the contrary, Winslow lets the apparent absurdity of Tisquantum's claim speak for itself, characterizing it as a "wicked practice."

One of the keys to understanding how this anecdote operates within a colonialist framework comes in the final lines, where an anonymous colonist appropriates and recirculates Tisquantum's narrative, only substituting God's divine sovereignty to send out the plague "at his pleasure" in place of the settlers' ability to do the same. Ultimately, the settler doesn't so much debunk Tisquantum's etiology, as he appropriates its chronology to consolidate colonial power on behalf of the English; Hobbamock is not fully disabused of his superstition that the English have the plague in their control—that power is only shifted to one remove, as it is the English God who maintains it. By narrating and then troping the story, Winslow defuses the significance of Tisquantum's observations to the end that they might naturalize and redeploy English assumptions about the epidemic's divine provenance, and in so doing, "possess" the Native Americans in fear of the Christian settlers and their God. This ventriloquizing function of Native American counter-epidemiologies is demonstrated at further length by Smith, who played on this very idea that epidemics sit at the nexus of human and divine power in a short doggerel that he composed to summarize the Native Americans' etiological explanation for these epidemics. Centering on a similarity between Tisquantum's name and that of a Penobscot god, the lines read: "They say this plague upon them thus sore fell, / It was because they pleas'd not *Tantum* well."[80]

A second crucial component of the counter-epidemiology emerges from Winslow's description of the causal force that drove Tisquantum to tell the

story—namely, his desire to "possess" his countrymen with fear of the English and of himself. Bradford, too, is fascinated by Tisquantum's motivation,
and his version of the story highlights the ideological framework of colonial
epidemiology rather bluntly:

> Squanto sought his own ends and played his own game, by putting
> the Indians in fear and drawing gifts from them to enrich himself,
> making them believe he could stir up war against whom he would,
> and make peace for whom he would. Yea, he made them believe they
> kept the plague buried in the ground, and could send it amongst
> whom they would, which did much terrify the Indians and made
> them depend more on him, and seek more to him, than to Massasoit.[81]

For Winslow and Bradford alike, Tisquantum seeks to establish his own authority over other Native Americans by cultivating a relationship between
himself and the English. Both suggest that the power of Tisquantum's narrative lies in its ability to inaugurate profitable transactions on the one hand,
and in its usefulness as an economic and political "game" to capture and terrify his Native American audience on the other. Ironically—and this is Bradford's blind spot—the very political and economic impulses that they accuse
Tisquantum of pursuing are at the heart of English epidemiologies, which
were written solely for the settlers' ends. Frank Shuffelton's reading of what
he rightly considers Bradford's overly simplistic representation of Tisquantum's behavior is quite useful in this regard, because it characterizes Bradford's attention to the economic stakes of Tisquantum's actions as a reflection
of his own colonialist stance. In other words, Shuffelton agrees that Tisquantum's actions were an "imaginative lever against his tribe's power structure,"
but he goes on to argue that "his demanding of tribute and gifts from the
Indians was not merely to enrich himself—he was not an Indian equivalent
of the Plymouth colony's London backers, despite what Bradford seems to
have thought. Giving gifts and tribute was for the Indian a token of respect
paid to men of spiritual and political power, and the giving affirmed both the
respect and the power. It was not capitalist accumulation."[82] Shuffelton's critique outlines two important dynamics in the narrative: first, he acknowledges that epidemiology can be used to leverage political power, implying
that this was Tisquantum's primary goal. Second—and without denying that
epidemiology can be leveraged for economic ends as well—he nonetheless
critiques Bradford's version of the story for its reliance on an analogy that
represents Tisquantum as an "Indian equivalent of the Plymouth Colony's
London backers."

What Shuffelton demonstrates is that although Tisquantum was perhaps not primarily interested in economic gain as an end in and of itself, Bradford's belief that he was marks the ideological referent that shapes his account of the New World. In other words, by representing Tisquantum's ends as selfish and economic, Winslow and Bradford appropriate his counter-epidemiology for their own ends, and displace their economic anxieties onto him, using him as a mouthpiece to naturalize English colonial acts. Ultimately, this means that from a narrative perspective, the figure we encounter in these counter-epidemiologies is not Tisquantum the Wampanoag, but "Tisquantum" the rhetorical figure who echoes the economic strategies behind early English epidemiology, and makes the genre's colonialist function transparent. Thus, what the circulation of Tisquantum's narrative in English texts demonstrates is that colonial epidemiology's usefulness lies in its ability to inaugurate economic transactions on the one hand, and in its power to create historical and political frameworks that can capture and terrify their audiences on the other. By troping the story, Bradford and Winslow—and the anonymous settler in the narrative itself—marshal these fears and behaviors for English ends so that the ability to effect economic and political gain—more so even than the ability to release buried plague—becomes the staging ground for colonial epidemiology in New England.

Thomas Morton would retell the Tisquantum story thirteen years after Winslow, and while his version is much the same, a few key details are different. First, Tisquantum is no longer present in the story, replaced here by a nameless "salvage"—a rhetorical substitution in which Morton generalizes the specificity of Winslow's and Bradford's stories to the universal case, and in so doing reveals the generic properties of the narrative itself. After the "salvage" facilitates a treaty between the English and a Sachem "of the territories," the Sachem catches sight of:

a place where a hole had been made in the grounde, where was their store of powder layed to be preserved from danger of fire (under ground) [and] demaunded of the Salvage what the English had hid there under ground, who answered the plague, at which hee starteled, because of the great mortality lately hapned, by means of the plague, (as it is conceaved). . . . Not longe after being at varience with another Sachem borderinge upon his Territories, he came in solemne manner and intreated the governour, that he would let out the plague to destroy the Sachem, and his men who were his enemies, promising that he himself, and all his posterity would be their everlasting friendes, so great an opinion he had of the English.[83]

Of the three versions, Morton's draws the most explicit causal link between the arrival of Europeans and the epidemics of 1616–19 by describing them explicitly as the source of the Sachem's fear. Morton further demonstrates the political force of epidemiology to forge alliances, as it is now the English—not Tisquantum—who benefit from their association with epidemics when the Sachem begs them to use the plague as a form of biological warfare against his enemies, promising friendship in return. Thus, what had been an oblique claim about economic and political stakes for Winslow and Bradford is now a central element in the narrative. Finally, and as with Winslow before him, Morton associates plague with "powder"—an association that is key for the Native American protagonists of the story, but which also turns out to be central to how this counter-epidemiology operates for the English.

Regardless of whether the Sachem (or Hobbamock) witnessed a store of gunpowder or not—and there is little reason to believe that he did not—it is difficult to ignore what a convenient trope the literalization of that powder as plague is. The central question when interrogating this scene thus becomes: What does this association mean for colonialism in New England? More particularly, how is a figure like gunpowder integral to these counter-epidemiologies, and how does it circulate as a generic or tropic convention of colonial epidemiology more broadly? Thomas Harriot's *Briefe and True Report of the New Found Land of Virginia* (1588) is a helpful point of departure for just such an inquiry because it outlines Native American etiologies for diseases that followed in the wake of the early English exploration of Virginia, and similarly associates those epidemics—albeit metaphorically—with powder. According to Harriot, the Natives "were perswaded that [the plague] was the worke of our God through our meanes, and that wee by him might kil and slai whom wee would without weapons and not come neere them."[84] As with the later Tisquantum narratives, Harriot also claims that Native Americans associated the arrival of the English with the onset of disease, although his language ("they were perswaded") is ambiguous enough to suggest that he and his companions might be responsible for that association, rather than relying on a Native American mouthpiece to do so.[85]

Harriot continues with one of his most famous images, which merges colonial fantasies of English epidemiological and technological superiority by reporting that some Native Americans apparently believed that English controlled disease by "shooting invisible bullets" at whomever they pleased, whenever they wanted.[86] The association to gunpowder here is tangential but striking, and offers a historical context for understanding the later New England narratives. While it is not clear whether the story that English guns (or powder) could shoot invisible epidemical bullets migrated from tribe to tribe

the full 600 miles from Virginia to New England in the early seventeenth century, Harriot's text was familiar to later English settlers (as witnessed by
Smith's reprinting of it in the *Generall Historie*), and very likely shaped their
own encounters in the New World.[87] Chaplin has written about the rhetorical
quality of the Harriot scene in ways that highlight its place within the ideology
of English colonial expansion, and her analysis clarifies the tropic quality of the
Bradford, Winslow, and Morton versions of the story, demonstrating how their
narratives naturalize English superiority as a function of the Native Americans' own susceptibility to, and observations about disease. Referring specifically to Harriot's contention that Native Americans associated disease with the
technology of firearms, Chaplin writes that "here is a tidy bundle of assumptions; natives recognize that English technology is superior to theirs, and they
react superstitiously to the new material conditions of colonization."[88] In other
words, even as Harriot describes a Native American etiology of disease, his
story is carefully calibrated for the European reader who will remark with him
about the unsophisticated nature of the Native, while simultaneously having
his own assumptions about English superiority confirmed by the narrative.

Harriot's assumption about the importance of European technological superiority carries through in the multiple incarnations of the Tisquantum narrative. In fact, to read Tisquantum's counter-epidemiology in the same context
as Harriot's invisible bullets metaphor is to recognize the narrative's colonialist implications as it circulates in English texts. And while Tisquantum's
etiology does appear to offer an alternative voice to English epidemiologies,
its contextual apparatus demonstrates that counter-epidemiologies still function within colonial generic conventions. Or, to think of it in the context of
Shuffelton's critique of Bradford, Tisquantum's leveraging of epidemiological
observations for political ends is being counterleveraged by English writers to
normalize their colonialist stance. As Chaplin argues, "When the English
appeared to be quoting natives, they were more likely engaged in
ventriloquism"—a process that was less associated with ethnographic accuracy than it was with English efforts to "assign [the Native Americans] statements that made more sense within English debates over nature than they did
within the conceivable field of Indian opinions."[89] Yes, these counter-epidemiologies ventriloquize Native American voices—and quite possibly, accurately
so—but even as they operate in tension with English reports of disease included in justification narratives, their generic and tropic conventions are
deployed by the English to establish the moral, technological, and biological
superiority of their bodies in the New World, to reify the narrative conventions of epidemiology for colonial ends, and to help secure the settlers' lawful
rights to property in New England.

The effectiveness of Tisquantum's counter-epidemiology becomes even clearer as it is further rewritten, troped, and redeployed in different contexts. In May 1637, during heightened tension with the Pequot Indians that would reach its violent crisis later that month at Mystic, Roger Williams wrote a letter to Governor Henry Vane and Deputy Governor John Winthrop of Massachusetts Bay in which he described his relationship to Canonicus, a potential Narragansett ally who was nevertheless "very sour, and accused the English and myself for sending the plague amongst them, and threatening to kill him especially." This charge is particularly notable because the Narragansett had reportedly been left unscathed by the 1616–19 epidemics. And yet, the narrative is uncannily familiar, as Williams goes on to write:

> Such tidings (it seems) were lately brought to his ears by some of his flatterers and our ill-willers. I discerned cause of bestirring myself, and staid the longer, and at last (through the mercy of the Most High) I not only sweetened his spirit, but possest him, that the plague and other sicknesses were alone in the hand of the one God, who made him and us, who being displeased with the English for lying, stealing, idleness and uncleanness, (the natives' epidemical sins,) smote many thousands of us ourselves with general and late mortalities.[90]

Again, the hallmarks of the Tisquantum narrative are present—or rather, a number of key elements are: the interlocutors are here, but the buried plague is not; the ability to "possess" others with the narrative is here, but its economic potential is not; Native American assumptions about the English power to deploy the plague are here, but Tisquantum is not. Indeed, Tisquantum's disappearance from the text is a function of two factors: first, what had by then become the utterly conventional mode of the story makes his presence unnecessary as a motive force, and second, by 1637, he had, like the rest of his Patuxet tribe, quite literally disappeared from the scene, having himself finally succumbed to illness at Manamoyick Bay a decade and a half earlier, in late 1622.[91] Here, finally, in Williams's letter, is the colonialist context for epidemiology in its clearest expression: epidemiology shapes and is shaped by perceptions of political and economic circumstances in the world, and it modifies specific behaviors according to its conclusions about how illness spreads. And while Williams doesn't accrue the power over epidemics to the English or to himself personally, he does point to its divine origins—a reflection of nearly two decades of Pilgrim and Puritan writings about "miraculous plagues" in New England. But Williams's epidemiology is a repetition with a difference, and he outlines the behaviors that cause sickness quite explicitly: no longer savagery specifically, but lying, stealing, idleness, and uncleanness are all "epidemical sins" that bring God's wrath.

By far the most noticeable difference between this and the prior iterations of the narrative is that the English now join the Native Americans as victims of epidemic. In the midst of New England's war with the Pequots, and of Massachusetts Bay Colony's internal religious and political crises, Williams finally turns Tisquantum's epidemiology inward, to warn *his* countrymen that their supposed technological and theological superiority would not inoculate English bodies against the moral and religious failings that threatened New England's communities from the inside. Even as he sketches the outline of Tisquantum's narrative, Williams reminds Vane and Winthrop that the English are not inherently immune to disease, but dependent on God's favor for survival. This, then, demonstrates the importance of reading across historiographic models like "virgin soil," and of considering immunological syntax as an alternative for understanding epidemiological history. This framework accounts for the ideological and generic implications of the epidemiologies and counter-epidemiologies popularized in early colonial texts, and it further situates these narratives within the temporal and spatial specificity of local histories. As Williams's letter suggests, the immunological disparities between Native Americans and English settlers that seemed so static in justification narratives were, in fact, far more dynamic than expected.

Over the next several decades, the patently deterministic epidemiological models found in first-generation justification narratives would become far too rigid to accommodate the unforeseen eruptions of epidemics and pathogens that struck New England communities. Even as epidemiological rhetoric would prove to be quite helpful in the mid-1630s during the Antinomian controversy—that "great and sore affliction"—when ministers and magistrates like Winthrop were able to look inward, and deploy tropes of infection to define, capture, and expel pathogenic agents that threatened the body politic, these models would continue to govern succeeding generations of New Englanders.[92] By the 1660s, however, immunological responses to the environment had shifted dramatically, and seemed to threaten the epidemiological logic of first-generation settlers. Williams's words would continue to echo as settlers succumbed to disease in far greater numbers than they had anticipated, and as ministers saw in these renewed outbreaks, the signs of declension.

2

Vectors of Dissent

As I was about to leave the plantation, a group of slaves came up to
me. I thought they needed treatment, women asking for potions,
children needing compresses for their wounds, or men showing
me their limbs crushed by the mills, for my knowledge of plants
had rapidly given me a reputation all over the island and the sick
would come up to me as soon as I appeared.
But this was another affair all together . . .
A man explained: "They say you've been carrying messages
between the field hands, helping them to plan revolts, and so
they're going to set a trap for you."

—Maryse Condé, *I, Tituba, Black Witch of Salem*[1]

I

In the summer of 1628, the Massachusetts Bay Company dispatched John
Endicott to New England in order to assert its rights over the Dorchester
Company, whose properties and privileges at Cape Ann it had recently
purchased.[2] Arriving at Naumkeag—soon to be renamed Salem—on
September 6th, Endicott's task was to prepare the ground for future settlers
and "to get convenient housing fit to lodge as many as [he] could."[3] The Company's desire to send more settlers to New England in the near future fueled
anxieties on two fronts: first, to protect its land claims from competing interests, and second, to ensure that the colony had a stable internal order.[4] Among
its many instructions to Endicott during his first year in New England, the
Company encouraged him to preempt social dissent before it manifested itself

publicly, and to be diligent in punishing offenses, rather than risk his government being "esteemed a scarecrow."[5] In offering this advice, the Company outlined a plan that would require its servants to be divided into "several families," appointing one member for each of these families to hold "a watchful eye [over it] . . . so disorders may be prevented, and ill weeds nipped before they take too great a head."[6] This mode of regulation, which focused the ruling council's gaze on its citizenry by relying on families to be simultaneously self-policing and responsible for communal discipline, reached its apotheosis in a proposed system of "overseers" who were to create a detailed record of labor production by keeping "a perfect register of the daily work done by each person in each family." Copies of these registers were to be examined by two to four "discreet persons," and sent to England "once every half-year."[7] In this manner, the regulation of labor and economic output for Massachusetts Bay colonists was bound within a system of order, and made transparent to inhabitants and government alike in an act of textual production that privileged the visibility of human actions over the individual autonomy of its workers.

At first glance, the justification for such watchfulness was primarily economic, rather than theological. Matthew Craddock wrote that because the Company assumed a "very great charge" for sending servants to the New World, a proper return on the investment depended on their "labor and endeavours," and was therefore to be one of the council's prime concerns.[8] This sense of economy runs throughout Craddock's and the Company's letters to Endicott, where time and again they give accounts of the various expenses involved in the colonial endeavor, paying particular attention to the cost of transport ships, and asking that he not detain them for "small matters," but rather ensure that "commodities [be prepared] in readiness against the ship's coming thither" so that they not return to England "wholly empty."[9] Craddock requested specific goods that already had a market in England, such as "wood," "beaver," "fish," "sarsaparilla," "sassafras," "sumach," and "silk grass," but also made an open-ended order for "aught else that may be useful for dying, or in physic."[10] The latter request defers to the colonists' local knowledge about the medicinal properties of New World plants in order to identify potential commodities of value to European consumers. By structuring his request this way, Craddock imagines America as a repository of as yet undiscovered pharmaceutics, and Colonial and Native American expertise as the medium through which raw goods could be transformed into marketable commodities in England. To this end, local botanical knowledge becomes a focal point in the production of transatlantic exchange, and appropriates a value inherent to itself; in a move that mimics the request to keep registers of human labor, Craddock asks

Endicott to marshal this knowledge for the Company's profit by creating an inventory of all such goods, and "to have some of each sent, and advice given withal what store of each to be had there, if vent may be found here for it."[11]

Despite the Company's optimism that the colonists could prepare enough goods to subsidize the cost of transport ships, Endicott's first winter in New England was almost as disastrous as the Plymouth colonists' had been a decade earlier. The second wave of settlers, who arrived in June of 1629 to help bolster the colony, discovered a community that had been devastated by famine, exposure, and scurvy.[12] While the Company's records of these events are spotty at times, the most explicit reference to the Salem mortality appears in William Bradford's history of Plymouth, as an oblique testimonial to the

> infection that grew among the passengers at sea, [and] spread also among them ashore, of which many died, some of the scurvy, others of an infectious fever which continued some time amongst them, though our people through God's goodness escaped it. Upon which occasion [Endicott] writ hither for some help, understanding here was one that had some skill that way and had cured divers of the scurvy, and others of other diseases by letting blood and other means.[13]

The pronoun shift between "them" and "our," centered as it is on the site of infection, already fractures any assumption about the homogeneity (immunological or otherwise) of English communities in New England. It marks the distinct geographic, political, and immunological boundaries between the two settlements, and figures local medical practice as a primary vehicle for the exchange of knowledge and services between communities—although it is worth noting that in this particular instance, such knowledge is represented as English, rather than Native American. The help that Endicott requested was certainly useful in treating and protecting his community, but it also provided a forum for the circulation of medical expertise within the colonies—a circulation that could have material economic significance in and of itself. In this instance, Plymouth settlers could introduce unnamed "other means" of treating illnesses to Salem's new colonists, helping to treat afflicted individuals, as well as producing and propagating markets of information that the Bay Company could then exploit to make trade with England more profitable, as Craddock had requested.

Bradford's note is also significant because it specifically (if somewhat obliquely) avoids attaching a divine etiology to the source of illness, though it situates God as the primary agent of protection against the infection. Bradford does not attribute a specific motive for the Salem illness, but Plymouth's status as a Separatist colony, and the fact that Salem did not have a minister at the time, would have intruded on the minds of settlers, who searched for providential meanings behind such events. Settlers wanted to understand why one community was touched by infection while the other was not, and what theological implications could be drawn from this difference; the description of "miraculous plagues" deployed in justification narratives certainly begs the question as to why similar etiologies weren't used in these cases.[14] The man who would guide this interpretive process in Salem was Samuel Fuller, Plymouth's physician and deacon, whom Bradford had sent at Endicott's request to treat the new colonists. Because it was not uncommon for ministers, teachers, and deacons to double as physicians in the seventeenth century, this dual role provided a ready conduit for theological doctrine to circulate in the wake of medical treatment.[15] Indeed, if the medical impact and success of Fuller's mission are uncertain, the importance of his visit in the eyes of New England historians lies in the opportunity it afforded him to talk to the Salem settlers about religious matters.[16] And despite the fact that the Salem Puritans were deeply suspicious of the Plymouth Pilgrims, Fuller and Endicott spoke at length about Plymouth's Separatism, and of the proper outward form of Christian churches. Endicott explicitly references these discussions in a letter to Bradford thanking him for the services of his physician:

> I acknowledge myself much bound to you for your kind love and care in sending Mr. Fuller among us, and rejoice much that I am by him satisfied touching your judgments of the outward form of God's worship. It is, as far as I can gather, no other than is warranted by the evidence of truth. And the same which I have professed and maintained ever since the Lord in mercy revealed Himself unto me. Being far from the common report that hath been spread of you touching that particular.[17]

This agreement was no less surprising to Endicott than it has been to modern critics versed in the fundamental differences between Separatists and the colonists who would go on to develop New England's Congregational Way. And yet the letter figures importantly as a sign that medical practices provided a powerful conduit for exchanging theological ideas in early colonial New England, and that communities which would otherwise remain theologically distinct were nevertheless bound by their shared commitments to health.

Williston Walker lends great weight to the impact of Fuller's visit to Salem in his history of American Congregationalism, arguing that Endicott would have been "readily impressed by the expositions of the Plymouth deacon."[18] More strikingly, Walker claims that Fuller was instrumental in moving the settlers toward Separatism during his visits, and was therefore "the man who was more than any other to be the means of transforming New England Puritanism into Congregationalism."[19] Hyperbole aside, if Walker places such importance on the verbal exchanges between Fuller and Endicott during the former's visit to Salem, it is because he reads in Endicott's letter a definitive change in opinion that was then communicated to future settlers. Perry Miller, on the other hand, points out that Walker's reasoning ignores considerable evidence that Endicott held Congregationalist beliefs prior to his meetings with Fuller, and that he was already "disposed to erect a Congregational régime."[20] Unlike Walker, Miller's analysis points not to a shift, but to a recognition of key similarities between Salem and Plymouth—a move that reflects the overall coherence narrative of the New England mind that is a hallmark of his work. For Miller, it is "inconceivable" that Fuller suddenly converted the Puritans. Although he acknowledges that the deacon may have provided the "little guidance [needed] to be translated into action," he maintains that it is "absurd to conclude that all later churches in Massachusetts followed the lead of Salem like so many sheep."[21]

While Walker focuses on the issues that were immediate to the New England settlers—essentially subsuming the influence of transatlantic exchange to that of intercolonial contact, Miller deals more closely with the interplay between Salem and the Massachusetts Bay Company still based in England at the time. From this perspective, an ironic reading of the Company's 1629 correspondence might suggest that it had worked out its church structure before the migration, because the letter's concerns were mainly economic, rather than religious. Tellingly, when the Company informed Endicott that Samuel Skelton, Francis Bright, and Francis Higginson were on their way to Salem to serve as clergymen, it remained silent about its intentions for the church's outward form, announcing cryptically that "we leave it to themselves, hoping they will make God's word the rule of their actions, and mutually agree in the discharge of their duties."[22] This apparent ambivalence is odd—particularly in the context of New England's mythologized religious origins, which, in Miller's version of events, point to a purposive teleological framework, rather than a haphazard evolution that followed the whims of bodily health. It hardly seems possible that the Company did not have some understanding with its clergymen, or that its silence on this score was not deliberate: this is Miller's point, and, in his inimitable style, he adds that if the Company "did not know what to expect of these men under such circumstances, then it was unaccountably stupid."[23]

And yet this teleological narrative is perhaps too easy as well, relying as it does on the fortuitous assumption that Skelton, Bright, and Higginson had the Company's full approval in the path they chose to follow. By all accounts, the system that the Salem settlers inaugurated was a radical departure from the Church of England's accepted practices, and if it was sanctioned by the Company, this implies a rather wide conspiracy in which the shareholders were willing to endanger their economic interests for religious principle—not impossible, but still a risky scenario, given the secular concerns of Craddock's correspondence with Endicott. The depth of Salem's unorthodox practices that emerged in the wake of Fuller's visit became clear in a letter from Charles Gott (who came to New England with Endicott) to Bradford, which suggests that the Salem church was founded with an eye toward pleasing its Plymouth neighbors, and closes with the hope that Bradford would "say that here was a right foundation laid."[24] The ceremony that Gott describes, including the election of Skelton as pastor and Higginson as teacher by the "imposition of hands," broke with the Church of England's system of Episcopal succession, and the candidates' admission that there existed a "twofold calling"—one inward from the Lord, and a second "outward calling which was from the people, when a company of believers are joined together in covenant to walk together in all the ways of God"—implied that individual congregations had the authority to ordain their own ministers; a practice that came dangerously close to Separatism.[25]

This foundation was viewed with great suspicion by a number of Salem settlers, most notably John and Samuel Browne, two brothers (one a lawyer, and the other a merchant), who arrived with Skelton and Higginson, and who took it upon themselves to organize meetings apart from the church, "in a place distinct from the publick Assembly" to read from the Book of Common Prayer.[26] Under the new powers granted to Endicott and his council to "remove or displace any unfit person or persons," the Brownes were immediately accused of spreading factionalism, and sent back to England.[27] Even if implicitly sanctioned, Endicott's actions marshaled the council's civil power to crush religious dissent, and were therefore potentially damaging to the Company, which worried that the Brownes might speak out against the colony, and accuse it of Separatism—a charge that could lead to the revocation of its charter.[28] As a precautionary move, the Company sent letters to Higginson and Endicott on September 16, warning them that the Brownes had been spreading rumors of "innovations" in the Salem church, which it nevertheless hoped were but "slanders."[29] The speed with which this factionalism spread in the colony complicates Miller's belief that the Puritans (and the Company) had a fixed notion of what the church structure would resemble in New England.

Adding to this doubt is the fact that on April 13, 1629, the Company explicitly approved William Backhouse's offer to ship the Book of Common Prayer as a gift to New England on the same voyage as Higginson and Skelton; if the Company knew that the book would cause such problems in the new colony, it would hardly have courted disaster by sending it.[30]

While Miller's argument leads him to read the Company's letters as a sign of astute political maneuvering—a public show of support for the king's sovereignty, rather than a heartfelt admonition—the Company still warned Higginson that if he was guilty of the Brownes's charges, he should "take notice that we utterly disallow any such passages."[31] In turn, it warned Endicott that Salem's close ties with Plymouth had led many to suspect that the controversy proceeded from "some undigested counsels [that] have too suddenly been put in execution, which may have ill construction with the State here, and make us obnoxious to any adversary."[32] Thus, even if Salem proceeded to develop its ecclesiastical system with the Company's full knowledge and acquiescence, the record reflects a strategic narrative decision to emphasize the dangerous, if not contagious, influence that communities could hold over each other at such a distance from England—as if either to inoculate the Company against charges that it approved of Salem's actions, or as evidence that it should be permitted to send the charter to New England in order to keep a closer watch over the settlers' actions. This concern was well-founded, as Plymouth's undue influence on Massachusetts Bay came to play an important role in the theological debates of the mid-1640s, and was subject to Robert Baillie's particularly pointed critique that the Plymouth doctrine of "liberty" spread quickly in the "free air of a new world."[33]

The Company's third major removal from England brought John Winthrop to Massachusetts with the colonial patent in the spring of 1630. Not long after their arrival, Thomas Dudley wrote to the Countess of Lincoln, telling her that as had been the case a year earlier, the new settlers found the community "in a sad and unexpected condition, above eighty of them being dead the winter before; and many of those alive weak and sick."[34] This report stands in stark contrast to the pamphlets that had proclaimed how healthful New England was for English bodies, but despite the link one might be tempted to draw between this English mortality and the "miraculous plague" of 1616–19—which the settlers nevertheless considered to be different in kind—their continued ill-health provided another opportunity for Fuller to treat and discourse with them on theological issues. Fuller wrote to Bradford on June 28 that while at Matapan (later renamed Dorchester), "[I] let some twenty of these people blood; I had conference with them, till I was weary," although "Mr. Warham [held] that the invisible church may consist of a mixed people, godly, and openly ungodly; upon which point we had all our conference."[35] This letter again reflects Fuller's practice of proselytizing to the Salem settlers, as well as his attempts to influence their ecclesiastical affairs. Meanwhile, in a move that shocked the new arrivals, and shows just how much Salem had strayed from familiar English practices, they refused to administer the Lord's supper to Winthrop, Dudley, Isaac Johnson, and William Coddington because these men were not yet attached to a local congregation—even if they were still members of the Church of England when they arrived. At the same time and for the same reason, they denied baptism to Coddington's child who was born during the crossing to America.[36] In and of itself, this refusal should have led to an immediate schism between the colonists. But perhaps because it was contemporaneous with the continued mortality that threatened them, the new settlers contextualized the disagreement through providential readings of their afflictions. In Charlestown, Winthrop (here transcribed by Fuller and Winslow) described that

the hand of God [was] upon them, and against them . . . in visiting them with sickness, and taking divers from amongst them, not sparing the righteous, but parting with the wicked in those bodily judgments, it was therefore by his desire, taken into the godly consideration of the best here, what was to be done to pacify the Lord's wrath; *and they would do nothing without our advice*, I mean those members of our church, there known unto them. (emphasis added)[37]

Given the apparent indiscriminate nature of God's judgment against individuals, Winthrop's desire to receive Plymouth's counsel is not surprising. The fact that the sickness was localized in new communities, and that Plymouth was again untouched, led Fuller and Winslow to map theological differences onto geographical locales, and had a likely influence on the formation of the congregations in Massachusetts Bay; Winthrop's refusal to proceed without Plymouth's counsel certainly lends credence to this assertion.

On August 2nd, Fuller again wrote to Bradford, relating the news from England that "the plague is sore, both in the city and country," and that "Bishop Laud is Chancellor of Oxford."[38] This juxtaposition conflates epidemiological and ecclesiastical threats to Plymouth, and is an obvious hint that the illness proceeds from a divine source—or is at least a punishment for doctrinal errors. Fuller mirrors this rhetorical move in the same letter by turning back to New England, and recounting the "sad news . . . that many are sick, and many are dead. . . . I can do them no good, for I want drugs, and things fitting to work with"; the implication is that the Company's continued afflictions proceeded from its errors. Yet in the midst of this desolation, Fuller announces that Charlestown had founded its church, and would surely soon return to health as a result.[39] The new congregation (which would come to be known as the First Church of Boston) was formed with extreme deliberation, admitting only four founding members: Winthrop, Johnson, Dudley, and the Reverend John Wilson.[40] Over the following weeks, these four would continue to admit new members, but kept strict controls over the process, maintaining a stranglehold on the form of worship in the colony. Less than a year later, in May 1631, this ecclesiastical control was formalized in the secular government, when the General Court agreed "that for time to come, noe man shalbe admitted to the freedome of this body politicke, but such as are members of some of the churches within the lymitts of the same."[41] Through this process, then, the religious cure to physical afflictions (i.e., the appropriation of specific doctrinal practices) was transmitted to the body politic as a way of consolidating disciplinary power, and effecting the Puritan elders' control over the community.

If Miller gives too much credit to his belief that the Puritans arrived in New England with a fully formed Congregationalist doctrine, Larzer Ziff and Slayden Yarbrough point out that the settlers' lack of practical experience in America—reflected, for example, in the disastrous first years of settlement— meant that "those who arrived in the New World, beginning with those at Salem, had no difficulty in adopting [John] Robinson's model of Separatism."[42] While these critics point to Walker's history of Congregationalism, it is only to reveal that this narrative had always been part of seventeenth-century historiography (to wit, the Company's fear of Plymouth's influence).[43] Half a century after Winthrop's arrival, William Hubbard would acknowledge the episode in his *General History of New England* (ca. 1682), explaining that the men of Salem:

> were not precisely fixed upon any particular order or form of government, but, like *rasa tabula*, fit to receive any impression that could be delineated out of the Word of God, or vouched to be according to the pattern in the Mount, as they judged. Nor are their successors willing to own that they received their platform of church order from those of New Plymouth; although there is no small appearance that in whole or part they did (further than some wise men wish they had done).[44]

If Hubbard's is a passive vision of knowledge production and the evolution of ecclesiastical practices among Massachusetts Bay Puritans, Edward Winslow's

1646 defense of Plymouth makes an important semantic distinction, denying that the Bay settlers "tooke Plimouth for their president," insisting instead that they had simply asked for advice about "how they should doe to fall upon a right platforme of worship."[45] The question of whether Fuller is the man most responsible for the development of Congregationalism in New England seems less interesting than the fact that he reveals conduits of narrative circulation; certainly, the founding of the Salem church points to a deep interpenetration of theological narratives with medical treatment, and whatever the ultimate degree of Fuller's influence, it is clear that his work in early Puritan settlements charts the intersection of illness and doctrine. Medical treatment becomes a vector for doctrinal dissemination, leaving an imprint of itself in the political and economic practices of colonial settlement.

To this end, I would quarrel with Miller's criticism of prior histories of New England, which he characterizes as having "stumbled over the seeming inconsistencies" of the Puritans. Miller's critique deserves to be quoted at length:

> To [these historians] the obvious explanation has always seemed to be the influence of Plymouth. If this be true, then indeed how can we have much respect for the intellectual development of these people when they did not seem to know where they stood or what they wanted, when the determination of the gravest problem lay at the chance mercy of a medical visit from Deacon Fuller? But if, on the other hand, the action at Salem can be seen to be the outcome of a long and matured program, the deliberate achievement of an objective deliberately sought after, then the religious history of the Massachusetts Colony is seen in an entirely different light.[46]

If it is somewhat sheepishly that I revive a debate more than fifty years in the offing, I do so to bring attention to the role of medical treatment as a vector for theological innovations in early colonial New England; where justification narratives carried their theological assumptions implicitly within the epidemiological frameworks they brought forth, my focus on Fuller describes the nexus of theological–epidemiological ideas as an active process that unfolds alongside the practice of medicine. It is not simply Fuller's work as a physician here that is important, but the specific conjunction of that work with the theological discussions that aimed to halt the progress of illness. My argument answers Miller's call for thinking of this history in a different light—not so much a return to Walker's narrative of Congregationalist history as an understanding of the interaction between medicine and theological doctrine. While illness and immunological responses to the environment are emphatically not the teleological outcome of "a long and mature program," the strategies deployed in the readings and treatments of epidemics (what I have so far called epidemiologies) do represent the "deliberate achievement" of understanding and shaping immunological interactions with the world for colonial ends. Fuller's role in this development may well be secondary, but his participation describes a dynamic that would continue to shape the Massachusetts Bay body politic over the next decade. If I resist Miller's teleological drive, it is because his focus on the colonists' intellectual development does not reveal a prescribed trajectory, so much as a static response to the constantly shifting nature of colonial environments. Rather than a dismissal of New England "mind," such an insight reveals the power of the colonial imagination to represent a radically new experience of the world in a coherent narrative that could be adapted to structures of political and religious order.

Despite the epidemiological rhetoric advanced in early justification narratives, it is clear that colonists were aware of the physical dangers of migration to the New World, and of the fact that establishing colonies was habitually marked by significant rates of mortality, which in some instances may have rivaled Native American epidemics. At the very least, this evidence underscores the rhetorical quality of justification narratives, which were, after all, less interested in divining the particular physiological mechanism of epidemics, than in deploying epidemiological rhetoric for colonialist ends. Of course, English mortality during this early period was often represented as a consequence of poor planning (and in any event unrelated to the Native epidemics) rather than as divine punishment—perhaps to avoid undermining the justifications that grounded the migration itself. For example, Dudley noted that at least two hundred of the settlers who had arrived with Winthrop died by December 1630, although most of them were of the "poorer sort, whose houses and bedding kept them not sufficiently warm, nor their diet sufficiently in heart."[47] Nevertheless, in order to maintain Native American and English mortality in distinct categories, colonists relied on alternate applications of epidemiological rhetoric to describe their experiences. Dudley was so touched by English mortality during the first months of settlement, that he felt compelled to draw an odd typological reference, comparing the colonists not to the Israelites, as was common practice, but, on the contrary, noting that "it may be said of us almost as of the Egyptians, that there is not a house where there is not one dead, and in some houses many."[48] The self-doubt in Dudley's comments is clear, especially as an echo of Bradford's earlier observations about Native Americans mortality. Any confidence he may have had regarding migration while still in England vanished as the settlers sought to understand the relation between their mission and the physical afflictions that surrounded them. And yet Dudley was firmly aware that he was not qualified to address the etiology of illnesses, a matter that he left "to the further dispute of physicians and divines"—again, a meaningful departure from the epidemiological rhetoric of Winthrop, who had no such compunctions at the time.[49] Even in his deferral, however, Dudley's emphasis on the inextricable link between religion and medicine offers a hint that this interplay would have ongoing significance for settlers, shaping their doctrines and nationalist historiographies, especially when illnesses forced them to look inward to their own bodies and communities.

But the colony's economic principles were never far from this intersection of medical and theological concerns. As Craddock's letters to Endicott indicate, markets drove the circulation of goods and medical expertise, and were produced by specialized knowledge of illnesses and their treatments in New England. Where markets were not centrally regulated, individual entrepreneurs could take advantage of prolonged illnesses, bypassing "legitimate" physicians like Fuller, and producing their own unauthorized treatments for settlers. The case of Nicholas Knopp illustrates such schemes. In March 1631, and doubtless in the wake of the great mortalities described thus far, he was "fined 5 pounds for taking upon him to cure the scurvy by a water of no worth nor value, which he sold at a very dear rate," and the Court imposed a sentence that he "be imprisoned till he pay his fine or give security for it, or else to be whipped and shall be liable to any man's action of whom he hath received money for the said water."[50] Knopp's punishment indicates the colony's desire to protect its citizens against quackery, and his example further demonstrates the speed with which such markets could propagate themselves in a new and potentially dangerous environment. If the economic nature of his impulse was subdued by the Court—if, in fact, the magistrates could regulate discipline and economics as explicitly communal projects—then more skilled healers (perhaps those like Anne Hutchinson, who knew how to exploit theological and medical conduits) could also take advantage of the central ambiguities of New England Puritanism, and threaten the colony's survival.[51]

II

The balance of this chapter focuses on the Antinomian controversy of 1636–38, and on the representational stakes that shaped its record over the following decade. Though the controversy is obviously better known to modern scholars than the debate about the influence of Plymouth's physician over church practices in Salem, I will be tracing conduits for theological discourse that operate in a parallel stream to Fuller's. Only here it will be vectors of dissent, as well as the means of representing that dissent, that I situate with respect to epidemiology. Antinomianism in New England is obviously not literally an epidemic, but my interest arises from the fact that men like Winthrop, John Cotton, and Thomas Weld used epidemiological rhetoric to assign specific meaning to the events that took place during those few years, and to regulate behavior in the colony. The epidemiological language that I examine ranges from the thematics of contagion, which include traditional images of healthful communities and contagious dissent, to a more narrowly focused attention on identifying and regulating the behaviors of dissidents as pathological. The most famous example of these thematics of infection arises from the title that Weld gave to Winthrop's account of the controversy—*A Short Story of the Rise, reign, and ruin of the Antinomians, Familists & Libertines, that infected the Churches of New-England*—which nevertheless only begins to hint at the ways in which epidemiology operates as an organizing principle for the victorious faction in the controversy.[52] So while this chapter does not trace the progress of a physical epidemic like smallpox or the measles, it does examine the magistrates' application of epidemiology in the political realm to define the terms of acceptable behavior, and to outline the contours of an ideologically healthy community in Massachusetts Bay.

It is because the subject of this chapter is not a literal epidemic that it clarifies epidemiology's narrative capacity for describing communities in ideological terms; a figural epidemic like the Antinomian controversy deliteralizes illness, but in doing so, redeploys epidemiological rhetoric with a vision of policing and regulating behaviors as a matter of communal (or national) security. For example, Winthrop's *Short Story* figures New England Congregationalism as a model of church polity to an English audience, but, just as significantly, it provides a platform for ministers and magistrates to cast themselves as a fundamentally healthful "Orthodox" core around which the larger community can cohere, and against which dissenting opinion can be abjected; it is the representational terms of this coherence that I examine here.[53] The fact that this chapter centers on a figural "epidemic" means that it is, perhaps more evidently so than any other in *Miraculous Plagues*, self-consciously invested in the linguistic stakes of epidemiology. This investment traces back to Patricia Caldwell's characterization that "whatever else it may have been, the Antinomian Controversy was a monumental crisis of language"—a claim that continues to resonate in the critical attention to the controversy, and that frames my own understanding of the historical record.[54]

Even as the Antinomian controversy has produced a vibrant body of scholarship over the past two decades, recent critical interest has fractured traditional histories of the controversy, which had previously tended to center on Anne Hutchinson as an early colonial model of individualism (or even Emersonianism), and proto-feminism. Janice Knight, for example, works against the "consensus" model of New England Puritanism to establish a plural vision of contested orthodoxies in place of long-standing narratives about a singular Orthodox voice. More recently, Phillip Round, Michael P. Winship, Elizabeth Maddock Dillon, and Jim Egan have situated the Antinomian controversy within a wider historical and geographic context to emphasize that it was not the product of a narrowly defined provincial debate, but emerged with a self-conscious attention to transatlantic audiences.[55] Winship in particular instantiates the recent critical approach to the Antinomian controversy by renaming it the "Free Grace" controversy, thus highlighting its place within a debate about Puritan theology that played out on both sides of the Atlantic. Perhaps even more radically, Jonathan Beecher Field has recently argued that "the Antinomian Controversy Did Not Take Place."[56]

Field, of course, does not literally mean that the events of the Antinomian controversy did not take place, or that its main participants did not exist, but he takes his cue from Jean Baudrillard's reading of the 1991 Gulf War to suggest that "what did not take place was the distinct, high-stakes contest for the future of the Bay Colony that is a staple of New England historiography from its earliest to its most recent iterations. Instead, these narratives of a crisis are an artifact of the historiography of the event."[57] Field's analysis engages the historiographic record as much as the controversy itself, and his argument is that early histories were, from the outset, committed to representing a coherent narrative of events that could project a consensus vision of Massachusetts Bay, and be circumscribed almost as easily as Winthrop and Weld would have us believe the magistrates dispatched Hutchinson and her followers to Rhode Island. And as Dillon argues, Winthrop's, Weld's, and Cotton's narratives were not "written for the sake of historical accuracy and rationality alone, but in order to make English readers believe that the Massachusetts Bay Colony was a thriving, godly enterprise that they might wish to join."[58] The upshot of Field's claim is that the narrative coherence that the record aims for should itself be a subject of analysis, as it is symptomatic of an emerging imperative for the Massachusetts Bay colony to define itself as a cohesive, stable community. Finally, if one is to consider the historiographic record within the trajectory of this imperative, then the recent critical fragmentation that I have alluded to ought to be read as the symptom of resistance to totalizing national narratives. I would like to situate myself within the trajectory of this resistance, and to consider how epidemiological analysis facilitates such a stance.

Field's argument stems from his recognition of the rhetorical nature of the historical record itself. By the same token, my analysis is less about the specific theological implications of the controversy than about the narrative framing devices that gave coherence to the events in question. To the extent that the Antinomian controversy "did not take place," I argue that epidemiological rhetoric is one of the strategic cornerstones used by men like Winthrop and Weld to establish that events did unfold in a very particular way, and, furthermore, to represent the controversy as a "singular crisis with Anne Hutchinson at its center."[59] This strategy produced a primary record of events that defined the behavioral boundaries of a healthy community, described an infectious threat to that community, prescribed the actions for restoring it to health, and established both the community and those behaviors as essentially Orthodox. In this manner, the concept of community that emerges in the wake of the controversy does so by projecting or positioning health as a timeless manifestation of "Orthodox" behaviors, which is to say that "community" is given shape insofar as it represents itself against (and as a cure for) the pathological behaviors of Antinomians. I will not argue for an Orthodox or consensus vision of seventeenth-century Puritan New England—on the contrary, I suggest that Orthodoxy and consensus are strategically projected into the historiographic record of the controversy, and are given voice with the help of epidemiological rhetoric; the record itself is designed as evidence that New England's Congregational Way is a self-regulating model of health to reassure the colony's Puritan supporters in England, as Dillon argues, "that justice and religious orthodoxy prevail in Massachusetts."[60] The images of community, of Antinomianism, and of Anne Hutchinson that modern scholars encounter when analyzing the controversy have thus been naturalized as the very terms through which the controversy constitutes itself as an historical event, and it is my claim that epidemiology helps to frame this process of naturalization.

If Weld and Winthrop represent Antinomianism as a figural epidemic that threatens New England's churches, I am interested in the depth of this representation, and in the rhetorical mechanisms that frame its cultural and ideological boundaries. As I argued in Chapter 1, epidemiology was central to the work of English colonialism during the first decade of migration insofar as it allowed settlers to deploy a rhetorical apparatus that represented English health in the New World as a sign of industry. In the years leading to the Great Migration, these epidemiological narratives focused primarily on dying Native American bodies by translating them into an historical European discourse, and facilitating the appropriation of North American lands within an English legal and theological order. But once the migration was well under way, the discursive power of epidemiology began to manifest itself in a reflexive turn, where English bodies and communities would become the site of the epidemiological gaze. This inward turn opened a space for figural epidemics to complement biological epidemics as sites of regulation, and to represent behaviors themselves as epidemical.[61] To this end, the relation between labor and property that marked the positioning of epidemiology as a colonizing tool in justification narratives later came to be subsumed to a relation between labor and discipline, as colonial narratives focused on representations of citizenship and community; in particular, the labor of medical practitioners such as Samuel Fuller plays an increasingly vexed role in discourses of communal identity, as they come to represent conduits—or vectors—of dissenting behavior. Because epidemiology highlights the behavioral differences between sick and well populations, the discursive strategies revealed by epidemiological narratives can be marshaled to regulate the behaviors of political subjects by defining the boundaries within which they are permitted to operate freely, and against which their transgressions will be marked as pathological.

To be sure, the figures most often associated with the pathologizing force of Puritan language in the first decades of settlement—and therefore most compelling to modern critics—are the "monstrous births" of Anne Hutchinson and Mary Dyer.[62] Winthrop's detailed description of the exhumed body of Dyer's child, and Weld's further fascination with it in the *Short Story* easily lend themselves to a medically inflected criticism, as does the overdetermined association that a number of seventeenth- and early-eighteenth-century Puritans made between those births and the "monstrous" errors of the Antinomians; in its clearest instantiation, Weld reads the monstrous births as the literal manifestation—or publication—of Antinomian error. Thus, the thematic of contagion that emerges from his obsessive cataloguing and pathologizing of the births manifests itself in a metonymic relation between those births and the monstrosity of Antinomian ideas; monstrous births offer a striking example of the symbolic force of pathology, and while this symbolism is important, it tends to obscure how broadly epidemiological rhetoric operates in the historical record by the very sensationalism that it represents. I would therefore like to defer such readings for the time being, if only to uncover and consider the significance of other examples of epidemiological thinking in the record.

The first such example is obviously the term "infected" that Weld uses in his title for the *Short Story*. The representation of community as a body politic, and of dissent as pathology was nothing new in and of itself, but Weld's words need to be contrasted with the opening sentence of his preface, where he writes that the controversy erupted "after we had escaped the cruell hands of

persecuting Prelates, and the dangers at Sea, and had prettily well outgrowne
our wildernes troubles in our first plantings in New-England."[63] The phrase
"wildernes troubles" is a compelling euphemism because it simultaneously acknowledges the difficulties that early New England settlers faced when they
arrived in New England, while deflecting the specifics of those difficulties—
namely, the high mortality reported by settlers like Endicott and Dudley when
they first arrived in New England, or the illnesses that led Fuller on his mission to help the Massachusetts Bay colonists. In this sense, "Wildernes troubles" represents Weld's deliberate epidemiological choice—his narrative
decision about how to represent the nature of that mortality. Even as it offers
a striking counterpoint to Winthrop's "miraculous plague," the phrase nonetheless recalls the epidemiological rhetoric of justification narratives by
pathologizing the wilderness as the site of those troubles. But the key here is
that by eliding settler mortality, "wildernes troubles" is deliberately ambiguous, and maintains the fiction of the English body's fitness in the New World
by withholding evidence to the contrary. Instead of highlighting any specific
behavioral trigger for illness or death, as would have been necessary had Weld
himself been more explicit about English mortality, the phrase renders that
mortality invisible to the historical record, thus normalizing the settler's body
as well-suited for New England's environment.

Because Weld uses the relatively neutral "troubles" instead of "death" or
"plagues" or "afflictions" to describe settler mortality, his epidemiological
choice is not invested in identifying the cause of an illness (as one would nor-
mally expect), so much as it is in erasing the mark of illness altogether, and in
reasserting the fundamental health of the colonial population. By implicitly
contrasting this health to the "infection" of Antinomianism outlined in the
title, Weld pathologizes Antinomian behavior, and represents the community
itself (the "Churches of New-England") as healthy. From a narrative point of
view, Weld also preserves the rhetorical force of "death" by avoiding any direct
reference to mortality until he deploys it at the very end of his preface, where
it becomes a clear sign of God's punishment against Anne Hutchinson. Finally, it is worth noting the further political stakes of this elision in a transatlantic context, insofar as it allows Weld to remain silent about the influence of
Plymouth settlers such as Fuller on the evolution of Congregationalist practices in Massachusetts Bay; without mortality, there is no need for Fuller's
treatment, and thus no controversy about his potential influence on church
doctrine. This is an important point with respect to the *Short Story*'s circulation in England as a defense of Congregationalism, where critics such as
Robert Baillie were well aware and suspicious of Plymouth's influence on Massachusetts Bay. At the very least, Weld avoids reminding his readers about

the potential connection between Plymouth's theological influence and Massachusetts Bay's susceptibility to Antinomianism.

Critical attention of this kind reveals that epidemiological rhetoric—even when it functions by indirection—sets the parameters for behaviors to be regarded as healthful or pathological, and naturalizes those behaviors in terms that manifest themselves politically and theologically. Thus, within the first pages of the *Short Story*, Weld represents Antinomians as an infection, and contrasts this infection to what he then projects as an essentially healthful Massachusetts Bay community, embodied by its magistrates and ministers. The operating metaphor of body and community is certainly not new to the Antinomian controversy, but it is central to the way that colonists like Winthrop described their place in New England, and as such was particularly suited for the application of epidemiological rhetoric. In *A Model of Christian Charity*, for example, Winthrop envisions the future colony as a cohesive body, and calls for settlers to unite themselves in a contractual bond of love through which "all the parts of this body . . . are made so contiguous . . . as they must needs partake of each other's strength and infirmity; joy and sorrow, weal and woe."[64] This representational pairing of strength/infirmity, joy/sorrow, and weal/woe helps to introduce a hermeneutics of discipline where public order becomes the normative sign of a healthful body politic in New England, while the colony's civil and ecclesiastical structures of power become the single body around which the community can cohere. Indeed, by situating God as the prime agent behind this move to unity, the sermon conflates civil and ecclesiastical authority, which means that heresy and sedition become coextensive; acts of sedition are potentially heretical, and vice versa.

At the end of *A Model of Christian Charity*, Winthrop revisits the relation between individual and community by explaining that for this bonded community, "The care of the public must oversway all private respects."[65] This statement implies that settlers must subjugate their individual (private) interests to those of the public, and suggests that no individual subject could pursue his or her own interests to the detriment of the community. To do so would be to undermine the contiguity of the corporate body, and to weaken the political viability of the state. This vision of community did not originate with Winthrop, as is evidenced by the Company's correspondence with Endicott a year earlier, which had outlined the mechanism for structuring the colony's civil and ecclesiastical order in terms of a disciplinary hermeneutic that required human actions to be visible to the community. Ultimately, what may have seemed to Winthrop to be a clear imperative for maintaining order was, in fact, deeply enmeshed in the local politics of that order: when the General Court limited the franchise to church members in May 1631, the Court's decision effectively excluded the vast majority of the population from participating in government because the bar for admission to church membership was so high. Indeed, settlers who had been church members in good standing before they left England often found themselves disenfranchised, and on the outside looking in when they arrived in the New World. Because this limitation on membership conflated secular and religious worlds, free grace, which was to be adjudicated by the church, provided a real temporal advantage to church members. The apparent arbitrariness of these exclusionary practices became all too apparent to those who could not—or would not—make the necessary professions of faith to be accepted into Massachusetts churches. To them, the particular branch of Calvinism that associated such temporal benefits with religious life came dangerously close to a covenant of works.[66]

As the early pressures of migration (or "wildernes troubles") eased after the first year of settlement, social and economic classes in Massachusetts Bay became increasingly polarized despite Winthrop's model vision of the colony. Settlers became more frustrated about being excluded from church membership, and being disenfranchised, so they sought new ways to describe the relation between individual and state. In particular, Louise Breen argues that this urge was largely driven by "cosmopolitan-minded individuals habitually called to play roles on a stage wider than Massachusetts."[67] And although the Antinomian controversy would find its voice in regenerate members of the church—their religious and political standing is what made their actions so threatening—it was particularly attractive to a wider circle that included merchants and military men because, in Breen's words, it "provided a theological discourse capable of underwriting a society more cosmopolitan, more individualistic, and more heterogeneous than orthodox Puritanism would allow."[68] Such a rearticulation would necessarily impact the colony's churches and government directly.

Winthrop's faction tried to frame the theological debate in secular terms, if only to defend itself against the charge of zealotry from English critics; the term "Antinomian" was helpful in this regard, because though the controversy ostensibly centered around a disagreement about the order in which faith and grace appeared in the regenerate soul, and whether sanctification (living a saintly life) could be used as evidence of justification, the Antinomians' uncompromising stance that sanctification had no role to play in conversations about regeneracy had important civil consequences. As Church elders saw it, once Antinomians accepted that good works and the rule of law were at odds with regeneracy, they had no reason to work within the bond of the community—in fact, they were bound to avoid it in favor of an ecstatic, unmediated relationship with Christ. Indeed, one tenet of Antinomianism that was particularly troubling to the emerging Orthodoxy was the fact that Antinomians apparently believed that a regenerate soul was in direct commu- nion with God—that it was gifted with an indwelling of the Holy Spirit (Win- throp would charge that Antinomians believed the regenerate soul to be given eternal life through salvation, such that "Christ is the new Creature").[69] Fur- thermore, the Antinomian argument that Christ was united to the regenerate soul seemed to remove any obligation to work toward saintly behavior. If there existed no inherent good in humans, but only in Christ, then humans themselves could not produce saintly behavior on their own volition, and it therefore "followed that man's unaltered sinfulness should be no cause for distress. There is no point in appealing for gifts or graces, but only for Christ."[70]

Shocking as this belief was to Winthrop and his faction, it crystallized the Antinomian threat, and pointed a way out of the controversy, as it highlighted the moral and disciplinary hazard presented by the faction. The basic com- plaint was that this belief freed the Antinomian from the burden of moral laws, but the corollary that justification was an intensely personal experience that could (only) be known with certainty by an individual who had received it, fundamentally transformed the Antinomians' relationship to language and authority. If the regenerate soul was literally sealed with Christ, and only then made immortal, the elders charged, this soul had access to God's word through immediate revelation, and would no longer be bound by scripture; eventually, this would lead to the conclusion that "the whole letter of the Scripture holds forth a Covenant of Workes," and that "All Covenants to God expressed in words are legall Workes" as well.[71] Indeed, for the Antinomians, human and divine things were ineluctably opposed to one another, so any claim by minis- ters to be able to read signs of grace—for example, through sanctification—as a means of adjudicating church membership was absurd. This understanding of grace precipitated a serious epistemological dilemma, the implications of which Winthrop grasped immediately. First, it threatened the Puritan order by apparently freeing human beings from obeying moral laws (hence the term "Antinomian"), which for Winthrop was evident in the breakdown of civil au- thority that appeared in Massachusetts Bay as soon as "many prophane per- sons became of [the Antinomians'] opinions, for it was very easie, and acceptable way to heaven, to see nothing, to have nothing, but waite for Christ to do all."[72] Second, it exchanged an order of communal discipline that had been based on labor and visibility for a model grounded on the inscrutability of human bodies. By internalizing language as the product of a direct union with Christ, the Antinomian drew a line between him- or herself and the external world, for which the regenerate's body was always illegible. In con- trast to this, Winthrop's stance toward the Antinomians is predicated on tropes of visibility and legibility—on the idea that truth will manifest itself publicly, and be legible to those who are properly trained. From this perspective, Winthrop's investment in drawing attention to and reading the bodies of Antinomians begins to make sense as a rejection of illegibility, and a reassertion of a regulatory hermeneutic stance toward language and meaning. The obsession with Dyer's and Hutchinson's "monstrous births" in the record of the controversy is symptomatic of this drive to visibility, so it is no accident that epidemiological rhetoric becomes a central component of reestablishing this regulatory gaze, and reasserting the legibility of bodies. Dyer's and Hutchinson's monstrous births were exhumed, brought into the open, and read as visible signs of Antinomian error—as if this simple act of reading would restore the colony's hermeneutic system, and bring it back to health.[73]

Though the controversy evolved over a period of years, the dramatic event that precipitated the final schism between the two factions in Massachusetts Bay occurred during the Fast Day of January 19, 1637, and played itself out as a debate over the use of language. Held under the pretense of reducing the mounting tensions in New England, John Wheelwright, who was Hutchinson's brother-in-law, and the man whom the Antinomians wanted as the congregation's teacher, was invited to deliver a sermon before the Boston congregation. But rather than preach a reconciliation of the two factions, he pointed out that "the only cause of the fasting of true believers is the absence of Christ."[74] This declaration was hardly meant to placate the ministers and magistrates, whom it implicated on either of two counts: first, for calling a fast when one ought not to have been called, or second (and taking the need for a Fast Day at face value), to bear responsibility for Christ's absence from the community. From here, Wheelwright's sermon only became more incendiary. He exhorted his followers to

> Prepare for a spirituall combate, [and to] put on the whole armour of God . . . [to have their] loynes girt and be redy to fight. . . . They ought to shew themselves valient, they should have their swords redy, they must fight, and fight with spirituall weapons, for the weapons of our warfare are not carnall but spirituall. . . . We must all of us prepare for battell and come out against the enimyes of the Lord, and if we do not strive, those under a covenant of works will prevaile.[75]

Whereas Wheelwright's emphasis on spiritual rather than carnal weapons overcompensates for the subtext of his message (the Antinomians had accused the Puritan elders of preaching a covenant of works, so they were clearly the intended target of this spiritual war), this image was all the more galling for the elders, to whom it appeared to be a cynical manipulation of language for political ends. In his call for all true Christians to identify the enemies of the Lord, and to rally "spirituall weapons" against them, Wheelwright insisted that he spoke "figuratively," whereas Winthrop believed that "he spake as he meant," and that his sermon was a deliberate call to arms against the government of Massachusetts Bay.[76]

Just three months earlier, in October 1636, when the Antinomian crisis was still taking shape, Winthrop had characterized the debates as a growing misunderstanding or miscommunication between the parties. At the time, he apparently still believed that tensions could be defused if the colonists paid closer attention to their use of language. He argued that the disagreement between factions had arisen from the use of a human language that failed to communicate God's word faithfully, so he spelled out the stakes of the debate:

> Seeing these variances grew (and some estrangement withal) from some words and phrases, which were of human invention, and tended to doubtful disputation, rather than to edification, and had no footing in scripture, nor had been in use in the purest churches for three hundred years after Christ,—that, for the peace of the church, &c., [I asked that] they might be forborn.[77]

The distinction between a divine language and a language of human invention puts the religious problem of Antinomianism in stark relief against the secular political issues in the colony. Or at least this is how Winthrop tried to represent the crisis in the short run. Both parties accused each other of misusing language, and Wheelwright's sermon was a play to set the terms for the linguistic schism. In contrast, Winthrop's insistence that Wheelwright spoke literally essentially charged the Antinomians with disrupting the order of secular and sacred unity in the colony, and propelled the crisis into the realm of civil discourse.[78] Winthrop's claim was a conscious attempt to restore the colony's hierarchy; this was so apparent to him, that in his *Short Story*, he complained that among the consequences of Wheelwright's sermon was that "all things are turned upside down among us."[79]

In Winthrop's eyes, Wheelwright's sermon crossed the boundary of scriptural debate, and became a secular issue in which the colony's security was at stake. The upshot is that Wheelwright was charged with, tried for, and convicted of sedition in March 1637. Amy Shrager Lang argues that the strategy of conducting Wheelwright's trial as a civil matter of sedition, rather than heresy, was "a response to English accusations that the colonists prosecuted cases of conscience as civil crimes, accusations [they] feared would be politically damaging to the Bay colony."[80] In order to further allay English skepticism, the Massachusetts Bay magistrates distanced themselves from the religious debate by charging that the Antinomians:

> miserably interrupt the civill Peace, and that they threw contempt both upon Courts, and Churches, and began now to raise sedition amongst us, to the indangering the Common-wealth; Hereupon for these grounds named, (and not for their opinions, as themselves falsely reported . . .) for these reasons . . . being civill disturbances, the Magistrate convents . . . and censures them.[81]

Wheelwright's trial marked an implicit admission that the Puritan search for their New Israel could not be separated from the political and economic exigencies of colonial administration. Pursuant to his conviction, Wheelwright's supporters signed a Petition of Remonstrance, again highlighting the rhetorical stakes of the controversy, as they asked the magistrates to reverse their decision because, among other things, they had "not heard any that have witnessed against our brother for any seditious fact."[82] Those who signed were effectively piggybacking on Wheelwright's defense, claiming to call the Court's interpretive ability—rather than its sovereignty—into question. But under the terms established during the trial, that claim was rejected. The status of Wheelwright's interpretive act had already been settled as seditious, and signing the petition was itself coextensive with his speech. At a set of trials held in October 1637, the remonstrants were given the chance to remove their name from the petition—in effect to reinsert themselves into the community by submitting to the magistrates' hermeneutic order. The reassertion of this order is evident in the acknowledgments signed by those who wished to withdraw their names. These documents largely make two points: first, that the remonstrants had transgressed "the Rule of due honour to Authority, and of the Modesty, and Submission in Private Persons" by quarrelling publicly with magistrates.[83] Second, as if to underscore the representational nature of their transgressions, that "as for the word remonstrance at which ofenc was taken I understood not what it meante."[84] It strikes me as no small coincidence that the acknowledgment required an explicit and public admission of linguistic failure—of failure to understand plain English—and that once the admission was made, reintegration into the community demanded a further submission to the government's political authority, as well as its linguistic and interpretive authority. Those who refused to make such acknowledgments were, like Wheelwright, tried, convicted, and disenfranchised.

III

The magistrates' decision to prosecute Wheelwright and his followers for sedition, rather than for any specific heterodox religious belief had important political implications for the colony, and for the historiographic record that emerged during the mid- to late seventeenth century. From a pragmatic standpoint, it brought the trials into a relatively straightforward civil arena, and protected magistrates against charges that they were persecuting religious dissent or matters of conscience; given the relative ease with which these trials were prosecuted, had Anne Hutchinson not been part of the Antinomian faction, the controversy itself may well have receded into the background as one of many theological debates about church polity and hierarchy during the first four decades of New England's history. But the very thing that made the early trials go smoothly also led to a difficult problem when it came to the prosecution of Hutchinson, whose trial seemed to spin out of control as soon as it started. Regardless of her actual role in events prior to her civil trial in November 1637 and her church trial in March 1638, I am interested in the fact that Hutchinson became the focal point for the epidemiological rhetoric that the controversy produced. Where a thematics of infection can be found throughout the records of the controversy, the full force of epidemiology as a means of regulating behavior only becomes evident when it is deployed against Hutchinson. While it is possible that Hutchinson was the primary source of factionalism and dissent in the colony, as Winthrop would eventually charge, the virulent rhetoric brought to bear against her suggests a deeper anxiety about her role. Indeed, I would describe my own approach to representations of Hutchinson in terms that echo Field's take on the controversy itself: If it did not take place, did Anne Hutchinson herself actually exist?

While religious dissent and heresy are not explicitly gendered acts, my own focus thus far on the controversy's male participants has been a self-conscious attempt to reflect the juridical status of sedition, which is a political act, and which, as my analysis of Hutchinson's trials will reveal, came to have specific gendered significance in the wake of Wheelwright's prosecution on civil grounds. By deferring my discussion of Hutchinson for so long, I have resisted the strain of criticism that reads her as the central figure in the events of 1636–38, and that underscores gender as a constitutive category for the controversy. Instead, I follow the lead of critics like Dillon and Ross Pudaloff, who examine the ways that the record of the controversy produced gender as a pathological category. My contribution to this discussion will be to outline the means whereby epidemiological rhetoric represents Hutchinson not just as a metaphorical illness, but genders her actions, and defines them as a contagious threat to the community—a threat that survives her, as it inheres in a set of gendered behaviors that must be regulated by the colony's disciplinary apparatus. As such, I am not making the case that gender doesn't figure obsessively in the record's most familiar documents—it does, though this obsessiveness is part of a retrospective attempt to control the terms of the debate. For example, Hutchinson is barely mentioned in Winthrop's *Journal* (a source used far less often than the *Short Story* for analysis of the controversy), and it is not always clear from the contemporary documents that her role in fomenting dissent was as large as, say, Wheelwright's, Henry Vane's, or even John Cotton's.[85] And yet, by the time Winthrop's history of the controversy was published in the mid-1640s, gender had become the focal point in representations of her transgressions, and she became the essential embodiment of Antinomianism in New England—a shift that I find quite compelling; and when Edward Johnson and Cotton Mather added their contributions to the historical record in the following decades, "Hutchinson" and "infection" were all but interchangeable, while Hutchinson's name was itself a synonym for Antinomianism.[86]

Although Hutchinson's gender was not the catalyst for her prosecution, it inflected the form and outcome of her trial. The fact that she was the last Antinomian to be tried, and that her trial turned out to be the most complicated of all the cases that went before the Court is a direct consequence of her being a woman, and of a gendered ambiguity that arose from the conflation of civil and ecclesiastical order—of heresy and sedition. While the civil matter was relatively easy for the magistrates to adjudicate while it involved men who had the political status to sign the Petition of Remonstrance, the case was altogether different when it came to Hutchinson, who did not. Whatever her relationship to the rest of the community, Hutchinson was a woman who had led conventicles in her home, and who had questioned the teachings of the Bay's ministers, but neither her words nor her actions constituted sedition; her demeanor and the tenor of her defense during the 1637 civil trial demonstrate that she knew this fact. As Mary Beth Norton explains the issue, "Because she was a woman . . . [Hutchinson] had not been involved in the formal protests against John Wheelwright's conviction. Accordingly, she was shielded from prosecution for sedition unless she explicitly aligned herself with the petitioners."[87] The most pressing issue facing the Court leading up to her trial was how to prosecute a woman who did not have the political standing to sign the petition—who had not, strictly speaking, committed sedition—but who nevertheless appeared to be in league with seditious citizens. This dilemma centered on the ambiguous political and religious status of women in the colony, and it is a critical point in the trial of Anne Hutchinson, as well as in the historical record itself, to the extent that it still confounds scholars who, with startling frequency, mistakenly assert that she was tried for sedition.[88] Had she been, the magistrates would have made short shrift of her, as they did her male counterparts, and the controversy as we know it would indeed not have taken place—certainly not with Hutchinson as its central protagonist. To the extent that we would still be paying attention to the controversy four hundred years after the fact, the primary actors would almost certainly be Wheelwright and Cotton.

On the other hand, the fact that Hutchinson was *not* prosecuted for sedition has everything to do with the rhetorical posturing that emerged in the wake of her trial, with the representation of her as an infectious agent, and with the emergence of gender as a pathological category the magistrates felt needed to be policed in New England. In this model of the controversy, the focus is not on Hutchinson per se, but on the narrative strategies that produced a shift from representing gender as an unspoken category for much of the controversy prior to Hutchinson's trial, to the embodiment of the way that Puritan elders talked about Antinomianism in Massachusetts Bay, and the very terms through which they imagined the healthful community. This representation of gender as a belated category of political identity is a position best articulated by Ross Pudaloff, who, in building on Caldwell's reading of the controversy's linguistic nature, suggests:

> The conflict between the elders and Anne Hutchinson, was not one more episode in a timeless struggle between the state and the individual, between objective rationality and subjective emotions, and between men and women. Rather, it was perhaps the first event in America that allowed those who have come after to recognize the struggle in those terms. The crisis constituted the individual, the subjective, and the female as separate entities, but did so by constructing these as culturally coded representations of powerlessness.[89]

For Pudaloff, gender is not an ontologically constituted category that produced the controversy, but a figure that emerged from it as an organizing principle of narrative coherence: an organizing principle that gave voice to the historiographic tradition, placing Hutchinson—autonomous female subject—front and center in the controversy. Likewise, Dillon's reading of the controversy stresses that gender "emerges as a category of knowledge through which liberalism effects social order on behalf of the Puritan fathers."[90] Both critics thus resist traditional temporalities that would cite gender as a catalyst for Hutchinson's prosecution to identify instead the ways that it emerges

from her prosecution as a political category defined (and made public) by
Winthrop to outline the boundaries of healthful behavior in Massachusetts
Bay. Put another way, Hutchinson was not prosecuted because she was a
woman, but her prosecution produced the terms through which to understand the status of womanhood in early colonial New England, as well as the
deployment of political power in the colony; this status was rehearsed in the
retelling and dissemination of the story, when what Pudaloff calls "the female"
quite literally became a pathological state.

From the earliest moments of Hutchinson's 1637 civil trial, it is clear that
her political status was problematic for the Court. As with the male Antinomians' sedition trials that immediately preceded hers, the magistrates tried to
secularize the religious disagreement by translating her transgression into
the civil realm as an act that struck at the heart of a well-ordered society. But
this translation was complicated by the fact that Hutchinson had not signed
the Petition of Remonstrance—that she had not, in fact, committed sedition
under the conditions established in the previous trials; as the opening remarks
in her trial demonstrate, Hutchinson was well aware of her prosecutors' dilemma, and she thrived on the fact that the charges against her were essentially incoherent. Winthrop's first question takes up where the earlier trials
had left off, asking whether she did not "hold and assent in practice to those
opinions and factions that have been handled in court already, that is to say,
whether [she did] not justify Mr. Wheelwright's sermon and the petition."[91]
But even as he tries to implicate her in the seditious actions of her male counterparts, he only arrives at this question after a rather convoluted speech that
lays out the breadth of her social transgressions in gendered terms, charging
that she committed "a thing not tolerable nor comely in the sight of God nor
fitting for [her] sex."[92] The awkwardness of this opening gambit highlights the
implicitly gendered status of sedition—and thus the central legal difficulty in
the case against Hutchinson. Two things stand out about her response: first,
she seemed uninterested in talking about gender during the trial; indeed, gender seems wholly irrelevant insofar as she fashions herself, in Dillon's words,
"as an authorized public speaker, contending that it is her godliness, not her
gender, that determines the authority of her actions and arguments."[93] Second, she was not afraid to confront the prosecutors by drawing attention to
the nature of their dilemma. Hutchinson famously opened her defense by
responding to Winthrop that "I am called here to answer before you but I hear
no things laid to my charge."[94] This was formally true, and her statement
echoes the male petitioners' claim against the Court that they had "not heard
any that have witnessed against our brother for any seditious fact." Thus, in
one brief moment Hutchinson simultaneously rejected the case against her,

and renewed the questions about language and interpretation that anchored the prosecution of Wheelwright and the petitioners—the same questions that were at the heart of the Antinomians' complaints against the Massachusetts Bay ministers.

Even as Hutchinson resists Winthrop's line of inquiry, he insists time and again that she answer his general (though never explicitly articulated) allegation of seditious behavior. The closest they come to settling the question is when she attempts to turn the table on Winthrop by asking him what the penalty would be if she had indeed "set [her] hand to the petition," to which he replies "you saw the case tried before"—a reference to the earlier guilty verdicts. This response delights Hutchinson, who retorts "but I had not my hand to the petition," thus seeming to end the case before it had even begun.[95] Here, Hutchinson makes it clear that any prosecution of her on grounds of sedition was inevitably headed for an embarrassing stalemate; her case *was* different from those who went before her, and so the Court would have to try her on different grounds. But Winthrop and the magistrates were not easily put off, as they went on to make a moral equivalence between the fact that she had "councelled" the petitioners (which Winthrop described as an implicit breach of the Fifth Commandment), and the seditious actions themselves. The redacted transcript of their exchange that is included in the *Short Story* goes further in drawing this moral equivalence, asserting that she could not "deny but [she] had [her] hand in the petition," despite the fact that she had not signed it—that her hand was, in a very literal sense, *not* in the petition.[96]

And yet Hutchinson did deny it until the frustrated magistrates moved on from their thinly veiled accusations of sedition. But as they pursued alternate lines of questioning, their attention to gender became increasingly insistent, perhaps because this was the source of their prosecutorial difficulties. When taken to task for the conventicles that she held in her home, Hutchinson pointed to the established tradition of women participating in weekly meetings to discuss sermons—a practice that she had been criticized for avoiding when she first arrived in New England, because she considered those meetings "unlawful" at the time.[97] And as the trial proceeds, the exchanges between she and the magistrates often come across as surprisingly petty to the modern ear, such as when Winthrop claimed that his biblical interpretations were more accurate than hers "because I have brought more arguments than you have."[98] These exchanges underscore the rhetorical rift between the two parties, as the more Winthrop pressed her, the more the linguistic artifice of the trial became apparent; as long as Hutchinson stood her ground, and demonstrated Winthrop's and the magistrates' inability to foreclose her interpretive agency, then their hermeneutic code risked falling apart. Hutchinson must have taken pleasure in showing up the magistrates for their inability to maintain control over the terms of their case, and demonstrates this in one of the few moments that she acknowledges her gender. She asks Winthrop whether "you think it not lawful for me to teach women and why do you call me to teach the court?" Winthrop's pointed rejoinder asserts the Court's power in hierarchical terms: "We do not call you to teach the court but to lay open yourself," and reminds her that "we are your judges, and not you ours."[99]

Even as Winthrop attempts to silence Hutchinson, he does so by calling attention to her gender, insisting that the Court does not "mean to discourse with those of [her] sex."[100] And yet the irony is that the entire trial is predicated on an attempt to "reduce" this woman—to grapple with defining the role of women in public spaces, to give voice to the boundaries for proper and improper female behavior, and to define those as coextensive with Hutchinson's actions.[101] As problematic as this proved to be, Hutchinson's success in changing the terms of the conversation, which would eventually lead to her conviction on religious grounds, pulls the veil from the magistrates' legal strategy—reveals it *as* a strategy built on the trope of a socially transgressive woman who must be reigned in by her elders. But for a surprisingly long stretch of the trial, Hutchinson's success in defending herself raised important concerns about the legal status of women in the colony, since the Court's initial failure to convict her on civil grounds (especially the "charge" of committing a thing not fitting of her sex) could encourage other women to strike out on their own in matters of biblical exegesis, giving them an implicit, if not explicit, right to speak publicly.[102] This is the crux of Dillon's reading of the controversy, insofar as Hutchinson "creates an oppositional public sphere within the colony; that is, she does not simply criticize the ministers, but on the basis of Puritan doctrine, mobilizes a public that operates outside state-sanctioned publicness."[103] For a brief moment between the beginning of the trail and her blasphemy near the end of it, the trope of transgression, and, by extension, the colony's gendered theological and political hierarchies remained perilously unstable, as Hutchinson maintained—and demonstrated—her ability to speak publicly in a way that the male Antinomians had failed to do. For Winthrop, the consequence of this unregulated speech was that Hutchinson's argument "overthrows all."[104] From this point forward, he and the other magistrates worked to back Hutchinson into a corner so that they could deploy the Court's full power against her.

The turning point of Hutchinson's civil trial occurred during the retelling of her spiritual autobiography, when she claimed an "immediate revelation" from God.[105] This confession gave her prosecutors the opening that they had been waiting for, and they lost no time in switching from the civil grounds that had given them such trouble to the religious grounds on which gender no longer presented a problem for the prosecution. Feeling it was safe to attack her, Winthrop pounced on Hutchinson's words, remarking:

> The case is altered and will not stand with us now, but I see a marvelous providence of God to bring things to this pass that they are. We have been hearkening about the trial of this thing and now the mercy of God by a providence hath answered our desires and made her to lay open her self.[106]

Winthrop identifies Hutchinson's admission as providential, but he also expresses relief that she finally "lay [herself] open," as the magistrates had hoped—and believed—she would do since the beginning of her trial. The "opening" was providential because it lay squarely within the magistrates' epistemological framework for the colony insofar as it dramatized the Antinomians' central error, which was their belief in an unmediated relationship to God that bypassed human language and scripture. Beyond this, however, Hutchinson's admission further confirmed the magistrates' power to produce a confession—to expose Antinomian belief as a visible heresy, and therefore to reaffirm the righteousness of "Orthodox" epistemologies. From this point forward, the Massachusetts Bay's emerging Orthodoxy set its full rhetorical apparatus in motion to define the terms of Hutchinson's transgression in unambiguous terms. If she had not been seditious, Winthrop eventually settled on calling her an "American Jesebel" at the end of the *Short Story*—a moniker that gendered her behavior with a vengeance, and cast it in sexualized terms; where gender had been a stumbling block for the prosecution early in her trial, it became shorthand for the magistrates' power to protect the community from this threat in the wake of the controversy.[107]

Although the verdict in Hutchinson's civil trial—like the Wheelwright verdict—called for banishment, she was allowed to remain in the colony until March 1638, when she was made to stand a second trial. This second trial, however, was a church proceeding arising from her blasphemy of the previous November, and was headed by Cotton, who was meant to demonstrate his own submission to and investment in the ruling faction by his treatment of Hutchinson. The church trial was initially intended as a means of further "reducing" Hutchinson, and admonishing her for her behavior, but also to give her the opportunity to return to the community by submitting herself to the church's authority—to move the debate over language and interpretation out of the civil arena, and back under the authority of church elders, much in the

way that the male Antinomians had been given an opportunity to recant.[108]
The end result of this trial is that Hutchinson could not—or would not—
subsume herself to the elders' interpretive authority, but instead compounded
her offense before finally being excommunicated and banished for good; famously, her failure in the church trial centered once again on an epistemological breakdown where she claimed a disjunction between inner belief and
human language—that is, as she tried to explain it, her beliefs were not in
error, though her expression of them was mistaken.[109] This claim infuriated
her prosecutors, who had no patience for revisiting an issue they thought they
had dealt with three months prior. By the end of Hutchinson's examination,
when it was clear that she had been defeated, and that she would not return
to the fold, the church elders launched a series of withering attacks against
her to define her transgressions in the starkest possible terms. Hugh Peter,
for example, described her as a woman out of place, telling her that she had
"rather bine a Husband than a Wife and a preacher than a Hearer; and a Magistrate than a Subject."[110] From here it was just a short leap to accusing her of
promiscuity, and while Cotton admitted that he had heard no evidence to sub-
stantiate such a charge, he was clear about the harmful effects of Hutchinson's beliefs on family and colony. He told her, "Though I have not herd,
nayther do I thinke, you have bine unfaythfull to your Husband in his Mar-
riage Covenant, yet that will follow upon it, for it is the very argument . . . that
which the Annabaptists and Familists bringe to prove the Lawfullness of the
common use of all Weomen and soe more dayngerous Evells and filthie
Unclenes and other sines will followe than you doe now Imagine or con-
ceave."[111] Cotton's comments fed into Winthrop's characterization of Hutchinson as an "American Jesebel," and had the further effect of locating the church
hierarchy—now reestablished as male and non-Antinomian—as the site for
curing the colony of this infection, and returning it to its well-ordered state.

The charges of promiscuity and of masculine behavior reveal a concerted
effort to ostracize Hutchinson, but these representations are only part of a
much broader strategy to publicly define the place and model behavior of
women in Massachusetts Bay. And though proper behavior is never defined
explicitly in the records of the controversy—except by negation of Hutchinson's actions—it emerges as a counterpart to the pathology she comes to
embody. It is here that I would like to focus directly on the broader effects
of epidemiological rhetoric that emerged from the Antinomian controversy.
That is, not just on the physical instantiations of pathology—for example,
Dyer's and Hutchinson's "monstrous births"—but on the ways that those
visible manifestations are assigned to specific classes of gendered behavior,
and given etiological significance that calls for new attention to policing

and regulating citizens. Where Hutchinson came to stand in for an infectious threat to the churches, texts like the *Short Story* generalize from her specific actions to set the parameters for future pathology in the colony, and to underscore the stakes of regulating behavior. This becomes apparent in the set of descriptions that Winthrop uses to introduce Hutchinson in the *Short Story*:

> The head of all this faction (*Dux foemina facti*) . . . the breeder and nourisher of all these distempers . . . a woman of a haughty and fierce carriage, of a nimble wit and active spirit, and a very voluble tongue, more bold then a man, though in understanding and judgement inferiour to many women.[112]

Winthrop's use of the term "distemper" relies on the trope of illness to characterize Antinomianism broadly. However, this description marks a move away from traditional thematic representations of disease (i.e., dissent and infection) toward a more transparent epidemiological narrative that identifies Hutchinson and her behaviors as the infection that courses through the community. More specifically, while the representation's pathologizing force seems to emerge from its attention to physical bodies ("The head," the "breeder and nourisher"), it comes to inhere in the particular behaviors that define her: her "carriage," her "wit," her "spirit," and her "very voluble tongue." I draw attention to this representational shift from body to behavior because it marks the moment of abstraction from a specific metaphorical pathogen (Hutchinson) to the set of behaviors that potentially endanger the community. This is precisely the move that I want to characterize in terms of epidemiological analysis, and it manifests itself in the way that Winthrop uses epidemiology (rather than simply allegory or metaphor) to circumscribe the controversy, and appropriate its history within a narrative of infection, containment, and regulation.

Winthrop's attention to behavior continues in the *Short Story* as he expands on his description of Hutchinson's infectious nature, revealing a compelling irony about the methods she allegedly used to spread dissent throughout the colony:

> Shee cunningly dissembled and coloured her opinions . . . and was admitted into the Church, then shee began to go to work, and being a woman very helpful in the times of child-birth, and other occasions of bodily infirmities, and well furnished with means for those purposes, shee easily insinuated her selfe into the affection of many.[113]

Here is Hutchinson at her most dangerous in Winthrop's eyes: an infectious healer, or, more sinisterly, infectious because she is a healer. The tension lies in the fact that Hutchinson's work during childbirth is both "helpful" to the community, but also potentially harmful, because, as Norton explains, "Only birthing rooms provided women with environments that consistently excluded men," and therefore existed outside of regulatory (male) supervision.[114] Under normal circumstances, Norton continues, midwives played a critical role in policing sexual practices because they "and their helpers often learned secrets that women would rather have kept hidden from view," and could therefore bring crimes like "bastardy, premarital fornication, adultery, or infanticide" to public view.[115] This function is predicated on the midwife and her assistant being aligned with the colony's disciplinary apparatus, and making the internal (or personal) realm of women visible. If, for whatever reason, they are not aligned, then the closed, unregulated space of the birthing room threatens the community precisely because it remains hidden from view. This anxiety is directly related to the broader fear of Antinomians, which Hutchinson embodied in her church trial, as she maintained a distinction between private, inner language, and public expression. In Winthrop's mind, Hutchinson was taking advantage of a hidden space, and of laboring women's susceptibility to insinuate her ideas far from the magistrates' and ministers' gaze, and to replicate the very epistemological disjunction that he and the magistrates were fighting against.

Cotton would repeat Winthrop's characterization of Hutchinson's helpfulness in his *Way of Congregational Churches Cleared* (1648), only being more explicit than Winthrop about her ability to exploit the conduits made available to her by her practical knowledge of childbirth. He writes that upon her arrival in Boston, Hutchinson

> did much good in our Town, in womans meeting a Childbirth-Travells, wherein shee was not onely skilfull and helpful, but rapidly fell into good discourses with the women about their spiritual estates.[116]

While Hutchinson is clearly the subject of Cotton's analysis, the suggestion that her nursing skills could be used to disrupt the ministry's hermeneutic order, and to undermine the community's social cohesion marks those activities as problematic in and of themselves—as potentially harmful, rather than nurturing for the community. Cotton identifies Hutchinson's "helpful acts," and her propensity to fall into "good discourses" positively here, but this identification only holds until the magistrates and ministers discover that she was using her work to operate as a vector of dissent, where she communicated her spiritual infection under cover of her medical skill, while remaining shielded from male supervision. Indeed, forty years later, William Hubbard would demonstrate how quickly such representations had become fixed into the historiographic record of the controversy, when he wrote that because of Hutchinson's ministrations, "the affections of those that labored under wants, and bodily infirmities, were notably prepared to become susceptible of any novel impressions."[117]

For Egan, the focus on Hutchinson's medical work demonstrates precisely the threat that Winthrop represented her as posing to the entire community. In this narrative, "a perfectly healthy woman 'contracts' the disease through contact with the Antinomian women attending at the birth of her child, and she 'carries' the disease back to her own home when leaving the birthing room, 'infecting' her own children in the process."[118] Thus, it is not simply the body politic in its corporate essence that is threatened by Hutchinson or by Antinomians, but each individual household that is at risk, so that one by one, as they succumb to infection, they endanger the "internal order of the body politic."[119] In Egan's model, Hutchinson's infectious threat figures beyond the theological boundaries of the controversy itself, but the consequence of this is that it permits the magistrates to recuperate the broader theme of sedition into their records of events. Indeed, where sedition was an inappropriate model for prosecuting Hutchinson because she had not signed the petition, the later representations of her nursing skills focus on the specific threat that she poses to the colony's bodily coherence and then moves the conversation back to questions about civil behavior. The upshot of Egan's reading of the controversy—and I agree with him here—is that by pathologizing Hutchinson's behaviors, regulating them, and banishing her from Massachusetts Bay, the magistrates and church elders represent the colony as fundamentally healthy, and themselves as physicians of the body politic. They have "disinfected the colonial body of the Antinomian plague by transforming themselves into a bureaucracy capable of examining and weeding out the sources of contamination, and thus making the body whole."[120]

As I tease out the way that epidemiological rhetoric functions in the historical record of the controversy, I would like to juxtapose Hutchinson's actions in Massachusetts Bay to Samuel Fuller's less than a decade earlier in Salem. If each has been treated differently by history, it is worth noting that both operated on parallel trajectories, using medical practice as a vector for disseminating theological opinions, which nevertheless had the potential to disrupt community. One of the distinguishing marks between the two, however, is that Fuller's medical practice fell within the colony's disciplinary hermeneutic order, as it was closely regulated and made public through the correspondence between himself, Bradford, and Endicott. Hutchinson, on the other hand, had an unregulated practice that her prosecutors represented as secretive and subversive; she, and midwives like Jane Hawkins practiced their skills outside of the medico-theological arc of the Puritan hierarchy—an arc embodied by Fuller in the late 1620s, and by John Eliot, Michael Wigglesworth, and Cotton Mather later in the century. And because Hutchinson's work was not supervised by male practitioners, it was not recognized as an acceptable formal conduit for theological doctrine. What the controversy teaches us is that even in light of the essential health services that midwives and their assistants provided to the community, there always remained a risk that subversive narratives could be transmitted along these vectors, which were free from the male regulatory gaze, and thus by definition always gendered female, and always potentially pathological.

The movement from an insistent focus on Anne Hutchinson's body to the identification of specific behaviors like nursing and midwifery as potentially pathological describes a key dynamic of epidemiological rhetoric that I have tried to underscore in this chapter. Cindy Patton describes this as the "performative aspect of epidemiology," which is to say its power to reassign meaning to social behaviors, and to mark

> spaces through describable trajectories of a disease phenomenon, performatively reinventing the meaning of quotidian acts by placing them in a model of transmissibility . . . where once-innocent or completely unnoticed acts are redescribed as "risk-taking behavior" only because a transmissible agent may now take advantage of—inscribe the very trajectory of—an already existing, but not "significant" conduit.[121]

Although Patton's analysis describes a particular moment in late-twentieth-century HIV/AIDS epidemiology that figures "risk," "movement," and "space" in relation to one another, I would like to argue that this, too, is at stake in the Antinomian controversy—or more accurately, in the historiographic trajectory of the controversy. For Patton, epidemiology's performative quality describes its regulatory practices, which is to say that by redefining behaviors as "risk-taking," epidemiology sets these apart as the object of the medical—and often the political—gaze. The transition that I would like to effect here with respect to the Antinomian controversy is one in which attention to the epidemiological practices of narratives like Winthrop's *Short Story* demonstrates how specific behaviors are transformed, with an eye toward focusing Massachusetts Bay's attention squarely on the regulation of those behaviors. And where so much of the debate that shaped the controversy was invested in bringing hidden heresy or hidden monstrous births to light, Winthrop emphasizes that visibility is central to the colony's regulatory apparatus; thus it is that Hutchinson's actions—because she has been pathologized—become the subject of epidemiological regulation, and identify those invisible spaces and behaviors that must be brought into the open for the sake of the colony's health.

I stated rather obviously when introducing the controversy, that Antinomianism was not a literal epidemic. But as I've tried to demonstrate, its figural status is irrelevant to the function of epidemiological analysis, which is, after all, invested in identifying and defining behaviors as healthy or pathological (i.e., "risky"), rather than in the ontological status of illness. What the various metaphors and tropes of infection arising from the Antinomian controversy hint at is the broader ideological investment at stake in regulating the citizens of Massachusetts Bay. Hutchinson's expulsion to Rhode Island, while an end-goal for Puritan elders in and of itself, held great significance (epidemiologically and otherwise) as a model for future behavior. Prior to the controversy, the position of women in Massachusetts Bay was largely unspoken (and unobserved in Puritan histories). In the wake of Hutchinson's activities, however, all of these acts came to be represented as risk-taking behaviors that had to be regulated in order to ensure the colony's survival. As Hutchinson was pathologized, so too were gendered activities in the colony circumscribed as potentially subversive. Here, I would pause for a moment to recollect Lang's reading of the controversy, which identifies American Antinomianism as being "gendered female from the outset" because of Anne Hutchinson.[122] I would amend Lang's statement, and invert its temporality to read that because of Anne Hutchinson—or because of the way that her prosecution and subsequent historical representation played out—American womanhood is figured as Antinomian from the outset. Such a description relies on a reading of gender as a performative category that emerges from the magistrates' epidemiological strategies for containing dissent and reasserting their sovereignty over representational modes in Massachusetts Bay.

When deployed against individuals, the colony's defense mechanism was brutally efficient: Mary Dyer, who gave birth to a "monstrous" child, was banished and eventually hanged in 1660 because she was a Quaker, who wouldn't stop returning to Boston. She transformed herself from a silent member of the controversy to a proselytizing female Quaker, representing Orthodox Puritanism's worst fears that Antinomianism would keep reinfecting the community, becoming more virulent over time.[123] Jane Hawkins, too, was banished: a midwife and associate of Hutchinson's, she was expressly forbidden to "meddle in surgery, phisick, drinks, plaisters, or oyels, [or] to question matters of religion" because it was assumed that she could use her

position as a means of influencing other women in the colony.[124] Anne
Hutchinson's fate is well known. After her banishment, the remainder of her
life was allegorized by Weld in his introduction to the *Short Story*, where she
served as the final providential evidence of the magistrates' righteousness in
prosecuting her. She suffered "30 monstrous births" that were said to represent her thirty errors; she was gradually forced into the wilderness like Jeze-
bel, going first to Rhode Island, and then to a small farm in what is now New
York. She was left to carve out her own space in the landscape, although
Weld's epidemiological rhetoric suggests that there was no place for her particular distemper in the New World; in 1643, just a year before the *Short Story*
was published, she and her family were killed by Indians, revealing, in Weld's
words, that "Gods hand is the more apparently seene herein, to pick out this
wofull woman, to make her and those belonging to her, an unheard of heavie
example of their cruelty above al others. Thus the Lord heard our groanes to
heaven, and freed us from this great and sore affliction."[125] It is no small irony
that the "cure" for the affliction popularly known as Hutchinsonianism proved
to be the victims of New England's first great recorded plague. As these epidemiological narratives came together, the records of Indian dispossession and
of Anne Hutchinson's sins remythologized the sacred and secular histories of
Massachusetts Bay.

But such acts were not simply directed against Hutchinson. These rhetorical strategies allowed Puritan elders to project themselves as the guardians of
the communal body, and as the guarantors of its health. Cotton used what is
perhaps the most explicit of all the infectious metaphors that emerged from
the controversy, when he charged that Hutchinson's opinions "frett like a
Gangrene and spread like a Leprosie, and infect farr and near, and will eate out
the very Bowells of Religions, and hath soe infected the Churches that God
Knowes whan thay will be cured."[126] Here, the rhetoric is unquestionably centered on illness, but Cotton's turn toward "cure" at the end of his screed presents the colony as a united corporation under attack from a diseased foreign
body. Furthermore, it suggests that this corporation will eventually be
returned to health (even if after a long delay) through the proper guidance of
its ministers and magistrates. Indeed, the trope of infection posits a healthy
colonial body against which dissidents like Hutchinson operate, and the narration of this relationship allows the elders to recreate the myth of an organic
corporate unity in Massachusetts Bay. Pudaloff argues that Winthrop's
language of organicism made "the analogy between a Family and a common-
wealth . . . and still thought of the family with the father as the head of a
body," thus creating a distinction between healthful, masculine care, and the
subversive, potentially monstrous care of women.[127] If masculine nursing

(figured by Winthrop or by Fuller) protects the colony, it does so by preventing further outbreaks of illness—whether caused by internal or external forces: after the election of Winthrop, who replaced Henry Vane as governor in 1636 (an election that began to mark the emerging Orthodoxy's ascendancy over the Antinomians), the General Court passed a law to limit the transmission of information in and out of the colony. It ordered:

> that no town or person shall receive any stranger resorting hither with intent to reside in this jurisdiction, nor shal alow any lot or habitation to any, or intertain any such above three weekes, except such person shall have alowance under the hands of some one of the counsel, or of two other of the magistrates.[128]

This law was specifically intended to halt the spread of Antinomian ideas, and functioned as a self-imposed quarantine to regulate mobility in the colony, and confine seditious acts to a specific location.

And if feminine nursing was subversive, the translation of Hutchinson's prosecution to religious grounds suggests that the remedy for a woman's lack of political standing in the colony lay in naming the church as the site of her transgression. But this split acknowledges that the secular law was unable to demarcate a woman's space in the colony adequately. Hutchinson's actions in Massachusetts Bay revealed the fundamental rift between the secular and ecclesiastical bodies that went far beyond the details of the charges and countercharges of the controversy: in August 1637, the Newtown synod declared that an assembly of women "where sixty or more did meet every week, and one woman (in a prophetical way, by resolving questions of doctrine, and expounding scripture) took upon her the whole exercise, was agreed to be disorderly, and without rule."[129]

Representations of the Antinomian controversy as an infection reflect a key assertion of Puritan epistemology. Where illness breaks down the boundary between internal and external bodies by manifesting observable (and readable) symptoms, so too is the epistemological gap that guarantees New England Puritan modes of governance dependent on a semi-permeability between the visible and invisible world—permeable, because it could provide knowledge of the invisible world, and semi-permeable, because the code for reading this information was not universally available. And if Hutchinson's theological ideas circulated in the same manner as Fuller's had, the difference lay in the fact that the Court could now marshal the full force of its representational practices to regulate these circulations. The gendered figure of the Antinomian is further evidence of the power that epidemiology has in the colonial field, and how it can be used to represent a community's ontological core even if no such core existed. The lasting image of the Antinomian controversy is revealed in Edward Johnson's providential history of New England. Citing the same epidemiological trope that he had used to justify the Puritan migrations, Johnson writes that "by the cunning art of these deceivers, were forescore grosse errours broached secretly, sliding in the darke like the Plague, proving very infectious to some of the Churches of CHRIST in their members."[130]

3

Puritan Immunology

I listen. I read. And now I know that they know it too. They know
they are unnatural. Their writers and artists have been saying it
for years. Telling them they are unnatural, telling them they are
depraved. They call it tragedy. In the movies they call it adventure.
It's just depravity that they try to make glorious, natural. But it
ain't. The disease they have is in their blood, in the structure of
their chromosomes.

—Toni Morrison, *Song of Solomon*[1]

I

Although the impact of early-seventeenth-century epidemics on Native New
England populations and the environment is familiar to historians, the place
and effect of diseases on the lives of English colonists later in the century are
far less likely to be included in histories of the New World, if only because the
story seems so deceptively straightforward: the common narrative trajectory
represents the transfer of pathogens as unidirectional (Europe to America)
and between two monolithic populations (Europeans and Native Americans),
with little regard for regional, national, or even generational differences
between either broadly defined demographic "group." This strategy may have
been useful for describing epidemics during the initial period of colonial
encounters, when Native Americans were disproportionately affected by
contagious diseases, but as these narratives were projected past the first
decades of settlement, accounts of immunologically homogeneous populations have flattened the relation between epidemics and colonial history. If
English colonists never experienced epidemics with the same intensity or
mortality as Native Americans did during the early seventeenth century, the

insistent focus on a virgin soil model of history to the exclusion of more nuanced descriptions of regional and generational immunologies has nevertheless fostered deterministic biological histories of colonialism, and forestalled further investigations into the complexity of epidemiological events in the region, particularly as these shaped English cultural practices over the next half-century.[2]

This master narrative has been handed down in one form or another for nearly four hundred years, from the earliest justification narratives to modern virgin soil theories, and it has proven to be so compelling that it often serves as the first and last word in New England's history—a history that is grounded on an exceptionalist vision of Puritan immunology. My drive to resist the virgin soil model of historiography in favor of immunological syntax in this chapter is therefore an attempt to move away from reading the bodies of first-generation colonists as exceptionalist in favor of a clearer delineation of the local historical and geographic specificities that shaped experiences of epidemic in New England.[3] In this manner, the immunological distinctions that I describe in this chapter follow a trajectory in which the English/Native American fault lines that are so evident in early justification narratives are subsumed to temporal categories of community. This trajectory begins with reports of the 1616–19 New England epidemics, which certainly helped early settlers to envision themselves as immunologically superior to Native Americans, and thus rightful heirs to the land. But significant as these early narratives were for setting the terms of New England's colonial legacy, they offer only a partial glimpse of the region's epidemiological history. I make this claim not to minimize the impact of epidemics on Native populations, which, as I've outlined in Chapter 1, were catastrophic, but to further interrogate the relationship between epidemiology and colonial history. That is, by displacing the virgin soil trope, I hope to better understand how seventeenth-century settlers came to terms with the status of their bodies in New England, and how this shaped their narrative practices in the colonial environment.

As a case in point, the dominant epidemiological narrative of the 1620s would be further consolidated in the 1630s, when smallpox visited New England, and decimated Native populations once again.[4] As was the case fifteen years earlier, first-generation English settlers were largely (though not universally) unaffected by the epidemic because many of them would have had smallpox in England when they were children, which means that they had already developed a lifelong immunity to the disease prior to arriving in the New World. So while English communities escaped this epidemic relatively unscathed, the high mortality among Native Americans helped settlers to reassert their sense of belonging in New England, and of their divinely ordained right to be there. As John Winthrop remarked in 1634, the recent epidemics only confirmed what the settlers believed about the earlier outbreaks, and reinforced English title to the land.[5] Also in 1634, William Bradford noted that in the wake of a particularly virulent outbreak of smallpox on the Connecticut River, the Natives feared the disease "more than the plague," and that "they die like rotten sheep." He contrasts this image to the fact that "not one of the English" colonists who tended to the dying Natives "was so much as sick or in the least measure tainted with this disease, though they daily did these offices for them for many weeks together."[6] Bradford's remarks reflect a vision of English healthfulness that must have struck him as remarkably providential, though he echoes comments made by contemporaries like William Wood, who noted how salutary New England was for English bodies: "The common disease of England, they be strangers to the English now in that strange land. To my knowledge I never knew any that had the pox, measles, green-sickness, headaches, stone, or consumptions, etc."[7] In light of these epidemiological patterns, it is not difficult to see why the large disparities that settlers observed between the effects of disease on Native American and English bodies helped to harden beliefs about their physical and religious superiority in New England.

And yet the truth of the matter is that despite the widely repeated epidemiological myth of New England's origins, New World epidemics were far more complex than the historically and geographically specific experiences of illness that settlers brought with them to North America could account for at the time of their arrival; even as Bradford celebrated English immunity to it, he noted that "upward of 20 [English] persons died" of the smallpox, and that among them was Samuel Fuller, the deacon and physician who had helped the Massachusetts Bay colonists during their first year in the New World.[8] It is clear that the English were not universally immune to disease, and this suggests that in the long run, the immunological disparities that were evident during the 1634 epidemic would prove to be the exception, rather than the norm. Again, this is not to minimize the impact of diseases on Native Americans throughout the century, but to argue that New England's physical isolation from Europe produced a distinct immunological history that would have striking consequences for the communal narratives and theological practices that evolved over the following decades—a model of transatlanticism built as much on the relative geographic isolation of its subjects as it is on the circulation of pathogens. Indeed, the roughly forty-year span from 1620 to 1662 would see a dramatic shift in the way that epidemics afflicted Anglo-American communities, calling the apparent immunological distinction between Native Americans and the English that had anchored the justification narratives into question. And because early epidemiologies were so closely bound to emerging juridical, theological, and colonial discourses, these new patterns of infection pushed settlers to reassess the relation between illness and community as a means of reasserting Orthodox Puritan theologies—or, more to the point—as a means of establishing an Orthodox tradition of Puritan theology in New England.

Even as the current generation of Early Americanists has focused on transatlantic networks and on the particularities of local experience to expand the field's geographic scope, and to develop powerful interdisciplinary tools for critiquing older monolithic models of exceptionalism, consensus, and orthodoxy, New England's early epidemiological history remains obscured by the more nuanced political, theological, economic, and cultural frameworks of criticism that have appeared over the last decade. This chapter seeks to redress the critical blind spot in New England's biological history by moving beyond the first generation of colonial experience, and reintegrating the experiences of mid-seventeenth-century colonists into the region's literary and cultural histories, because their relationship to epidemics in the New World was radically different from their parents' and grandparents' generations. For these later settlers, epidemics were far more likely to strike English communities than they had in the past, so that the epidemiological association of health and land rights that had been so formative earlier in the century was no longer particularly useful. Nevertheless, these were important differences that demanded an appropriate shift in epidemiological rhetoric to account for new patterns of infection.

Though this shift would not specifically address questions of land rights, it influenced the political, social, and theological debates that shaped practices such as the New England jeremiad and the halfway covenant later in the century. This is not to say that the halfway covenant and jeremiad emerged fully formed out of an American wilderness, or operated independently from the theological debates circulating among the colonists and across the Atlantic World, but that these debates were inextricably linked to the changing face of local colonial epidemics. I will not argue that epidemics produced the halfway covenant or the jeremiad, but that epidemiology provided midcentury colonists with a vocabulary that helped them account for the changing nature of epidemics, and allowed them to consolidate their new theological practices. Emphasizing the importance of colonial epidemiology to the lives of second- and third-generation settlers will demonstrate how shifting patterns of illness and immunity pushed them to look inward to themselves for the source of epidemical outbreaks, rather than projecting those causes onto external pathological forces such as Native American savagery or Antinomianism, as had been the case with their forebears. Moreover, the critical and historiographic impact of such an inward turn maps epidemiology's shifting role within the grammar of colonialism—a role that calls for rethinking the ongoing influence of epidemics within the theological and cultural discourses of early New England communities, and accounting for that influence by examining the relation between immunology and rhetoric.

First-generation epidemiologies shared a common structure insofar as they visualized epidemics in terms of their ability to reorganize and redefine geographic spaces. This is evident in the way that justification narratives represented landscape as a vacant wilderness in order to establish English rights to property in the wake of Native American epidemics, or even in how magistrates deployed epidemiological rhetoric during a figural illness such as the Antinomian controversy to represent their community as an inherently healthy space under attack from pathogenic agents that needed to be expelled—or banished—for the common good. What makes these epidemiologies so powerful in terms of their colonialist implications—the one for appropriating land and the other for centralizing political power—is their ability to quickly and efficiently delimit the boundaries of healthful behavior, and to map those boundaries on a spatial plane. By the same token, this strength also points to a broader limitation of early epidemiologies: namely, that as with the virgin soil model of colonial history, these mappings provide only a synchronic snapshot of epidemics, where susceptibility and immunity are assumed to be timeless manifestations of a body's essential constitution, thus binding immunology ahistorically to location, rather than representing it as a mutable function of demographic shifts and changing behaviors over time. Justification narratives describe health as a static feature of a body's civil or savage state, and make few, if any, temporal allowances for English bodies to fall sick and die on their own—or indeed, for Native Americans to be immune to illness. So long as epidemics strike well-defined, homogeneous population clusters in relatively consistent and predictable patterns—as occurred through the mid-1630s—the physical and behavioral boundaries that colonial epidemiology helped to construct remain coherent, and perhaps more importantly, can be redeployed and reproduced as needed; colonial communities project themselves against a background state of health, while savagery and Antinomianism become coextensive with illness and pathology. But when these early epidemiological patterns fall apart and become unpredictable—when diseases target English in addition to Native American communities—the synchronic snapshot blurs; familiar behaviors no longer protect against illness, well-worn narratives no longer account for epidemical outbreaks accurately, and bodies once intuitively considered healthy fall sick.

In order to decipher the trajectory of New England's epidemiological history, then, one must complicate early synchronic mappings with a diachronic perspective of immunity and susceptibility that traces these shifts over time—on generational, or even cross-generational, scales.

I argue that this diachronic perspective is provided via the framework of immunological syntax, which resists reading epidemics as static historical events in favor of tracing the cross-generational currents of epidemiological history. For example, instead of representing the immunological distinction between Native American and European bodies during the first two decades of settlement strictly as the internalized manifestation of a timeless geographic and cultural isolation, as is the case with the virgin soil model, immunological syntax pushes us to think about these distinctions on a temporal axis as well—namely, to consider geographic isolation (and its immunological consequences) as an ongoing function of colonial life. Such an analysis is initially occluded in cases like the 1616–19 epidemics precisely because these outbreaks were so virulent, and occurred in such a brief period that for all intents and purposes, they did act homogeneously, decimating Native populations while apparently leaving English communities unscathed; in this historical trajectory, virgin soil really is the simplest and most elegant explanation. But if we resist thinking about these populations in homogeneous terms, and if we project forward half a century, a new frame of reference comes into focus. That is, we come to see first-, second-, and third-generation English colonists as distinct demographic groups in and of themselves, each with its own immunological history despite their shared ancestries. The kind of analysis that I undertake here overlays a geographic understanding of epidemic with a temporal framework to reveal the immunological difference between generations of settlers, and to fracture genealogical bonds where nationalist histories would seek to shore them up by modeling communal narratives according to an internally coherent and consistent trajectory.

In this manner, it is possible to think about the ways that a third-generation settler living in 1662 might have had as much (if not more) in common, immunologically speaking, with a Native American from 1616, than with his or her own grandparents. This observation describes an important factor in the evolution of New England's epidemiological history, and it reorients our own critical relationship to early colonial practices. By uncovering the immunological distinctions between the various generations of English settlers, and by contextualizing these distinctions within the divergent experiences of illness and epidemic that evolved independently on both sides of the Atlantic, this chapter will investigate how mid-seventeenth-century epidemiologies helped colonists come to terms with an unexpected and deeply unsettling immunological shift in which they saw themselves becoming the victims of epidemics that had seemed to leave prior generations untouched. Furthermore, by revealing the biological and demographic mechanisms that account for this turn, I use the concept of immunological syntax to analyze how mid-century theological innovations like the jeremiad and halfway covenant serve as textual traces of New England's epidemiological history.

The path for such an analysis of the generational dimensions of colonial immunology runs through a discussion of smallpox—one of the most terrifying diseases of the seventeenth century, and one that was experienced in a radically different manner in North America, than it had been in England. The key to understanding this difference within a colonial setting lies in a 1716 letter from Cotton Mather to John Woodward of the Royal Society, in which Mather discusses the disease and the potential benefits of an emerging treatment known as inoculation. Mather describes his anxiety about the virulent effects of smallpox in New England, and gives a brief history of its appearance in Boston, explaining that it was a central recurring preoccupation throughout the seventeenth century:

[We] even suspect a peculiar agency of the invisible world in the infliction of the smallpox upon our city of Boston, when we saw that from the first foundations of it, in the year 1630, down to the year 1702, it observed the precise period of twelve years in its mortal visits unto us. Now and then a vessel would in the intervening space bring in the distemper among us. However, it would not spread. But on the twelfth year, still no precaution would keep it off. In the twelfth year it must be epidemical. So raging, so reaching, that it may come at unborn children; they have been born full of it upon them.[9]

Epidemiological records for the first half of the seventeenth century are difficult to piece together accurately because diseases were frequently confused for one another, and because the information was not collected systematically in New England, as it was in the London *Bills of Mortality*. Nevertheless, after the 1634 outbreak recounted by Bradford and Winthrop, English communities faced epidemics in 1648–49, in 1666, again from 1677–79, from 1689–90, in 1702, and, most famously, in 1721—roughly one to two decades between visitations. And while there is general agreement about the timing of the last four epidemics, there is a good deal more ambiguity about the prior outbreaks. For example, John Bonner's 1721 map of Boston lists epidemics in 1640 and 1660, rather than 1648 and 1666—a slight, but not trivial difference.[10] If Mather fudges details slightly in favor of the symmetry that a "precise period of twelve years" offers his narrative, he is not far off the mark, and his observation provides important details for understanding the history of smallpox in seventeenth-century New England, and this for a variety of reasons: first, because it puts the lie to any notion that English settlers were unaffected by the diseases that struck Native Americans so severely in the years leading to colonization, or that there was an essential immunological difference between them; second, because the twelve-year cycle suggests a quasi-generational interval between successive outbreaks of the disease that bears further inquiry; third, because Mather identifies the disease as epidemic in Boston rather than endemic (the town being relatively free from infection during the intervals); and finally, because this epidemical nature of smallpox is directly related to the severity of the illness, as well as its cyclical patterns (although Mather had no way of knowing so at the time).

Aside from the obvious physical hardships that colonists would have contended with during these epidemics, the cyclical recurrence of virulent smallpox left communities to explain an apparent shift in God's will. If the migration to New England had been justified with legal and theological arguments grounded in Native American susceptibility as opposed to English immunity to disease, then these same illnesses logically undermined those justifications when Anglo-Americans succumbed to them on a large scale later in the century. Not surprisingly, then, this shift repositioned the colonists' epidemiological stance in a fundamental way: where first-generation narratives stood on the apparent distinction between Native American and English bodies during the 1620s and early 1630s, the second and third generations had to reexamine the distinction between English and Anglo-American bodies as time wore on. My use of the hyphenated term "Anglo-American" is deliberate at this stage, and I intend it to highlight an important generational distinction that bears emphasizing. As epidemiological patterns changed during the first half-century of settlement, the apparent immunological gap between Native American and English bodies tended to narrow, given that the English began succumbing to disease in a way that they had not earlier. At the same time, a gap between North American settlers and their countrymen in England (or their grandparents' generation) grew, as the former succumbed to diseases in patterns that were unfamiliar to the latter. Immunologically speaking, the settler's body in midcentury New England was no longer the same as the one that had arrived thirty years earlier. Thus, the hyphenation is intended as a syntactical marker to denote an immunological evolution that mirrors a geographic and temporal displacement, and that can be traced rhetorically, according to the shifting experience of epidemics in the New World.

Modern epidemiological theory explains the initial discrepancy in immunological sensitivity (and the subsequent shift in susceptibility) through a series of factors that include a community's ability to support disease endemically, and an individual's prior exposure to pathogenic agents (which, in the case of smallpox, triggers lifetime immunity by stimulating the production of antibodies to the variola virus).[11] Further refined, these two issues—the one individual, and the other communal—rest on a question of demographics and population distributions, and, even more specifically, on the relative population densities of England and America.[12] To illustrate this point, I turn briefly to seventeenth-century London, which was a densely populated city that supported diseases like smallpox endemically.[13] With a pool of susceptible people that was continually replenished through birth and migration, London's concentrated population acted as a reservoir in which variola could survive and reproduce, passing from person to person, from house to house, crisscrossing from one end of the city to the other, and coming into contact with new potential victims every day. Any Londoner who was susceptible to smallpox lived in an inherently dangerous environment, at constant risk of being infected during the course of daily life. By the same token, because smallpox was an ever-present danger, and because it was quite contagious, most susceptible individuals could not avoid the virus for long. As a result, infection usually occurred during early childhood rather than adolescence or adulthood for native-born Londoners, so the illness came to be known as a "disease of children," who, if they survived, went on to become immune adults. This effect was so powerful, that "nearly all native inhabitants of London had been infected by the age of seven."[14] Although endemic smallpox invariably meant that infant mortality rates were high, the adult population remained largely resistant to the disease precisely because the overwhelming majority had already been infected in childhood. For this very reason, the frequency and severity of smallpox epidemics in the adult population were comparatively low against this endemic background presence of infection, and Londoners would have been well aware of this fact.

Of course, London was unique in terms of its size and population density, so using it as the basis for generalizing about England's experience with smallpox in the seventeenth century is problematic. Certainly, there were isolated English towns and villages—especially those with populations under 2,500—where smallpox was not endemic, and where the experience would therefore have tended to skew differently.[15] And yet, because trade and market routes were sufficiently well developed, the low population density of these smaller towns was often offset by their relative proximity to larger cities, where smallpox was endemic. This proximity—measured geographically and temporally by the number of miles or the number of days it took to travel from point A to point B—ensured a constant circulation of pathogens and contagious bodies throughout the country.[16] Rural villages where smallpox was not endemic nevertheless did experience cyclical smallpox epidemics—especially if they found themselves on market routes, but these epidemics ranged in fairly short five- to seven-year periods—less than half the interval Mather reported for Boston.[17] Thus, despite pockets of localized sparseness, England could be considered "nationally dense," meaning that even in isolated rural locations, smallpox remained predominantly a disease of young children throughout the seventeenth century.

This, then, was the immunological pattern that most first-generation settlers were accustomed to when they left for New England. And while not all of those settlers were from large cities, and certainly not all of them were immune to smallpox, the majority would have been infected with the disease early in life, and would have known smallpox as a childhood disease.[18] This fact helps to account for the difference between Native American and English susceptibility to smallpox in the first third of the seventeenth century—a temporal and *temporary* function of population density and prior exposure to pathogens. But as Mather would indicate nearly a century later, Native American susceptibility represents only one aspect of New England's epidemiological history. Unlike England, which was nationally dense, New England populations were both locally and regionally sparse: towns were small, and few and far between, and their distance from Europe was measured in weeks and months rather than days, so the problem that cropped up for settlers over the succeeding decades was that these much smaller communities did not have the critical population base to support smallpox endemically. Because immunity was high among first-generation adult settlers (who were therefore not carriers of the variola virus), there simply wasn't a significant enough reservoir of susceptible colonists for the virus to survive for long, and gain a permanent foothold in the region. As a result, second- and third-generation children born in New England had no regular exposure to pathogens like variola early in their lives, and were therefore much more likely to reach adolescence and adulthood while still susceptible to smallpox than were their parents and grandparents who had been raised in England; what had been a childhood disease in England was no longer obviously marked as such in New England. Indeed, New England would have felt particularly blessed by the fact that smallpox was relatively rare in childhood, and this would only have confirmed their sense of being on a righteous mission.

The flipside of the colony's early immunological condition, however, is that New England's population as a whole—which had been relatively immune during the first years of settlement—became increasingly susceptible to smallpox with the birth of every child—a factor that, if not significant on a case-by-case basis, nevertheless increased the risk of epidemics exponentially when considered in the aggregate over a period of years. Ironically, the very demographic and immunological conditions that produced a discrepancy between English and Native American mortality between 1616 and 1619, and then again in 1634 (and labeled by historians as "virgin soil" in indigenous populations) were replicated by New England's Anglo-American communities later in the century, as these became increasingly susceptible to smallpox en masse. Virgin soil is obviously not the right term for describing Anglo-American communities at midcentury—in part, because epidemics were never quite as devastating as they had been for Native Americans—but this unfitness, I argue, also points to the phrase's problematic relation to Native American populations. Certainly, by the end of each twelve-year interepidemic cycle, Anglo-American settlements were ripe for dramatic epidemics, which would then be followed by periods of relative healthfulness, because each outbreak essentially reset a community's immunological clock to zero—to what it had been for the first generation. People who were susceptible prior to an epidemic outbreak either escaped uninfected, succumbed to smallpox and died, or became immune and went on to have their own children. In this context, the twelve-year interval that Mather described highlights a key feature for understanding the colonial experience in North America, because it illustrates a cyclical demographic shift from communal resistance to susceptibility, and back.

The process of communal susceptibility and resistance that I have been describing is tied to what modern epidemiologists call *herd immunity*, which Priscilla Wald describes as "an epidemiological concept that focuses on the biology of a population rather than of an individual or a disease."[19] Put briefly, herd immunity refers to a community's collective (rather than individual) immunity, and helps to derive the probability of epidemic outbreak for a given ratio of immune to susceptible inhabitants.[20] When that ratio is high—when immune people outnumber the susceptible in a community by 4, or even 5 to 1—the risk of epidemical outbreak decreases precipitously, and vice versa. In other words, even if a specific individual is susceptible to smallpox, he or she can be protected from infection if enough of his or her fellow community members are themselves immune; the individual benefits from the community's relative immunity. Likewise, the community as a whole can be protected from epidemic when herd immunity is high, even if some of its inhabitants are susceptible to infection. The reason for this is a simple numbers game: when herd immunity is high—meaning that there are considerably more immune people than susceptible ones—a contagious carrier of variola is far less likely to come into contact with susceptible individuals during the normal course of daily events, than with immune people. Because immune individuals do not incubate or pass on the virus, they act as dead ends in the chain of infection. The more dead ends, the lower the rates of transmission and infection, and the less likely an epidemic will erupt. On the other hand, when herd immunity is low, a contagious carrier will almost certainly come into contact with several susceptible people, each of whom has a chance of being infected, then incubating and passing on the virus to others, setting off an epidemic chain reaction in the process. Herd immunity is a fundamental concept in modern public health policy because it allows officials to manage and monitor vaccination programs; it is often not essential to vaccinate every community member against specific pathogens, because communities themselves can be considered "sufficiently resistant" to a disease when enough citizens are vaccinated.[21] But while herd immunity is not a widely used historiographic concept, I deploy it as such here because it offers a powerful framework for understanding the mechanics of colonial epidemics, and it creates an immunological framework for visualizing community.

Projected back onto the seventeenth century, the concept of herd immunity allows us to make a number of claims. In London, for example, where smallpox was endemic, the disease nevertheless cycled in two- to three-year epidemic intervals.[22] But as the disease's endemic nature would predict, adults were largely immune to smallpox, so epidemics generally struck children, which further suggests that herd immunity among that particular age group was extremely low (as one would expect, given that children are not born with natural immunities to the disease), while it was much higher among adolescents and adults (who had most likely survived it in infancy). Taken in the aggregate, London's herd immunity was stable enough that it did not produce dramatic epidemic swings as in New England, but low enough that variola remained a constant endemic presence throughout the seventeenth and eighteenth centuries. In New England, on the other hand, there were two significant factors at work: low population density prevented smallpox from becoming endemic, and this low density manifested itself through dramatic cyclical swings in the level of herd immunity, where large segments of the population would either be susceptible or immune at the same time. When Mather wrote that "now and then a vessel would in the intervening space bring in the distemper among us. . . . However, it would not spread," a modern epidemiologist would decipher this comment by indicating that the virus was being introduced to the region while herd immunity was high, so that outbreaks of smallpox would remain fairly localized and trail off quickly.

These events in all likelihood occurred on the front end of the twelve-year interepidemic cycles, when the community as a whole was "sufficiently immune" to the disease. At the end of these cycles, however, herd immunity would have been significantly lower, setting the stage for a new epidemic to erupt—just as Mather describes.

It is important to emphasize that herd immunity does not actually prevent individual infections, but that it merely regulates the periodicity and virulence of epidemics. Generalizing from these demographic and immunological effects, William McNeill explains that high-density populations tend to "settle toward endemicity," whereas low-density areas tend to experience higher frequencies of epidemics—patterns that reflect the relative experience with smallpox in both England and New England.[23] This notion is most clearly illustrated in practical terms by John Duffy, who points out that overall eighteenth-century death rates from smallpox were actually *lower* in America than they were in England. However, the epidemic nature of smallpox in America led to the misconception that "smallpox was peculiarly fatal to Americans," a pattern that had its roots in seventeenth-century demographics and immunology, and which was magnified by the fact that smallpox fatalities in England concentrated on relatively invisible populations like infants and small children.[24] Duffy goes on to suggest that the fear of smallpox infection preyed heavily on the minds of Anglo-Americans, and that travel to Europe—whether for business or education—was surprisingly dangerous for young adults, who could often expect to encounter smallpox for the first time during their travels.[25] Although the concept of herd immunity is crucial to the development and management of modern immunization programs, it is also a useful model for describing the disparate effects of smallpox in Europe and North America prior to the advent of inoculation and vaccination in the eighteenth century.

Ultimately, Wald's description of herd immunity as a way to think about the biological basis for imagining community is extremely helpful because it allows her to figure community as an "immunological ecosystem," which is to say a system that regulates and transforms itself to "precipitate new communal affiliations" when epidemics disrupt the immunological equilibrium of a community.[26] In the context of the colonial era, I argue that the trajectory of these affiliations is marked by the set of narrative and theological practices that emerged in the wake of midcentury epidemics. Given this elaboration of herd immunity, I would like to return briefly to discuss the distinction between virgin soil and immunological syntax as two paradigms for considering New England colonial epidemics, because this distinction is central to revisiting the relationship between epidemiology and narrative history in the mid-seventeenth century. As I've outlined in Chapter 1 with the help of David Jones's work, while virgin soil does offer a simple and dramatic metaphor for describing Native American susceptibility to European pathogens, the term imprints a biological homogeneity on disparate populations, and tends to produce immunologically deterministic histories of the New World.[27] And while it is clear that virgin soil depends on the mechanism of herd immunity, what lies at the heart of this determinism is a fundamentally ahistorical assumption that generalizes from an immunological condition at a given point in time, to project a broader historical truism about the effect of diseases on specific populations. This is not to deny the undeniable: diseases like smallpox and the measles were absolutely devastating to indigenous populations throughout the Americas, and continued to be so for centuries. But rather than fixating on what is ultimately a metaphor of limited value, it might be more productive to consider the epidemiological history of colonialism in terms of cyclical, rather than essential, immunological conditions. Indeed, the reason that early epidemics seem to have fascinated English explorers and settlers so much was not only the number of Native Americans who died, but also the fact that those deaths ranged across the age spectrum, including adults as well as children; such a cross section of mortality was uncommon enough for the English, whose radically different experience of diseases like smallpox leant significant providential weight to the scenes they encountered in New England, and therefore had a great impact on their early narratives.

If, instead, we were to conceive of these epidemics using a model informed by a longer view of herd immunity, two fundamental differences would shape our understanding of colonial history: first, where virgin soil offers an essentially static model of disease, immunological syntax provides a way to understand epidemiological history dynamically, as a process that responds to demographic changes over time. In temporal terms, this means thinking about the disparate immunological factors that might shape epidemics at a specific point in time, but also about how those factors are part of an ongoing cycle that is dependent on the relation between the materiality of local histories and of transatlantic circulations; it means thinking about epidemics as cyclical rather than singular events, and, more importantly, thinking about immunological responses to the environment as a dynamic rather than fixed function of individual and communal bodies. Such a model resists determinism by suggesting that immune systems operate in spatially and temporally heterogeneous patterns, so that the 1616–19, and the later 1634 epidemics were not timeless manifestations of the inferiority of Native American bodies, but vivid snapshots of comparative immunological conditions over time—a snapshot that is replicable in other locations, and among other peoples. This observation leads to a second crucial difference from the virgin soil model—namely, that immunological syntax asks us to consider mid-seventeenth-century Anglo-American epidemics in parallel with the earlier Native American epidemics, and subsequently to reposition our understanding of the ways that epidemiological rhetoric shaped the colonial world. Herd immunity explains the initial disparate reaction of Native American and English bodies to pathogens, and it properly contextualizes later Anglo-American smallpox epidemics as a reflection of similar (if less severe) demographic and immunological patterns that occurred in Native American communities. In other words, where virgin soil implicitly posits an essential immunological difference between Native Americans and English colonists, immunological syntax tropes that difference, and recasts it as a similarity that only becomes visible over time; immunological syntax reveals parallel epidemiological patterns where virgin soil tends to obscure them. More pointedly, the issue is then to think about the critical impact of an immunological syntax model on the genre of seventeenth-century New England epidemiology. As a starting point, cyclical epidemics are significant because they invert the patterns of infection and immunity with which first-generation settlers were familiar. The remainder of this chapter investigates how colonists adapted to such inversions in order to reconsider the temporal relations that informed their epidemiological rhetoric.

II

To be sure, immunity and immunological sensitivity are easiest to consider in terms of individual responses to disease. Exposure and susceptibility to pathogenic agents determine the effects of illness, and these effects are generally conceived as personal events. As the 1616–19 epidemics and the Antinomian controversy suggest, diseases leave legible imprints on communities as well as individuals. The nature of contagion and of epidemics means that these personal events are deeply implicated in public health concerns and, by extension, in communal histories. Quarantines, vaccination programs, and similar public policies are most effective when they negotiate the intersection between public and private realms—when the community's interests dovetail with the individual's. Modern medical discourses abstract the communal effects of epidemics from their effects on private bodies, and represent these as functions of population density, the mobility and mutability of pathogens, as well as the ratio of immune to non-immune individuals. This is perhaps the distinction between illness and epidemic: as illnesses act on individuals, so epidemics act on communities. Ultimately, the concept of herd immunity suggests that to speak of immunity is to consider the dynamic relation between personal and communal bodies—a relation that, if not particular to seventeenth-century New England Puritans, is certainly central to the tensions at the heart of Puritan rhetoric. For this very reason, herd immunity and the cyclical patterns of smallpox in New England become useful staging grounds for imagining how Puritan communities relied on epidemiological observations to constitute themselves around shared responses to disease— conceived both geographically and generationally (or spatially and temporally)—over the first half-century of colonial history.

Drawing on Benedict Anderson's work, Wald has coined the term "imagined immunities" to describe just this ideological function of illness, summarizing the relation between health and the "strategy of community" succinctly: "The inextricability of disease and national belonging shapes the experience of both; disease assumes a political significance, while national belonging becomes nothing less than a matter of health."[28] New England's early epidemiologies are perhaps not constituted in terms of nationhood, but they reflect a clear link between political and theological practices, on the one hand, and health, on the other; it is this filiation that I now propose to investigate. As Mather's brief history of smallpox suggests, "health" would become an increasingly unstable ground for political identity in the latter half of the seventeenth century because immunological and epidemiological patterns began to shift in important ways. Where the boundaries between health and illness had been clearly delineated along savage and civil (or Antinomian and Orthodox) axes in early colonial epidemiologies, Mather's suspicion that cyclical smallpox epidemics were regulated by the "peculiar agency of the invisible world" displaces "health" as a coherent organizing principle for community and "national belonging." Or, if it doesn't quite displace health, it nevertheless requires a patient epidemiological elaboration of how health, behavior, and illness stand in relation to emerging structures of community. Indeed, if health and political character are intertwined in the way that Wald suggests, these shifting patterns called for a careful reassessment of the first generation's epidemiological narrative conventions. Second- and third-generation colonists were thus compelled to grapple with the problem of their bodies' frailty in an environment they had supposedly been destined to populate, and in so doing, to reimagine the way that health and immunity constituted their place in the world.

Although it is clear that seventeenth-century New England settlers could not possibly have understood the modern demographic and immunological mechanism of herd immunity, I want to suggest that they nevertheless recognized that familiar epidemiological patterns were changing around them, that their experience with epidemics was starkly different from those described in justification narratives, and different, too, from their parents' and grandparents' experiences of illness in England. Mather certainly had the benefit of hindsight when he wrote about the cyclical nature of smallpox in his 1716 letter to Woodward, but it also appears that midcentury settlers paid close attention to diseases around them, as they debated political and theological issues publicly. Where epidemics did break out in Anglo-American communities, ministers, magistrates, petitioners, and poets alike quickly drew on the tropes of New England's early epidemiologies to frame political and theological debates so that they could reassess the community's fundamental health, and narrate its history. As they did so, the balance between the individual and the communal—between responsibility and reward—weighed heavily on their minds.

By the time Massachusetts Bay was well into its second decade, the colony had survived the dangers of the initial migration, the Antinomian controversy, and the Pequot war, and had fostered an economic climate where trade flourished, and new classes of wealth began to emerge, if not intermingle. Whereas first-generation settlers had found epidemiological rhetoric to be effective in justifying colonial expansion, the story began to change when illness and infection seemed to erupt from within the borders of Anglo-American communities. Wherever they looked, settlers encountered the limits of their providential rhetoric in the face of an unrelenting assault: here, factionalism, sedition, heresy, earthquakes, drought, famine, and even epidemics announced themselves at every turn, and reminded colonists that this New World was not exactly the place they had imagined for themselves before embarking on the migration. Providential readings aimed to make sense of singular catastrophic events by thematizing them within a conventional logic of exceptionalism and declension—the "strategy of community" elaborated by first-generation colonists in their justification narratives, and in their responses to the Antinomian controversy. Nevertheless, shifting epidemiological patterns required colonists to reconsider the behavioral causes of New England epidemics as a means of accounting for God's changing judgment, because savagery could no longer be used to explain these later outbreaks. By the mid-1660s, these shifts would begin to imprint themselves as a generational paradigm on New England's new class of epidemiological narratives, as epidemics themselves appeared to discriminate between children, their parents, and their grandparents.

These strategies shaped communities in a number of ways, often emerging as public practices designed to centralize political and juridical power, as was the case during the Antinomian controversy. But they also often proved to be problematic, as when settlers struggled to make sense of their status in New England, given the sometimes bewildering array of civil and ecclesiastical rules enacted by the government and churches. One striking example occurred in relation to the May 1631 decision by the Massachusetts General Court to limit the franchise to church members—a rule that flew in the face of the then prevailing custom in England, where "every man was accounted of the church by reason of his membership in the state." In place of this system, the Court offered a model of governance in which "a voice in the state was now conditioned on membership in the church."[29] The decision to limit the franchise may not have been so problematic in and of itself, but it was magnified by the particularly restrictive process of election to Congregationalist churches, which, if not explicitly intended to produce a perfect church on earth, did, in the words of Edmund Morgan, imply "a departure from the world and a closer approach to perfection than others had attained."[30] It is this desire to depart from the world—to escape the corruptions of the body— that compelled Congregationalists to mimic the invisible church as closely as they could on earth. New applicants for membership to Congregational churches were required to undergo a rigorous examination by elders, to give an accounting of the inner workings of grace, and to make a public profession of faith.[31] This process set the standard for election extremely high, as the goal was to prevent hypocrites from getting a foot in the door, and threatening the churches from within. The worldly consequence of these strict requirements was that this system frustrated settlers who had been church members in good standing back in England, but now suddenly found themselves debarred from taking communion, prevented from baptizing their children, and, to add insult to injury, disenfranchised. Indeed, Massachusetts's Congregational churches were so restrictive that by 1646, roughly four out of every five settlers were still not elected, and therefore could not vote, legislate, or adjudicate laws.[32]

The relationship between church membership and voting rights became increasingly vexed during the 1640s, as the system's defenders—including Winthrop and John Cotton—found themselves participating in a heated transatlantic debate about Congregationalist practices.[33] Their histories of the Antinomian controversy were clearly written as part of this debate with an English audience in mind, but this did not slow down the internal dissension in New England itself. While the defenders of Congregationalism tried to mute any charge that the New England Way was a challenge to English authority, their defense took on an added air of urgency after the Westminster Assembly of 1643, when Presbyterians became increasingly powerful in

England. Even if they saw themselves as non-Conformists rather than Separatists, Congregationalists worried that Presbyterians would try to assert a centralized power over New England communities—which was anathema to the very concept of Congregationalism—and that the parliament might try to establish conformity and unity among New England churches, as they had in England and Scotland.[34] On a local level, the tension between Congregationalists and Presbyterians revolved around the structure of church hierarchies: Congregationalists rejected the formal power of a centralized authority like the Church of England, as well as concepts like a "Presbyteriall Church" or "Ministers at Large" who could dictate actions to communities.[35] As it was, individual congregations were formed by distinct covenants between members, and continuity did not necessarily hold from one congregation to the next.[36] Although congregations could join together in federations, and could seek advice from their neighbors if they wished to, they tended to guard their autonomy jealously, being particularly sensitive to the election of local officers and the administration of church discipline.

Linking the franchise to church membership proved to be highly problematic by the mid-1640s, particularly when coupled with the fact that a number of local communities chafed under the centralized authority of the Massachusetts General Court. In 1645, the issue of church membership and local election of officers erupted when the citizens of Hingham, upset at the Court's reluctance to accede to their wishes in appointing a new militia commander, filed a petition against the magistrates, and threatened to take their complaints to the English parliament if their concerns were not addressed.[37] Hot on the heels of this dissent, Doctor Robert Child and six of his associates submitted a Petition and Remonstrance to the General Court in May 1646, under the pretext of asking the Court to extend political rights to a greater percentage of the population, and of bringing religious toleration to the Bay. If the petition reminded magistrates of their troubles with the Antinomians a decade earlier, they were dismayed to discover that simultaneous to submitting it, Child and the remonstrants circulated copies throughout North America and the Caribbean colonies, and had it printed and distributed in England by Child's brother in 1647. The Court took both the petition and its circulation as the clear affront that they were, and marshaled its political power to quash the dissent as quickly as it could.[38]

The petition's opening lines are a witty send-up of Winthrop's *Model of Christian Charity*, which famously begins with a spirited defense of social and economic hierarchies, explaining that "God Almighty in His most holy and wise providence, hath so disposed of the condition of mankind, as in all times some must be rich, some poor, some high and eminent in power and dignity;

others mean and in subjection."[39] In contrast, the petitioners subvert Winthrop's hierarchical model of community with the revolutionary observation that the lowly are actually in a better position to protect the ship of state than those currently at its helm: "Those who are under decks, being at present unfit for higher imployments, may perceive those Leaks which will inevitably sink the weak and ill compacted Vessell, if not by your Wisdoms opportunely prevented."[40] There are two important details to note about the petition's use of "ill compacted vessel" as an opening trope. First, it offers a critique of the fundamental building block of New England communities—the compact— suggesting that Massachusetts Bay, as presently constituted under the leadership of Winthrop and the magistrates, had been ill conceived and poorly established from the outset. Second, the reference to a vessel recalls the famous metaphor at the end of *A Model of Christian Charity*, in which Winthrop speaks of the figural shipwreck that threatens to destroy the colony if settlers turn away from God (and even more pressingly, the literal threat of a shipwreck if God did not approve of the settlers' articles before they landed in New England). But unlike Winthrop's sermon, which projects this shipwreck into the future as a punishment for potential misdeeds, the petitioners charged that the danger to the colony was at hand, and they lay the blame for this fact squarely at the magistrates' feet: they were the ones who were elected to steer the vessel safely, and yet it appeared that they could not. Turning back to Winthrop's defense of hierarchy, the petition makes a show of preserving the distinction between the rich and the poor, the powerful and their subjects, only to upend them by emphasizing that the poor and mean have the best vantage from which to guide the colony through future perils.

Bringing Winthrop's threat of future punishment into the present, the petitioners go on to charge that the community's affliction was already well under way, and thus that the turn from God has already taken place:

God who through his goodnesse hath safely brought us and ours through the great Ocean, and planted us here, seems not now to be with us, nay rather against us, blasting all our designs . . . by which many of good estates are brought to the brinks of extreme poverty; yea, at this time laying His just hand upon our families, taking many away to himself, striking others with unwonted malignant sicknesses and noysome shamefull diseases.[41]

Once again, the petitioners tweak Winthrop's defense of social and economic hierarchies by pointing to the "many of good estates" who have been made poor in New England, and they offer this observation in partial evidence of

God's displeasure with the colony. While the petitioners' critique is predicated here on providing a specific case in response to Winthrop's general vision for the colony, the parallel between these texts is unmistakable. Furthermore, the petition goes for the jugular by calling on familiar epidemiological tropes to identify the specific affliction that God sent to punish the colony for the magistrates' misdeeds. The reference to "noisome shamefull diseases" reminds us once again of the shipwreck that Winthrop had threatened in his sermon, but what is particularly interesting in this case is that the petitioners use a very recent outbreak of illness to literalize that rhetorical threat; Winthrop confirms in his journal that during the spring of 1646, Boston was visited by a "malignant feaver," and by a "loathsome" outbreak of syphilis which "raysed a scandal upon the Towne, & Countrye."[42]

The peculiar thing about the outbreak, if not the reports of its progress, is that Winthrop cites it so matter-of-factly, making no attempt to read the disease providentially. Foregoing the opportunity to represent the illness as a communal punishment (as the petitioners do), he explains instead that the magistrates examined the infected woman who was the supposed "patient zero," and concluded that the disease was spread because she nursed several neighborhood children. Unsure of how this woman first contracted syphilis (her husband, a sailor, was apparently uninfected), Winthrop seems surprisingly naïve, as he defers to those with medical expertise, writing that "this is a question to be decided by Phisitians"[43] It is hard to imagine Winthrop having this reaction to Anne Hutchinson, so it may be that he downplayed the outbreak to avoid raising a scandal—or to avoid drawing attention to their dissent—but the petitioners do not let the chance slip, making the most of the opportunity to embarrass the magistrates by associating them with the disease. Where Winthrop had merely anticipated future national traumas and insisted on their sacred meaning in *A Model of Christian Charity*, Child and his associates reassert the worldly import of epidemics by assigning a clear temporal significance to them. Yes, diseases were a sign of divine displeasure directed against the colony, but this danger was tied to abuses by the magistrates who lived "above-deck" on the "ill compacted vessel" rather than to the impiety of those who lived below; redress could only be had through a wholesale reorganization of the government.

The petitioners' use of illness as a mediating figure during this moment of social unrest demonstrates that they had assimilated the lessons of the previous decade well, and that they understood the narrative force of epidemiology in the political arena. The magistrates had used illness as an effective figure for dealing with dissent during the Antinomian controversy of 1636–38, but their representation of dissidents as a health risk for the body politic took its most explicit form in Winthrop's *Short Story of the Rise, reign, and ruine of the Antinomians, Familists & Libertines, that infected the Churches of New England*, printed in England in 1644 as a transatlantic defense of New England Congregationalism in the wake of the Westminster Assembly. Although it would be speculation to assume that Child, who arrived in New England in September 1645, had read the *Short Story*, his role in submitting the petition less than a year after his arrival suggests just such a connection. In the words of George Kittredge, Child was an "ardent Presbyterian" and a disciple of Robert Baillie, himself a key figure in the attacks against New England Congregationalism.[44] Furthermore, Child had first visited New England in the late 1630s, at the tail end of the Antinomian controversy, and was a correspondent with John Winthrop Jr. in the years between his visits, so it is not difficult to imagine him being intimately familiar with the details of the controversy.[45] Certainly, his fellow petitioners would have been aware of the magistrates' representations of Antinomianism as an "infection" in Massachusetts Bay when they submitted their document to the Court. I make this suggestion because the *Short Story* illustrates that well into the 1640s, the trope of infectious disease helped to secure the Puritan elders' hold on secular power by labeling dissident citizens as the site of a figurative illness, and by positing themselves as a core Orthodox body around which to build a cohesive community; the petition picked up on this rhetorical strategy, and turned it back on the magistrates themselves.

For the elders, Antinomianism was a disease that could be treated through quarantine, banishment, and excommunication, so it would have been especially galling to see epidemiological language deployed against them in this way. Nevertheless, the petitioners found that in combination with the recent outbreak of syphilis, epidemiological tropes were impossible to pass up. But instead of reading Congregationalism itself as a social ill, their representations signal a turn away from Winthrop's and Cotton's narratives of the Antinomian controversy's figurative illness by mapping a *physical* epidemic onto its alleged ideological source: here, dissent is not a threat to the community, but a democratizing instinct posited as the cure to a very real public health threat posed by the magistrates. In making this claim, I don't want to insist on the specific herd immunity response that I've outlined above in relation to smallpox, because syphilis is, first and foremost, a bacterial (rather than viral) infection. Nevertheless, the petition's opening figure of the colony as an "ill compacted vessel" leans on epidemiological readings of syphilis to charge that the very premise behind the colony's civil and ecclesiastical government— indeed, the premise at the heart of Winthrop's *Model of Christian Charity*— was flawed. That this was highly offensive to the magistrates is clear, and much as it had done with the male Antinomians, the Court charged the petitioners with sedition. Winthrop went on to complain about the petitioners' reading of the syphilis outbreak, seemingly mortified by their attempt to publicize it. He writes that they "laye open the Afflictions, which God hathe pleased to exercise us with, & that to the worst appearance, and impute it to the evill of our Government."[46] With a final flourish, he goes on to reestablish, once and for all, just who had the power to define the boundaries of community in Massachusetts Bay. The petitioners, Winthrop writes, tried to persuade the "people" that "the libertyes & priviledges in our Charter belonge to all freeborne Englishe men, Inhabitants heer: whereas they are granted onely to such as the Governor and Company shall thinke fitt to receive into that fellowshippe."[47]

Winthrop's tone in these remarks touches on one of the primary complaints made by the petitioners—namely, that the magistrates had created an "arbitrary government" with the attending "non-certainty of all things we enjoy, whether lives, liberties or estates." Other complaints include the fact that many free-born English countrymen were "debarred from all Civil imployment," and lived in fear of "perpetuall slavery and bondage"; and, significantly, that "righteous, and godly men" were being:

> detained from the Seals of the Covenant of Free-grace, because (as it is supposed) they will not take these Churches Covenants, for which as yet they see no light in Gods word, neither can they cleerly perceive what they are, every Church having their Covenant different from anothers, at least in words, yea some Churches sometime adding, sometimes detracting, calling it sometime the Covenant of Grace, sometime a Branch of it, sometime a Profession of the Free-Covenant, &c. Notwithstanding they are compelled . . . to contribute to the maintenance of those Ministers, who vouchsafe or not to take them into their Flock. . . . Whence (as we conceive) abound an ocean of inconveniences; Dishonour to God and his Ordinances, little profit by the Ministery, increase of Anabaptism.[48]

This last remark serves as the pivot on which the petitioners turn from their complaints against government, to their problems with Congregationalism itself. Of the many issues they had—including the restrictive, inconsistent, and incoherent barriers against church membership—the charge of Anabaptism resonated loudly, and is the one that I would like to pursue at length because it involves questions of generational inheritance that paralleled New England's changing immunological properties as the century progressed.

Whereas Presbyterians in England tended to offer church membership to all baptized adults able to make a profession of faith, and had liberal rules for baptism itself, Congregationalists struggled to maintain the purity of their churches in the face of demands that they baptize all children.[49]

The importance of baptism in Christianity need not be belabored—it mirrors circumcision as the seal of the covenant between God and Abraham. The point that would prove critical in New England is that this Old Testament covenant included Abraham's "seed," and descended through the generations of the house of Israel. Congregationalists widely held that this intergenerational promise to Abraham was mirrored in the Christian church, and could be extended to the children of regenerate church members through baptism. Strictly speaking, these children did not enter the church by virtue of being baptized, but were baptized because they had inherited church membership at birth.[50] Simple as this concept of inheritance would seem to be, it nevertheless conflicted with Calvinist notions of unconditional election, which held that humans were powerless to effect their salvation, and could never know the state of their soul with certainty; in other words, claims to direct (i.e., genetic) inheritance of grace undermined the doctrine of God's absolute sovereignty, and implied a worldly assurance that had never been intended—a claim Morgan further dismisses as "an arrogant and inconsistent expectation, for it implied a presumption that every child of a saint was destined for salvation and such a presumption was obviously wrong. No Christian could believe that grace was really hereditary."[51]

Faced with this dilemma, Congregationalists maintained that baptism was not efficacious—that it neither conferred nor guaranteed grace, but signified only an "external" or "provisional" membership in the church—still subject to its disciplinary authority, but not yet permitted to participate in the Lord's Supper. This compromise meant that children of church members could be baptized under the assumption that they would likely eventually demonstrate the requisite signs of saving grace as they grew older, and be admitted as full members when they finally did so. By the same token, children of nonchurch members (even those who had previously belonged to a church in England), while not precluded from eventually receiving grace, were nevertheless refused baptism in Massachusetts, because congregations had no legible sign on which to base their judgments, one way or the other. Presbyterians, who were much less discriminating when it came to the rites of baptism, saw the Congregationalists' practice as an egregious abuse of power—hence the charge of Anabaptism in the remonstrants' petition.[52]

My specific interest in the petition derives from its use of epidemiological language, on the one hand, and its focus on baptism, on the other.

Although I am not arguing that the petitioners were consciously drawing attention to a link between syphilis and baptism in 1646, I do want to raise the issue here because the relation would come to cast a long shadow over the next twenty years of Puritan history in New England. Clearly, neither the petitioners nor the General Court recognized the significance of herd immunity or the cyclical patterns of smallpox that would later appear, but as virulent epidemics began to strike Anglo-American communities, ministers came to see in their troubles evidence of a cultural shift that they characterized as a sign of declension, and this declension was, as far as they could tell, the behavioral trigger for new epidemiological patterns. The point I want to argue is that the emergence of this epidemiological shift occurred in tandem with ongoing concerns about baptismal inheritance, and the association between the two had significant formal consequences for New England's narrative practices. During the middle decades of the seventeenth century, for example, the question of baptismal inheritance became increasingly difficult to avoid, as churches faced declining membership that was most easily measured in generational terms: where baptism had been used to signal provisional church membership for the children of first-generation congregants, problems began to arise when these external members failed to give the adequate professions of faith that had been expected of them once they reached adulthood; the fact that so many of these external members were not giving their professions of faith was read as a troubling sign that this younger generation was not living up to the promise of its parents.[53] This specific issue had further worldly consequences that would put increasing pressure to bear on the Congregationalist system itself. The central question concerned how to treat the children of provisional members. Would they be barred from baptism like the children of nonmembers were, or could they skip a generation and inherit their grandparents' baptismal rights directly?

This question was to be taken up by the 1646 Cambridge Synod, which was called to settle questions of church polity, and to reconcile Congregationalism with the Westminster Assembly. The call to the synod reflected the diverse rules of baptism then in effect in New England, noting that the majority of churches

> do baptize onely such children whose nearest parents, one or both of them, are setled members, in full comunion with one or other of these churches . . . [but] there be some who do baptize the children if the grandfather or grandmother be such members, though the immediate parents be not.[54]

The synod was held over two years, and periodically interrupted by epidemic outbreaks, such as in the spring of 1647, when an "epidemicall sickness" erupted among "Indians & Englishe, Frenche & Dutche," killing forty to fifty people in Massachusetts, and as many in Connecticut.[55] These epidemics loomed large in the minds of synod participants, who could not help but notice that among the victims were Thomas Hooker, and "the Governors wife," Mrs. Winthrop.[56] As a response to crises such as Child's petition and ongoing uncertainty about baptismal rights, the *Cambridge Platform* attempts to articulate a consensus notion of the first twenty years of Puritan experience in New England, and to provide a vision for the community's future. But because the Presbyterian influence in England had already begun to wane by this time, the synod managed to skirt some of the most contentious issues. Where the call asked the synod to address the question of inheritance of baptismal rights directly, it merely reaffirmed that baptized children were required to give a profession of faith in adulthood, and that "if not regenerated, yet [they] are in a more hopefull way of attaining regenerating grace, & all the spiritual blessings both of the covenant & seal," but it deferred the main question for another generation.[57]

Sacvan Bercovitch visualizes the question of baptismal inheritance in pragmatic terms as a "widespread generational rift" that threatened to shut churches down if membership continued to be as restrictive as it had been during the colony's first years. Indeed, if the baptized children of the regenerate did not themselves become full members in adulthood, it was clear that churches would disappear as the first generation of colonists died out.[58] And because liberalizing the requirements for election was not a viable option at this juncture, the most direct doctrinal solution to this problem came via the halfway covenant—a loosening of baptismal requirements that permitted third-generation infants to skip over their parents, and inherit their grandparents' membership directly. The halfway covenant has long fascinated critics—some, like Bercovitch, seeing its roots early in the history of New England, while others, like Morgan, seeing it as "neither a sign of decline in piety nor a betrayal of the standards of the founding fathers, but an honest attempt to rescue the concept of a church of visible saints from the tangle of problems created in time by human reproduction."[59] I find Morgan's emphasis on the biology of human reproduction over and against the rhetoric of declension to be particularly interesting, as it parts with Perry Miller's earlier characterization of declension as an historical force that shaped New England's intellectual history, and substitutes, in its place, an attention to the materiality of human bodies. And while I am not interested in turning back to Miller's analytical model, I would like to dwell on the tension between the rhetoric of biology and declension that Morgan seeks to pass over, because it makes room for a clear articulation of New England's immunological syntax at midcentury.

Morgan's biological rhetoric naturalizes the evolution of the halfway covenant even as it creates an artificial distinction between reproduction and declension that Congregationalist thinkers would not have recognized. My point here is to expand on Morgan's understanding of biology, and to highlight the ways that it operates in tandem with declension—to look at how Puritan thinkers used declension as a rhetorical strategy to account for the pressures of biology. In substituting a biological narrative for that of declension, Morgan wants to read the halfway covenant as the unavoidable compromise that made allowances for human reproduction in the face of Congregationalism's otherwise unyielding exclusionary practices. Indeed, by focusing on reproduction, Morgan explains that "the world had its own ways of controlling those who propel themselves too far from it; and the New England churches were eventually brought back to earth, not by the corruptions of the flesh, but by its biology," and he goes on to claim even more forcefully that "the Puritans had in fact moved the church so far from the world that it would no longer fit the biological facts of life."[60] While Morgan's analysis of biology provides deep insight into the "natural" forces that shaped theological thought in the mid-seventeenth century, it remains strangely ambivalent as it replaces the corporeality of sin ("corruptions of the flesh") with the corporeality of reproduction and birth. This substitution represents sin and declension as incorporeal, so I would like to push his insight further, and make biology account for more than the simple fact that human beings procreate; I would like, in other words, to foreground immunology and epidemics in the biology of the halfway covenant because these provide a way to talk about declension while offering a deeply embodied understanding of disease as the literal manifestation of sin.

Even as I remain beholden to Morgan's biological reading of the covenant, I will split his ideas about human reproduction along two axes: the first, which is his, identifies reproduction in its most basic mathematical sense, and argues that every time an external member of the church had a child, the Congregation took one step closer to an inevitable reckoning whereby it would have to loosen membership and baptism requirements, or face ever-declining enrollments. In this sense, the halfway covenant is a pragmatic response to the numerical certainty that excluding these children was a sure way to destroy New England's Congregational system from within. The second axis looks beyond birth to the immunological consequences of reproduction in colonial New England. That is, the birth of every child (provisional church member or not) lowered New England's herd immunity, putting communities under increased threat of epidemic. Indeed, by the time the halfway covenant was endorsed at the synod of 1662, New England communities had already begun to experience new cyclical patterns of disease that confounded their assumptions about how epidemics and illness functioned during the first decade of settlement. Because these cycles were driven by "biological facts of life" such as birthrates and herd immunity, they disproportionately affected children, adolescents, and young adults—a pattern of infection that colonists could not help but read in generational terms as punishment for these younger colonists' sins (or their failures to join the church). In this context, the halfway covenant should be understood in the context of the changing epidemiological patterns that second- and third-generation settlers experienced at midcentury, and thus it acts as a doctrinal response intended to forestall future punishments; an epidemiological model where declension is the behavioral trigger for illness.

Where "human reproduction" may have set in motion the demographic imbalance that would eventually threaten church rolls and lead to the halfway covenant, I argue that processes like herd immunity produced the epidemiological shift that made those demographic imbalances legible within a narrative of declension. The important point here is that diseases like smallpox were epidemic rather than endemic in New England, and the long interepidemic cycle between outbreaks ensured that these illnesses would no longer be read primarily as children's diseases, as they often had been in England; instead, cyclical outbreaks trained settlers to read disease and sin as intertwined *generational* issues when they observed the effects of epidemics on an entire cohort of descendents at a time. Morgan rightly discounts declension as a factor in the decrease of midcentury conversion experiences, but the move strikes me as too far-reaching, because it oversimplifies the extent to which biological effects could be read in terms of illness and immunity, and it obscures the ready analogue between illness and sin that is bound in New England's epidemiological cycles. In other words, epidemiological analysis reveals that the generational issues that played into the evolution of the halfway covenant encompassed both the number of new members who could potentially join the church, as well as their susceptibility to illness—and that both could be read as reflections of one another. Thus, what I am arguing is that the halfway covenant was, like Morgan claims, a doctrinal solution to a biological issue, but a solution that nonetheless accounted for the "tangle of problems created in time by human reproduction" via the immunological experience of epidemics in the New World. The halfway covenant offered anxious ministers a ready model for bringing the colony back toward piety through its commitment to health by allowing Puritans to claim an intergenerational lineage for the covenant of grace.[61]

Even as the halfway covenant presented a solution to a thorny theological problem, it accounted for phenomena such as communal susceptibility to epidemics by dramatizing the internal and intergenerational inheritance of grace and of sin. This internal shift is the genesis of what Bercovitch has called the "Genetics of Salvation," which acts as the "doctrinal counterpart to the concept of errand," and "confirms the Puritan mission from within."[62] I would first point out that Bercovitch's construction parallels Morgan's turn to biology and reproduction, and then suggest that what Bercovitch reads as a metaphorical process that provides "'internal evidence' of generational succession" certainly functions in that strain, but also provides an immunological model for the evolution of communal narratives in New England.[63] This is a model that helps shape the temporal and geographic effects of epidemics into cultural and ideological frameworks, and through which, as Wald suggests, identity can be imagined as a shared immunological response to the world. In this sense, my argument has been that the "internal evidence" that Bercovitch points to in his analysis of the halfway covenant is not simply tied to cultural models of inheritance and succession, but encompasses the "invisible" process of herd immunity that regulates susceptibility to epidemics, and which critics can make visible with an analytic model of immunological syntax. In the remainder of this chapter, I describe the way in which immunological syntax is not simply a model that accounts for dynamic shifts in New England's epidemiological history, but leaves a narrative imprint on its epidemiological histories.

III

What is so striking about Bercovitch's "Genetics of Salvation" is the way that it describes an historical shift while already taking its cue from a lineage of Puritan studies that draws on Miller's "Genetic Study" of Orthodoxy in Massachusetts.[64] Like Morgan, Bercovitch's insight in troping Miller's phrase was to claim a physical (and temporal) correlation to what his predecessor had characterized as a willful intellectual project. Thus, this genetic imprint on Puritan studies—exemplified by the inward trajectory from Miller to Morgan to Bercovitch—reveals the interrelated biological and intellectual processes that anchor the trope; significantly, this inward turn to genetics mirrors the internalizing movement made by mid-seventeenth-century Puritans to account for the inheritance of grace and sin through baptism and the halfway covenant. But I would like to expand the scope of what Morgan understands as biological to include the dynamic patterns of immunity and susceptibility that midcentury colonists faced. Thus, I read Bercovitch's and Morgan's parallel turn as something more than metaphor, and ask how it might be made to account for a genealogy of New England Puritanism in terms of its immunological history. Indeed, by taking this inward turn as the foundation of my own analysis, I hope to make clear that our historiographic models of colonialism are very much structured by the stance critics take toward biological processes, whether they attend to these or not, and whether they intend them as metaphorical or something other than that. In this manner, models of intellectual consensus, exceptionalism, and declension are framed by determinist accounts of biological history, where immunology is imprinted as a timeless property of monolithic populations; it matters, then, whether our engagement with narrative and theological practices in New England is informed by a virgin soil model of colonial epidemics, or by immunological syntax, so my own inward turn toward a genealogy of New England Puritanism is informed by the long view that herd immunity and other epidemiological narratives provide.

To be sure, virgin soil is a masterfully elegant trope for describing immunological distinctions between English and Native American populations in the early period of colonial history, but this trope characterizes as timeless and inevitable that which New England's immunological syntax reveals to be mutable and contingent. By appropriating an epidemiological mode of analysis into literary and historiographic criticism, we begin to see how public practices (such as the halfway covenant) and narrative forms (such as the jeremiad) emerge in relation to New England's history during the first half of the seventeenth century. Because illness and epidemics were so readily adaptable to providential Puritan rhetoric—where diseases act as belated signs of sin, and take their place in a teleological history of New England rather than being the consequence of immunological and demographic shifts over time—it is all too easy for modern critics tracing the genealogy of New England Puritanism to work within this rhetorical tradition, and to understand the historical role of disease in the allegorical or thematic contexts that they were constructed. Epidemic becomes, in this instance, one of any number of substitutable signs of God's displeasure with the colonists (such as famine, Indian attacks, earthquakes, flood, drought), thus flattening out the dynamic interaction of humans and pathogens within local landscapes. The historiographic effect of such readings, however, is that as the local specificity of epidemics recedes into the background in favor of broader social and intellectual histories, so too do the effects of epidemics and epidemiology on the evolution of communal narratives tend to be elided from the critical discourse. Taking this elision as the motivation for my analysis, I ground my understanding of immunological syntax in a recognition of both the thematic and the formal spaces in which seventeenth-century epidemics operate on texts.

Read thematically, epidemics do not appear as dynamic historical events, but as markers pointing to a predestined historiographic record—a record that descends to us through the biological determinism of virgin soil models. That God would ease the Puritans' way into the New World through the use of a "miraculous plague" becomes a normalizing sign of colonial discourse in which immunological differences between populations are subsumed to trans-historical nationalist projects. First-generation justification narratives thematize Native American susceptibility and English immunity to disease as the foundational event guaranteeing property rights in the New World, and these themes carry over into the political and theological rhetoric deployed during the Antinomian controversy to advance an Orthodox vision of community. Thus, thematic readings of disease shape colonialist discourses by offering communal coherence as the core body on which epidemics can signify meaningfully. The ontological status of such claims assumes fixed boundaries (on territorial as well as human bodies) to set the communal imaginary at work. In this context, illness and epidemics draw attention to what is alleged to have been a timeless immunological bond within populations—immunity is not dynamic in these readings, but purports to reveal essential national and cultural kinships. In contrast to this thematic elaboration of epidemics, the formal reading practices of immunological syntax reveal the shaping influence of thematic readings *as* thematic (rather than essential or timeless) by investigating the links between a given region's historical experience of epidemics and the narrative properties of epidemiological texts and conventions. The inward turn of immunological and epidemiological analysis that I propose here precipitates a critical reexamination of the relation between health and narrative traditions in early New England, and in so doing produces reading practices that map the colonial experience of disease onto the formal conventions that emerged in theological and narrative traditions. Thus, one would consider the midcentury move by Congregationalists to accept the cross-generational inheritance of baptismal rights as the formal manifestation of immunological conditions experienced by second- and third-generation settlers, whose susceptibility to epidemics came to be read as widespread declension.

If communal susceptibility and immunity to smallpox in colonial New England are not, strictly speaking, shared hereditary traits, they nevertheless proceed from specific local experiences of disease, and manifest themselves on a generational scale that colonists deciphered in providential terms. This movement is straightforward: the unanticipated failure of many second-generation settlers to relate their conversion experiences in adulthood was extrapolated as a sign of national declension, and these failures became legible as failures when communities were afflicted with the diseases that had previously aided their migrations. In this context, illness and sin imprint generational differences onto communal narratives; they stand in for each other because they operate on the ambiguity of personal and communal bodies. Whereas herd immunity reflects a communal dynamic dependent on rates of individual susceptibility to disease, national sin is an abstraction of individual failures to be pious. Both manifest themselves generationally in early New England when the immunological dynamic of seventeenth-century communities inserted itself into the consciousness of Puritan ministers so that individual failures to enter into church membership could be punished as a breach of the national covenant. For this reason, the mid-seventeenth-century debate over inheritance of baptismal rights lies at the nexus of medical, theological, and nationalist discourses, even if this relation is not always self-evident.

By midcentury, colonists could recognize a definitive shift in the way that diseases such as smallpox and the measles infected Anglo-American communities. Unexpected epidemiological patterns such as these were enough to force even the stoutest of minds to reevaluate its body's place in the world, and to reconsider the relation of theology and health in communal rhetoric. If changing epidemiological patterns subverted the colonial expectations imagined by first-generation settlers, they provided later colonists with the tools to adapt their rhetorical practices to changing historical events. That these practices would lead to a theological development like the halfway covenant is hardly surprising, given that the covenant itself combined individual and generational concerns, and blended what Bercovitch refers to as the "heterogeneous covenants of community and grace."[65] Bercovitch's claim begs a shift toward an examination of the genetics—or genesis—of the New England jeremiad, for which, he argues, the "motive and substance . . . [was] to obviate [the] division" between the two covenants.[66] Significantly for my own analysis, Bercovitch suggests that the rhetorical and historical ambiguities that Puritans faced in New England helped give rise to narrative forms like the jeremiad, which "was born in an effort to impose metaphor upon reality . . . [and] was nourished by an imagination at once defiant of history and profoundly attuned to the historical forces that were shaping the community."[67]

When Bercovitch describes the jeremiad as an effort to impose metaphor on reality, he neatly circumscribes the thematic narrative concerns about epidemic and illness in Puritan rhetoric, but what I would like to suggest is that by recognizing this thematizing impulse within a broader immunological history of New England, critics can now consider the evolution of the jeremiad form within parallel theological and epidemiological trajectories. This is to say that when Bercovitch points to an imagination that was simultaneously defiant and attuned to historical forces, we must consider those forces beyond the traditional intellectual history of Puritan studies to account for the corporeality of biology; that imagination was responding as much to the body's shifting immunological condition in New England as it was to the pressures imposed by Calvinist theology. For first-generation settlers like Winthrop and Cotton, epidemiological rhetoric provided a way to mediate those pressures, while second- and third-generation settlers, who experienced a dramatic shift in the way that epidemics targeted Anglo-American communities, found themselves adapting their practices to evolving immunological conditions. The narratives that describe and account for these shifts emerged from a particularly rigid attempt to read illness as metaphor, but the critic's task is to decode the general thematics of declension within their etiological and epidemiological contexts.

To frame this argument, I will focus on Michael Wigglesworth's "God's Controversy with New England"—a poem that traces the first half-century of New England settlement, beginning with an off-handed remark about the 1616–19 epidemics, and ending with "the great drought . . . [of] 1662"—the year in which the halfway covenant was accepted as doctrinal in New England.[68] Although the poem is less well known than *The Day of Doom*, Miller long ago suggested that "God's Controversy" was the first text to "fully set forth" the theme of the New England jeremiad, so its primacy in this area provides an opportunity to consider how the poem's generic qualities are tied to its dramatization of the anxieties that illness and infection engendered in New England—particularly as large-scale epidemiological patterns shifted over a period of four decades.[69] The poem signifies meaningfully both in its generic literary form, and as a model of epidemiological historiography; taken together, these literary and historiographic qualities intersect to provide insights into the role that immunology plays in shaping New England's political and theological landscapes. More to the point, the poem exploits a fundamental rift in New England's epidemiological history, and attempts to reconcile this rift within orthodox theological rhetoric.[70]

As the poem's title suggests, "God's Controversy" relies on a premise that is familiar to any modern reader of mid-seventeenth-century New England religious texts: God is unhappy with the backsliding settlers, and threatens to punish them if they do not mend their ways. The narrative opens with a human narrator who gives a brief history of New England, praising Winthrop's stewardship during the colony's first years. He emphasizes God's central role in the colonists' survival, and describes Winthrop's generation explicitly, saying that "This was the place, and these the folk / In whom he took delight" (131–32). While the poem's opening stanzas reflect on the glory of New England's early history, things quickly take a turn for the worse, as one would expect in a jeremiad. The narrator is interrupted by darkening skies, which are soon followed by God's "awfull . . . thundring" voice (155–56). The narrator then disappears for the middle third of the poem, his voice replaced by God's, who then provides a divine providential reading of history. Eight of the first ten stanzas that God speaks are punctuated by rhetorical questions that ask whether these present-day New Englanders (i.e., the second and third genera- tions living in 1662) could possibly be the same "folk" with whom He had so recently made a covenant. The central of these stanzas rehearses New England's by then mythic history. God asks:

Are these the folk . . .
I brought and planted on the Western-shore,
Where nought but bruits and salvage wights did swarm
(Untaught, untrain'd, untam'd by Vertue's lore)
That sought their blood, yet could do them no harm?
My fury's flaile them thresht, my fatall broom
Did sweep them hence, to make my people Elbow-room. (169, 175–80)

Paraphrasing earlier justification narratives, this section of the poem domes- ticates civil law discourse by framing New England as a space that God had swept clean in order to create "elbow room" for English settlers. Of course, the "fatall" nature of God's broom is meant to recall the epidemics of 1616–19, a point further figured in the act of threshing Native Americans with "fury's flaile." While New England's earliest justification narratives represented Native Americans as incapable of properly cultivating the land, Wigglesworth takes this representation a step further by abstracting the "salvage wights" as grain to be threshed—as the agricultural products of God's labor.[71]

Bracketed as they are by rhetorical questions, it is clear that the primary subjects of these stanzas are the English rather than the Native Americans: yes, these are the folk for whom God has toiled, and no, they have not lived up to their parents' promise. Indeed, the poem goes to great lengths to high- light the claim that epidemics were not an arbitrary event sent merely because the Native Americans were Native American, but because they were "untam'd by vertue's lore"—a fatal flaw that readers are left to assume is not genetic, insofar as it could potentially describe the English settlers if they were to backslide (which they do by line 259 of the poem). Just one hundred lines after describing the Native American epidemics, God denounces the settlers in terms that echo his characterization of Native Americans; only this time it is the English who are faulted for not listening to "vertue's Lore" (271). Instead of "Heaven-reaching hearts, and thoughts, Meekness, Humility," these settlers display:

> ... a sensuall Heart all void of grace,
> An Iron neck, a proud presumptuous Hand;
> A self-conceited, stiff, stout, stubborn Race,
> That fears no threats, submitts to no command:
> Self-will'd, perverse, such as can beare no yoke;
> A Generation even ripe for Vengeance stroke. (289–94)

This stanza serves as the pivot on which the narrative turns from its backward glance at providential history toward its concern with the present, and the future—a hallmark of the New England jeremiad. If "vengeance stroke" acts as a pointed reminder of the "flaile" that had threshed the Native Americans earlier in the poem, so too do God's subsequent threats of turning "glorious noon-day light" into "a dark Egyptian night" (318), and of delivering an "All-Consuming stroke" (341) warn settlers of the plagues that will visit them if they do not amend their ways. By centering the threat of vengeance on the current "Generation" specifically, Wigglesworth reveals a temporal rift that is central to both the poem and to seventeenth-century New England communities. On the one hand, this threat represents New England as a homogeneous community ("Generation" describes the entire community collectively), while on the other, it announces a temporal fault line in the colony (the present "Generation" is distinctly different from the colony's first generation "Who, Ruling in the fear of God, / The righteous cause maintained" [121–22]). As convoluted as the poem's temporal structure is, the significance of this rift does not simply lie in the broad rhetoric of declension and punishment that it calls forth, but in the platform it provides for narrating the generational dynamic that drives New England's immunological syntax in the second half of the poem.

In the poem's third, and most literal section, God's voice recedes almost as abruptly as it had arrived, marking the return of the human narrator, who informs his audience that God's threat had in fact already materialized in an ambiguously recent past—a narrative shift that echoes the move offered fifteen years earlier in Child's petition—and that New England was currently suffering for its sins. Not surprisingly, the narrator points to a recent upsurge of illness as evidence for his claim, further contextualizing this historical shift in a theological narrative that is consistent with the poem's first half. He laments:

> Our healthfull dayes are at an end,
>   And sicknesses come on
> From yeer to yeer, becaus our hearts
>   Away from God are gone.
> New-England, where for many yeers
>   You scarcely heard a cough,
> And where Physicians had no work,
>   Now finds them work enough.
>
> Now colds and coughs; Rhewms, and sore-throats,
>   Do more and more abound:
> Now Agues sore & Feavers strong
>   In every place are found.
> How many houses have we seen
>   Last Autumn, and this spring,
> Wherein the healthful were too few
>   To help the languishing.
>
> One wave another followeth,
>   And one disease begins
> Before another cease, becaus
>   We turn not from our sins. (359–78)

The image of the healthful being too few to help the ill is eerily reminiscent of Bradford's descriptions of Native American epidemics thirty years earlier. This is not to suggest that Wigglesworth had read Bradford's account of the ravages of smallpox on Native American populations, but that these images carried an important narrative currency in New England, circulating broadly as part of its seventeenth-century myth of origin. And even as the originating myth is turned on its head at this juncture of the poem, with English settlers now becoming the victims of disease, this echoing image provides a striking platform for updating the narrative. No longer merely a threat, the waves of disease washing over colonists reflect a dramatic immunological shift. Where epidemics had once helped support the migration to New England—where Winthrop's generation "for many years / . . . scarcely heard a cough, / And where physicians had no work"—they now endangered the colony's very survival. As a result of this shift, second- and third-generation New Englanders like Wigglesworth found themselves compelled to reassess the relation between illness and community established in the colony's first years, and adapting a narrative tradition that more accurately reflected New World experiences in the middle of the century.[72] When disease patterns shifted from their familiar English forms, New England communities were forced to look inward, to rethink communal narratives, and to reimagine how their theological apparatus might reflect a history that no longer followed its initial trajectory.

Wigglesworth's reading of this shift in theological terms is not all that surprising, but "God's Controversy with New England" nevertheless provides evidence that the figure of illness functions as something more than a thematic element in the poem. Ministers like him recognized shifting disease patterns, and tried to reconcile them within an orthodox Puritan rhetoric, seeing in their troubles evidence of a cultural shift that they characterized as a sign of declension. As a man with a life-long interest in medicine, Wigglesworth would have been familiar with New England's patterns of illness, while his ministerial work would have led him to revert to theological models of declension for his etiological frameworks of disease. Indeed, Wigglesworth, who is just as well known for his private diary, rehearsed these kinds of reading in late 1653 to early 1654, when a "plague" afflicted both he and his compatriots. Structuring his lamentation about the effects of plague in terms of declension, Wigglesworth writes that "My soul longeth for the Lord, not onely for pardon from him, when my sins beset me roundabout and the tokens of gods displeasure are upon me and the country, but also for his sweet soul satisfying presence which is the life of my heart, Lord pardon my sin and heal my backslidings and love me freely."[73] In the poem itself, the projection of theology and medicine continues, as Wigglesworth internalizes both illness and declension, writing that "one disease begins / Before another cease, because / We turn not from our sins." Here, Wigglesworth provides evidence that Morgan's reading of "corruptions of the flesh" as a figural term for sin resonated just as loudly along immunological lines for seventeenth-century spiritual divines, carrying with it the deeply embodied understanding of disease as a literal manifestation of internal sin. To be sure, diseases retained their theological valence as signs of divine punishment despite the immunological shift, but the struggle to understand new epidemiological patterns was circumscribed by a need to represent disease as a very real sign of God's anger with the colonists, rather than support for their migration. And although this representational shift falls within traditional Puritan theology, it would nonetheless test the limits of early epidemiological narratives by bringing great pressure to bear on static accounts of otherwise dynamic historical events.

After all, the settlers were unlikely to argue that their new susceptibilities to disease negated prior legal claims to land in North America.

   While Wigglesworth's poem doesn't address the halfway covenant specifically, his representation of illness as a divine response to New England's "sensuall Heart" highlights the fact that immunology and theology have strong generational dynamics in the seventeenth century. Here, then, epidemiological thought does not replace all other analytical models as a framework for understanding the halfway covenant, but it does provide a method for thinking about the relation between theology and cultural practice by focusing on the specificity of local and temporal experience. "God's Controversy with New England" bookends two distinct eras in New England's immunological history in order to make a broad point about the behaviors of second- and third-generation settlers. To this end, Wigglesworth focuses on illness as a means of dramatizing the supposed spiritual declension that mid-seventeenth-century New England ministers rallied against. But his formal arrangement of illness in the text is more than merely a thematic tool to drive the narrative, as it articulates New England's immunological syntax in ways that complicate first-generation narratives. In this vein, I would categorize the poem itself as an epidemiological narrative that struggles to give formal and thematic coherence to what, by then, had become New England's problematic immunological history.

   The poem's final optimistic turn toward the future is a last attempt to stamp a thematic imprint on New England's epidemiological history by projecting a healthful future that is also a return to the glories of the past. In this way, "God's Controversy with New England" reflects the typically "American" qualities of this jeremiad form while highlighting ambivalence about the ultimate meaning of epidemics in New England. The narrator informs his audience that if they "Repent, and turn to God" (436), then "Still in New-England shall be my delight" (446), an implicit promise that projects a background state of health against which New England communities can measure their temporal and spiritual progress in the future. Thus, the jeremiad is not simply an exhortation bemoaning declension or the sins of a generation as it would be if disease were merely a thematic marker, but it naturalizes the relation between English bodies and American land by looking forward, and holding out the promise that immunity to illness would once again become the sign that Puritan settlers belonged in New England. And yet, one is left to wonder about the poem's reliance on disease to propel the story. On the one hand, early epidemiologies consistently held disease out as a threat against those whom God wished to punish. However, the immunological shift that proved Anglo-Americans could be susceptible to the same diseases and in similar patterns as Native Americans undermines the assumed moral and physical superiority that grounded the colonial project, thus shining a light on the contingent nature of English land claims, and on their increasingly vexed status as a chosen people in the New World.

Epidemiology provides a useful framework through which to reconsider the physical effects of diseases in seventeenth-century New England, but the impact of epidemics on narrative forms cannot be fully understood without investigating how cultural discourses appropriated the generic conventions of epidemiological analysis. For example, if Michael Wigglesworth simply used illness as a thematic marker of divine wrath in "God's Controversy with New England," then the figure is not much more interesting than any other symbol that could have been substituted for it (for example the drought of 1662 that he alludes to in the poem's subtitle). But if disease is a critical catalyst for propelling the poem, then a deeper relation between New England's experience of epidemics and its communal narratives exists, suggesting that epidemiological thinking may have helped to structure the terms through which important theological and cultural practices voiced themselves for Puritan settlers. While providential readings of illness have reduced the meaning of epidemics to thematic signposts—like heresy, sedition, Indian attacks, droughts, earthquakes, etc.—the experience with viral diseases like smallpox in seventeenth-century New England complicated the colonial project significantly, and so should prompt modern critics to reassess the ways in which we understand illness to operate narratively in texts. Immunological syntax reveals New England's epidemics to have been cyclical (rather than one-time events), and their periodicity asserted itself in an overarching generational dynamic—the very dynamic that operates at the heart of the jeremiad, and that is crucial to the development of the halfway covenant.

From this perspective, I would argue that it is no mere historical accident that 1662 marks the advent of both the halfway covenant and Wigglesworth's early formulation of the New England jeremiad; both are actively working through a complex network of theological issues, and each finds its voice in the generational patterns of New England immunology. Unlike heresy, sedition, Indian attacks, drought, and earthquakes, epidemics inscribed themselves on Anglo-American colonial bodies as generational events by virtue of New England's herd immunity and demographic patterns. "God's Controversy with New England" gives voice to those patterns by representing the first generation of settlers as fundamentally healthy (and righteous), while their children and grandchildren—who remained susceptible to disease on a broad scale—represented the generation of declension. As this declension came to be thematized in midcentury narratives, epidemics took their place in a teleological history of New England as anticipated signs of national affliction. But by refocusing our attention on immunological syntax and epidemiological analysis, we reconsider this narrative trajectory *as* a trajectory, and better understand the evolution of communal and national discourses in relation to immunological and demographic shifts. I would further argue that the ambivalence second- and third-generation Puritans had for the particular meaning of illness reflects the fact that epidemics behaved in ways that were neither familiar nor predictable to them. This unpredictability is both a consequence of New England's demographic history, and a factor that shapes how we are to understand immunological syntax. Narratives like the jeremiad were certainly influenced by emerging disease patterns, and reflect an attempt by Puritan writers to project communal coherence where little seemed to exist.

My analysis suggests that Puritan readings of epidemics in the first three generations of settlement in New England describe an ongoing strategy for communities to visualize illness and health as functions of a communal identity, and for situating citizenship as a shared immunological response to the world. However, as disease patterns changed from the forms predicted by the experience of first-generation settlers with illness in England, communities were forced to look inward, to rethink this narrative, and to imagine how their theological apparatus might reflect an apparently incoherent history. Ultimately, it is my argument that the halfway covenant and the New England jeremiad emerged from these shifting epidemiological patterns as a way of imposing order on a disordered world. Wigglesworth's poem is not simply a cry against declension, but an attempt to make sense of immunological events that were threatening to derail New England's colonial project at midcentury. The poem's convoluted temporal structure is indicative of Wigglesworth's struggle to understand how epidemics functioned during the first years of settlement, and it is only through an understanding of New England's immunological syntax that this ambivalence can properly be positioned as a narrative manifestation of shifting disease patterns.

"God's Controversy with New England" uses its epidemiological observations to glance backward at the region's early colonial history, and to project thematic coherence onto current events. As the coincident development of narrative forms such as the jeremiad and cultural practices like the halfway covenant reveal, New England's epidemiological history was a central shaping event in seventeenth-century life. And because the generic terms of epidemiology call for an assessment of behavioral differences between sick and well populations before identifying a cure for illness, shifting epidemic patterns compelled mid-seventeenth-century theologians to rethink the etiologies of divine plagues. Disease-causing behaviors came to be imprinted within second- and third-generation colonial bodies as declension, while both the jeremiad and halfway covenant offered prescriptions for countering disease by looking inward, troping illness, and drawing attention to the intertwined effects of epidemic and sin on the communal body. Radical shifts in immunological susceptibility to disease are a pointed reminder that familiar trajectories of history are subject to the interdisciplinary reading practices that interrogate the significance of local geographic and temporal experience in early colonial histories. Immunological syntax asks us to reconsider how tenuous a category like "good health" is in relation to communal identity in seventeenth-century New England, and to think about the very real implications of reading health in formal and generic terms that shape literary and historical discourses, rather than as idealized thematic representations of communal and national spaces.

While the formal structures of the halfway covenant and the jeremiad parallel New England's epidemiological history (read through the dynamic of herd immunity), I am not arguing that New England's epidemiological patterns *produced* either one, or that neither would have evolved in the absence of illness. Instead, what I have argued is that the halfway covenant and jeremiad—which I very much think of as early epidemiologies—make New England's complex immunological history legible. This legibility is mediated through immunological syntax—the analytical model that seeks to push aside static and monolithic biological histories in favor of recognizing the demographic and generational dynamics that shaped immunities and susceptibilities in the colonial context. In terms of how immunological syntax imprints itself on narrative history, I would suggest that the shift from thematic to formal analyses of epidemics is perhaps the clearest manifestation of the reading practices that it encourages. So with this in mind, I would begin to characterize immunological syntax in terms of its inquiry into the formal literary elements of epidemiological texts—or the formal epidemiological elements of literary texts. Thinking of epidemiology in this way creates an avenue for critics to deploy the tools of literary analysis toward uncovering the complex relation between language and form, on the one hand, and epidemiological history, on the other. By 1721, when a smallpox epidemic would infect half of Boston's population, the jeremiad had been codified as a traditional narrative form. And though this form did once again figure in epidemiologies of the outbreak, immunological syntax made itself legible in the formal and stylistic elements of the print debate that raged between Boston's ministerial elite and a new class of professional physicians.

4

Technologies of Inoculation

Some advantages of a peculiar character are connected with this
institution, which it may be proper to point out. No place in the
United States offers as great opportunities for the acquisition of
anatomical knowledge. Subjects being obtained from among the
coloured population in sufficient numbers *for every purpose*, and
proper dissections carried on *without offending any individuals in
the community*!

—William Wells Brown, *Clotel; or, The President's Daughter*[1]

I

On the 22nd of April 1721, the H.M.S. *Seahorse* set anchor in Boston Harbor
at the end of an inbound voyage from Saltertudo, only to have an African crew
member fall "sick with the smallpox."[2] Within a week, a second crew member
had been infected, and by mid-May no less than eight people showed symptoms of the disease.[3] The town selectmen quickly mobilized to quarantine the
infected crew, and made "a strict search and enquiry of the Inhabitants at
their respective Houses, touching the Small-pox, and found none Sick of that
Distemper, but a Negro Man at the House of Capt. Paxton near the South
Battery, being the House that was first visited therewith: The Negro is almost
Recovered."[4] By the 3rd of June, *The Boston News-Letter* reported that "we
have had but one Person taken Sick of the Small-Pox since Saturday last, and
those that were then Visited with that Distemper are all in a likely way to
recover, most of them being up and about their Chambers."[5] This news was
particularly welcome to Bostonians, who had every reason to be alarmed by
the appearance of the disease in their midst. The town had not experienced a
significant smallpox epidemic since 1702, and herd immunity was so low that

more than half the population (including virtually everyone under the age of twenty) was now susceptible to the disease. But despite the selectmen's precautions and the optimism expressed in the *News-Letter*, the quarantine failed to hold; the variola virus spread from household to household, and raced through the community. By late June, the epidemic had taken on a life of its own, and by the time it receded later that year, roughly 6,000 of Boston's 11,000 inhabitants had been infected; nearly 850 of those had died.[6] If any event in the first century of New England's colonial history could be interpreted as an unambiguous sign of national affliction, this was it. Desperate to fend off the scourge, ministers and laypeople alike turned to the familiar rhetoric of the jeremiad for refuge, and to account for the epidemic that raged around them.

But the legacy of the 1721 epidemic does not lie in the general incidence of smallpox or in its rate of mortality. Instead, it lies in what Carla Mulford has described as a collision between the competing scientific technologies of print and of medicine—a collision that was fundamental to how Western medicine came to understand the modern relation between disease and self, and that proved to mark a "crossroads in the formation of liberal subjectivity."[7] Specifically, this epidemic set the stage for the first widespread and widely publicized Western uses of a procedure known as inoculation (or variolation), and the use of this procedure was framed in a print debate— known as the inoculation controversy—that took place during an unprecedented period of liberalization for the New England press. Unlike Edward Jenner's discovery of the smallpox vaccine at the end of the eighteenth century, inoculation was not the product of Western scientific experimentation, but had been imported into the consciousness of English physicians through the Royal Society's *Philosophical Transactions*, where Jacob Pylarinus and Emanuel Timonius each described the procedure as they had witnessed it in Constantinople; perhaps the most famous early proponent of inoculation in England was Lady Mary Wortley Montagu, whose husband was the British ambassador in Turkey. She wrote back to England about the procedure in 1717, and had her son inoculated in 1718; her family physician in Constantinople was the same Dr. Timonius who had written to the Royal Society in 1714. The Montagus returned to England in 1718, at which time she continued to tell her friends (including the princess of Wales) about inoculation until a major outbreak of smallpox erupted in 1721, at which time inoculation was tested on a number of Newgate prisoners.[8]

Inoculation involved making an incision into the arm or leg of a patient who had never been infected with smallpox, and inserting into this incision the pustulent matter from someone who had recently contracted it in the

"common way" (i.e., naturally). Although the immunological mechanism
behind inoculation was not understood, its effects were startling, given how
lethal the disease could be; inoculees generally developed mild symptoms of
smallpox, and subsequently recovered with what was assumed to be life-long
immunity (although this latter claim was by no means certain to Western audiences at the time of the controversy). For inoculation's proponents, the
results proved to be irrefutable. Where 14 percent of Bostonians who had
been infected by smallpox in the "common" or "natural" way died in 1721, less
than 2.5 percent of those who were inoculated (6 out of 247) succumbed to
the disease, despite the risk that they had taken on themselves.[9]

The man who first publicly advocated for inoculation in Boston, and who
lobbied Boston's physicians to adopt the procedure during the epidemic was
Cotton Mather. But Mather took pains to highlight a slightly different history
of inoculation, as he claimed to have learned about it from his slave Onesimus
prior to reading about it in a copy of the Society's *Transactions* borrowed from
William Douglass—Boston's only European-trained physician at the time.[10] In
a 1716 letter to John Woodward of the Royal Society, Mather underscored the
broader implications of inoculation, reporting excitedly that if it worked (and
he seems not to have doubted it for an instant), then the practice would "save
more lives than Dr. Sydenham," later adding in his diary that "some hundreds
of thousands of Lives, may in a little while come to be preserved" by it.[11] But
Mather's unrestrained enthusiasm troubled a number of Bostonians, not the
least of whom was Douglass, who quickly emerged as the leading voice aligned
against inoculation. As a trained physician, Douglass's words carried considerable weight in the community, and so too did his resistance to Mather's unwa-
vering—and seemingly uncritical—faith in the *Transactions* and in Onesimus's
testimony. Douglass questioned whether the procedure was safe, ethical, or
even legal. He argued that left in the hands of an amateur, inoculation could
do more harm than good, giving patients a false sense of hope, and fanning
the flames of epidemic; he worried that the procedure had not been properly
tested or its effectiveness demonstrated; that it was not being performed
safely or consistently; and, finally, that it was helping to spread rather than
curb the epidemic, because contagious inoculees were left free to wander
about in public, thus endangering their fellow townsfolk. Douglass wasn't
against inoculation in and of itself—he would come to advocate its use later in
the decade—but he believed that Mather's advocacy was irresponsible, and
derived as much from superstition as it did from reason and rational judgment.[12] It seemed obvious to him that fighting an epidemic by deliberately
spreading the disease among the population was reckless, to do so in an inconsistent, haphazard manner without extensive observation or follow-up was

even more dangerous, and to do so while Boston was in the grips of its worst affliction in a generation, threatened the town's very survival.

Because the stakes of this debate were so high, the inoculation controversy exploded onto the pages of newspapers and pamphlets published on both sides of the Atlantic, and lasted well into 1722—longer than the epidemic itself. Curiously, the debate's focus shifted almost immediately from questions about inoculation's effectiveness to the role of the clergy in advocating for it, to the proliferation of the press and of printed material in discussing it, and to the debate's linguistic forms and conventions; it was as much about public discourse as it was about public health. The controversy pitted the six "inoculation ministers" who, under the prodding of Cotton Mather, wrote a letter of support for the procedure that was published in the *Boston Gazette* on July 31, against Douglass and a heterogeneous group of allies who were drawn together by a fear of inoculation, a suspicion of the clergy's authority, and a general dislike of Mather.[13] Among the most important anti-inoculation voices was James Franklin, who founded *The New England Courant* at the height of the epidemic in August 1721. While the *Courant's* editorial policy encouraged both pro-and anti-inoculation submissions, the paper served as a mouthpiece for critics of Mather, and was more broadly aligned as a counterweight to "authorized" publications like the *Boston Gazette* and the *Boston News-Letter*.[14] Reading the debates makes it seem that "anti-inoculation" stood for "anti-Mather" at times, and the attacks against him were deeply personal, as the anti-inoculators insisted that he had little business inserting himself into the world of medicine. Gone were the early colonial days when ministers regularly practiced theology and medicine, replaced by a new era that increasingly privileged specialization and professionalization.[15] Douglass praised this shift as a sign of the colony's maturity, noting that Massachusetts had finally "come of age" in the early eighteenth century, and arguing that ministers "should cease pretending to Physick, there being Practitioners sufficient in Number and Qualifications to supply the Place."[16] Citing the professional boundaries of medicine (which included "Physicians, Surgeons, Apothecarys, [and] Chymists"), Douglass asked of Mather, "How can we suppose, a Man of a Vocation, which requires all his Time conscientiously to discharge the same, should pretend to a Business of so great Extent?"[17]

The anti-inoculators ridiculed the ministers for meddling in affairs that were supposedly beyond their professional scope, and for putting their community in peril. These anti-inoculators had a field day taunting Mather for what they saw as his scientific pretensions, which included signing his name as a Fellow of the Royal Society, despite the fact that he did not appear on the Society's official rolls. In what must have been a particularly galling attack,

Douglass drew attention to this clerical error, using it as an opportunity to suggest that the Society had "disown[ed] him for a son," going on to call Mather a man of "Whim, Credulity and Vanity" who made absurd observations about the natural world.[18] Among these absurdities, Douglass charged, was Mather's description of the twelve-year cyclical recurrence of smallpox epidemics in New England's history.[19] Although these cycles were based in fact, Douglass upbraided Mather for his seemingly superstitious belief that the patterns were meaningful. The introduction to one of Douglass's anti-inoculation pamphlets mocks "Dr." Mather by calling attention to other "infatuations" that possessed the colony with a similar periodic regularity:

> All Countrys, or Bodys Politick, (our own Mother Country not excepted) have been subject to Infatuations: These in this Country seem always to have proceeded from some of those who call themselves Sons of Levi. The Persecution of the Quakers about the Year 1658, the hanging of those suspected of Witchcraft, about the Year 1691, &c. and Inoculation, or Self-procuring the Small Pox, in the year 1721; and to speak like an Astronomer, or rather in the manner of Dr. C.M. Infatuation seems to return to us after a Period of about Thirty Years, viz. from the Massachusetts-Bay being colonized Anno 1628, to the Persecution of the Quakers, Thirty Years; and so from Infatuation to Infatuation.[20]

The hostility in these remarks is barely contained beneath the surface, and although Mather's observation was correct—the cycles would eventually prove to be significant in and of themselves—the criticism of his analysis rests on a deeper suspicion of New England's ministerial elite. The introduction to *Inoculation of the Small Pox as practiced in Boston* suggests that if Mather was to use New England's history to shape his understanding of smallpox, then he (as a representative of the ministry) had much to answer for: it was one thing to perform providential readings in the name of national historiography, but to draw medical insight from providence was another matter entirely. By putting inoculation in a direct line with the Quaker persecutions and the witchcraft trials, this passage implicates Mather in the deaths of those who were hanged in 1692, and holds him responsible for any additional deaths resulting from inoculation. And in a rhetorical revision that overturns the traditional logic of those events in the seventeenth century, neither Quakerism, witchcraft, nor smallpox is figured here as a grave danger to the colony. Instead, it is the ministers who are the source of affliction, and who bear responsibility for the very maladies they sought to treat.

The rhetorical appeal of this critique rests on its appropriation of the narrative tropes and conventions that had been worked out in New England's epidemiological history over the previous century, as once again, the community—figured here as the "Body Politick"—coheres around a sense of shared affliction. Douglass takes this point up in considerable detail when he dissects the tensions between private and public concerns that are raised by the issue of inoculation. In his mind, the danger is twofold: patients endanger their own lives when inoculated, while the community also faces a higher risk of epidemic when inoculators spread the disease. The anti-inoculators made this point explicitly in the very first issue of the *Courant*, printing a piece of doggerel that referred to the inoculation ministers as a "certain set of men . . . Who like faithful Shepherds take care of their Flocks, By teaching and practicing what's Orthodox, Pray hard against Sickness, yet preach up the POX!"[21] The key, once again, is that unlike traditional treatments that focus on the symptoms of a disease, inoculation required patients to infect themselves with smallpox deliberately. And while Mather highlighted the number of lives that would be saved by the procedure, Douglass maintained that these lives would potentially come at a great cost, because despite the fact that inoculees tended to develop an attenuated form of the disease, he believed that they could pass virulent strains of smallpox to others. He was appalled that inoculees were not quarantined, and was certain that the infection would spread as they wandered the streets of Boston, endangering friends and strangers alike. Douglass recognized that this presented a serious public health dilemma, and framed the argument as one in which inoculees placed their own self-interests above those of the community.[22]

What seemed so extraordinary to Douglass and the anti-inoculators was that the ministers' advocacy of inoculation required a wholesale reformulation of New England's epidemiological narrative—negotiated over the previous century—by shifting the ground from which to speak of contagion. Where the relation between individual and communal immunity drove New England Puritans to adopt the halfway covenant and develop the jeremiad as a means of rallying communal penitence to combat affliction half a century earlier, Douglass flipped the terms of the discussion in 1721 by charging that individuals who inoculated themselves under the advice of Boston's ministers were placing their own personal interests above the community's. In other words, inoculation meant thinking about illness as a personal rather than national affliction, which if not medically problematic in and of itself, clearly subverted earlier models of communal authority. Douglass addressed this point insistently, charging that the decision to inoculate oneself was not simply an attack on public health, but one on public order as well—that "if a Man may make free with his own Body Natural, because in Conscience he thinks he ought to do so, this . . . is also a considerable Step towards the making free with the Body Politick."[23] The interplay between "Body Natural" and "Body Politick" is not new to the inoculation controversy, but Douglass's use of the phrase literalizes the metaphor, and casts the decisions that individuals make about their physical health in terms of the national good. If individuals have the right to consider their own health without regard to the community, then civil authority is meaningless. Samuel Grainger would make the point succinctly in a pamphlet titled *The Imposition of Inoculation as a Duty Religiously Considered* (1721), where he juggles religious and secular concerns in building his anti-inoculation argument:

> Common Justice and Charity forbid the Use of any Means, which may hurt or prejudice our Neighbour. The Laws of Nature and Nations, oblige Mankind to consult the good of the Community whereof they are Members; and not to offer any Violence or Injury to the Publick Good, upon any private advantage whatever.[24]

Reminiscent of John Winthrop's rhetoric in *A Model of Christian Charity*, Grainger subverts the theological order represented by ministers like Increase and Cotton Mather by figuring them as dangerous innovators who ignore New England's rhetorical, medical, and religious traditions.

Although the anti-inoculators were allied against Boston's ministerial elite, they did not confine themselves to secular argument. Instead, the rhetoric of the jeremiad had been so successful in mobilizing metaphors of communal space, and in articulating an ideology of cultural cohesion in the seventeenth century, that it was deployed by and against ministers during the controversy. Grainger took up the issue where Douglass's analysis left off, criticizing inoculation from a familiar theological stance, and promising to consider two questions: "What are the Means which may be lawfully us'd for our preservation FROM [God's] desolating Judgments?" and "Whether the new Method of Inoculation is a lawful means."[25] Not surprisingly, Grainger addresses these questions by turning to Jeremiah (Chapter 18), and to God's announcement that "if that Nation against whom I have pronounced, TURN FROM THEIR EVIL, I will repent of the Evil that I thought to do unto them."[26] These words are standard fare in any jeremiad, and Grainger's audience would not have missed the point. He places smallpox in its epidemiological framework as a "Judicial National Sickness," and considers inoculation within this context.[27] Significantly for Grainger, the rhetoric of the jeremiad demands that such national judgments be treated through "National Repentance and Reformation" rather than human medicines, because repentance "removes the Cause which brings the Judgment," while medicines simply treat the temporal symptoms.[28] In other words, just as afflictions are a belated sign of divine wrath, so must appropriate treatment be given after the onset of illness, and after the providential signs have been deciphered correctly. Grainger argues that inoculation contradicts this temporal order, as it consists of deliberately making oneself sick *before* God has passed judgment. He goes on to write that during moments of such national judgment, "We are no where directed to Humane Means to anticipate, prevent, or over-rule" them, for to do so would further anger God.[29] Grainger thus places the inoculation ministers in a defensive theological position that requires them to explain why they would advocate a procedure that was so clearly antithetical to the national good, and why they would stray from the narrative mode that they had helped to shape.

Whereas the jeremiad obviated the distinction between the national covenant and the individual covenant of grace, inoculation only made it more apparent. Regardless of its effectiveness (indeed, the very mention of its "effectual" nature went against the grain of Calvinist theology), inoculation left ministers open to the charge that they had deserted the community in its time of need. Given the opportunity, anti-inoculators refused to grant Mather any quarter. For Douglass, John Williams, and James Franklin, the crux of the issue was not religious; each found the debate to be readily adapted to his concerns. In Douglass's case, this was taken up in questions of public health and public order. It was clear to him that despite Mather's argument, a community could not survive an epidemic if each citizen acted in his or her own self-interest, rather than in the interest of the community. Even more forcefully, Grainger implied that Mather's advocacy of inoculation undermined the jeremiad, and was a hypocritical reliance on human means to alleviate divine affliction. For Perry Miller, this is one of the essential problems that arose from the controversy. In surveying the rhetorical landscape, he would lament that by early 1722, when the epidemic came under control, the debate still raged, but "the whole formula of the jeremiad, with its cosmic threats, was reduced to nonsense."[30]

While Grainger mounts this criticism, he acknowledges that medicines and other physical means such as bleedings and purges are permitted in the treatment of "pestilential sickness," but the distinction he makes between these means and inoculation is significant.[31] What so worried the religious anti-inoculators about the procedure was that it was preventative rather than curative—that inoculation meant taking smallpox onto oneself, in anticipation of God's judgment. Not only did inoculees deliberately put themselves in harm's way, as Douglass had charged, but this was also a direct challenge to

God—"a Tempting of the Lord," as Edmund Massey put it in a London sermon—to intervene on their behalf.[32] Such an act placed the "Supream Providential Will" in a subservient relation to the "Becks and Appointment of the Humane Will," which was clearly blasphemous.[33] Here, in a nutshell, the anti-inoculators tried to undermine Mather's reasoning. In their eyes, it was impossible for him to simultaneously affirm traditional Puritan theology, and to deny it by advocating inoculation, which he was nevertheless rightly convinced would save lives. Although Mather was clearly not antireligious, he found himself caught, arguing for the public good in a way that was difficult to articulate, and at a time when his moral and religious authority was no longer powerful enough to stand on its own as evidence. Indeed, even as the anti-inoculators railed against the procedure, they deliberately questioned ministerial authority in medical matters; Increase Mather recalled a time when this authority was taken at face value, suggesting that it still ought to stand as evidence in favor of inoculation:

> It cannot be denied but that some Wise and Judicious Persons among us approve of Inoculation, both Magistrates and Ministers. . . . But on the other hand, tho' there are some Worthy Persons, that are not clear about it; nevertheless, it cannot be denied, but that the known Children of the Wicked one, are generally fierce Enemies of Inoculation.[34]

Whereas such an argument might have carried the day during the Antinomian controversy a century earlier, the anti-inoculators were not to be intimidated by this line of reasoning. They gleefully responded by publishing their own parodies in the *New England Courant*, reveling in the absurdity of grounding logical arguments on the self-proclaimed merits of one's character. In the very first issue of the *Courant*, an anti-inoculator wrote that "I think their Character ought to be sacred, and that they themselves ought not to give the least Occasion to have it called into question," while another tweaked the Mathers several months later, adding that "a method of preventing Death, which is approv'd of by Magistrates and Ministers, is not only lawful but a Duty. But, Magistrates and Ministers do approve of inoculating the Small Pox. Therefore, it is not only lawful, but a Duty."[35] It became a game for the anti-inoculators to print satires and burlesques of the Mathers's pamphlets, inventing empty syllogisms to the point of distraction. This is perhaps what makes the inoculation controversy such a fascinating event in Boston's history: quite apart from the ravages of smallpox, arguments about the practice eventually deteriorated into the equivalent of a schoolyard spat. At every opportunity, Mather's language, his style, and his education were parodied. But what are we to make of such arguments? On the one hand, they were central to a crucial moment in the history of New England and the history of medicine, while on the other, they tended toward the absurd.

II

I am drawn to the inoculation controversy because of the way that it has traditionally been framed in twentieth-century Early American studies. References to the epidemic and controversy have long focused on whether Mather was "right" in his advocacy of the procedure, on the power struggle between religious and secular forces in Boston, on providing evidence of New England's relative position with respect to medical and scientific innovations, and, more recently, as evidence for the potential influence of African practices on Western medicine, and the evolution of creole identities and racial discourses in the Atlantic World.[36] Delving a little deeper into the criticism, one is struck by how little attention has been paid to the event by *literary* critics, an oversight that I would like to correct here because the two technologies that were so central to the controversy itself—inoculation and print—are deeply implicated in our notions of what it means to be, and how we talk about being modern Western subjects. In this vein, I take my cue from Miller, whose characterization of the controversy drips with the disdain that he reserved for what he saw as the most egregious cases of small-mindedness. Referring to the ongoing newspaper and pamphlet war between pro- and anti-inoculation advocates, Miller lamented that "what had begun, under the shadow of pestilence, as a grim struggle for the mastery of New England's soul . . . petered out, by the next spring, into a tiff about style," where "the point of attack [shifted] to language."[37]

It is easy to sense Miller's disappointment that the New England mind he so deeply admired would stoop to express itself in what he believed to be such an unflattering manner. He certainly has a point: to read the arguments and counterarguments about the legality and usefulness of inoculation is to submerge oneself in the absurdities and ambiguities of public debate. At a time when half of Boston's population was either sick or dying, the ministers and physicians seemed to expend as much energy on parody, satire, and burlesque as one would expect on the victims of smallpox themselves. Nevertheless, Miller's off-handed comment is fascinating to me because if not exactly a deliberate act of literary criticism, it does express a clear judgment about the insignificance of language and style relative to "serious" theological and medical issues. The struggle for New England's mind and soul is, for Miller, vastly more important than the struggle for its body—or for the bodies who perished under the "shadow of pestilence"—and more important too, it would seem, than the terms through which that struggle was narrated. I disagree. Even if the tail end of the controversy could be dismissed as a "tiff about style," as Miller would like, it was no common tiff, and its principals were no ordinary men. Although the controversy carried into the streets of Boston—sometimes with violent results—the main disputants included university-trained ministers, physicians, and professional tradesmen who had the opportunity, as well as the capital, to disseminate their ideas widely through the explosive and exploding medium of print.[38] As fanciful as some of the arguments on both sides of the debate were, the disputants' self-conscious concern with style implies access to certain linguistic forms and conventions that are neither transparent, nor universal; despite Miller's characterization, the pamphlets and newspapers that circulated during the controversy performed important ideological work in shaping the grammar and syntax of eighteenth-century colonial identity, and in producing the terms through which health and illness—but also knowledge—were categorized and transmitted in public. A closer attention to the structure of this tiff—to the forms and meanings of its satires, its attention to style, and to the channels it traveled in making its way through Boston—gives deeper insight into the community of letters that these men were in the process of creating. And it is worth remembering that if Benjamin Franklin was to become the representative man of letters in America by the end of the eighteenth century, he first sharpened his skills at his brother's press during and in the immediate aftermath of the inoculation controversy.

Rather than pushing Miller aside, my instinct is to follow his lead, to use his critique as an impetus for introspection, and to uncover the alternate critical pathways that are made available to literary critics by focusing on the formal, stylistic, and rhetorical issues that arise from medical crises like the inoculation controversy. I'd like to interrogate his assertion more fully, to ask what is at stake in his dismissive nature, and to consider the ways in which concerns about style and language are not merely the by-products of an overwrought public health debate, but integral to the underlying tension between increasingly polarized disciplines seeking to define and resist the limits of their respective boundaries, and integral, too, to the way that these Bostonians saw themselves in the world. Although inoculation carried the day, comments like Miller's reflect a deep ambivalence about the controversy's ultimate significance. The representation of style as secondary to scientific and theological matters is part of a vision that accepts the conventions of specialized discourses as foregone conclusions rather than the product of contested epistemologies. I am therefore interested in the linguistic stakes of the controversy, which in this instance I measure by reading Cotton Mather's knotted rhetorical posturing as an attempt to reintegrate the growing schism between science and theology. Finally, I am curious about the limits of Mather's rhetorical affect: Where do his representational practices cleave to—and depart from—the formal structures of public health debates? The broader claim of this project is that such concerns are not peripheral to medical and epidemiological discourses, but constitutive of the very means through which medicine envisions the body, the patient, and the community; that in early-eighteenth-century New England, these visions are negotiated publicly, and in print; that the printed nature of these debates matters because it tests the limits of how language produces, represents, and even erases knowledge; and finally, that attention to style and language reveals to us the ideological pressures that come to bear on national, literary, and print traditions, as well as on medical and scientific ones. Insofar as I resist Miller's dismissive tone, I like to linger on his characterization, because examining style is, after all, one of the things that literary critics do.

Because Cotton Mather is the person who was responsible for a significant portion of the written material that circulated during the controversy, and whose personality became its central focus, I continue my investigation into the rhetorical posturing at the heart of the inoculation debates with him. In both his contemplative and polemical writings on the subject, his self-conscious struggles with language, with style, and with metaphor shaped the way that the controversy played itself out on the public stage. But just as significantly, they underpinned his medical and theological models of the human body. His medical writings reflect a lifelong interest in the subject—an interest that is not all that surprising, given the habit of seventeenth-century New England Puritan ministers to tend to settlers' health when the need arose, and which meant that because he was not formally trained as a physician, he was left to build the case for his authority rhetorically, rather than on the basis of any professional experience. Of course, this is the very practice that Douglass and the anti-inoculators rejected as outdated and dangerous in the early eighteenth century, but despite what his critics charged, Mather's approach to medicine is inextricable from his theological training, and his overarching interest in finding a link between spiritual and physical health. Indeed, his long treatise on "the common maladies of mankind" titled *The Angel of Bethesda* is heavily invested in producing a model of the human body that accounts for just such a link, and it guides physicians in how to treat diseases ranging from infantile sickness to the gout, melancholy, dropsy, and madness. *The Angel of Bethesda* is an amalgam of natural philosophy, medical history, aids to prognostication, and home remedies, all culled from such diverse sources as the Bible, Homer, Hippocrates, Plato, Aristotle, Galen, Plutarch, Boyle, Harvey, and Sydenham, among others.[39]

To be sure, Mather's approach to aggregating information suggested that an educated layman could assimilate disparate theories, and minimize incongruities through painstaking analysis. In this case, it produced a heterogeneous body of knowledge that allowed him to draw his own conclusions about the function of the human body, and to free himself from the two standard models in operation at the time, neither of which he fully accepted or rejected. These were the iatrophysical model, which considered the body to be a mechanical apparatus that could be restored to balance via purges, bleedings, sweats, etc., and the iatrochemical model, which, as the name suggests, sought chemical means such as herbal remedies to treat illness.[40] Instead, Mather drew on his reading of classical medicine to posit a mystical "Middle Nature, between the Rational Soul, and the Corporeal Mass" that he called the Nishmath-Chajim, or "Breath of Life."[41] Among other things, Mather believed the Nishmath-Chajim to be responsible for such acts as the "Several Digestions in the Body," as well as "muscular motion," and the functions of the human body that other theories failed to explain.[42] Vague though many of his assertions on the subject are, Mather further suggests that "there are indeed many Things in the Humane Body, that cannot be resolved by the Rules of Mechanism. Our Nishmath-Chajim will go very far to help us, in the Solution of them. Indeed we can scarce well Subsist without it."[43] He goes on to say that the Nishmath-Chajim is the "Seat of our Diseases, or the Source of them," and that physical illnesses can therefore be traced back to imbalances and weaknesses in it.[44] And yet despite his promise to explain its mechanism more fully, Mather never completely clarifies how the Nishmath-Chajim operates, or how, exactly, to restore this spirit to balance when a patient is ill. He speculates that physicians who treat illness through physical means might find "Remedies (particularly in the Mineral or Vegetable Kingdome) that shall have a more Immediate Efficacy to Brighten, and Strengthen, and Comfort the Nishmath-Chajim," and that whoever makes such discoveries "will be the most Successful Physician in the World"—a concern with fame that colors a number of his medical texts, particularly those dealing with inoculation.[45] But the key point for Mather lies in his belief that the Nishmath-Chajim is a middle ground between body and soul, which means that the best cures for illness are likely to be found in treatments of the mind (via agreeable conversation), and in piety. The "Rational Soul," he remarks, "in its Reflections has Powerful and Wonderful Influences on the Nishmath-Chajim."[46]

As mystifying as the Nishmath-Chajim proves to be, it offers Mather an elegant organ for mapping a patient's spiritual estate onto his or her physical health. Just as significantly, this model, which remains rooted in ancient theories of the body and of selfhood, provides him with a unifying theory for grounding his medical readings in a familiar theological context. For example, his extended meditation on the causes and treatments of smallpox is heavily invested in what he calls the "Sentiments of PIETY to be raised in and from this Grievous Disease," and these sentiments negotiate the familiar conflict between individual and community that were visible in seventeenth-century New England Puritan Rhetoric.[47] Beginning broadly with an address to "Mankind in general," he uses tropes of the jeremiad to explain why the smallpox afflicts them:

Ah, Sinful Generation, a People Laden with Iniquity, a Seed of Evil-doers, Children that are Corrupters; They have forsaken the Lord! And Why are ye Stricken more, Even with Strokes that were unknown to the more Early Ages? Tis because ye Revolt more and more![48]

Even as he deploys this language, Mather effects a rapid transition, moving from the general to the particular in order to explain how individual patients can alleviate this divine scourge. What emerges from this transition is that "treatment" does not operate within communal, cultural, or generational frameworks here. And while the treatment he calls for is spiritual rather than physical, the shift from generational to individual sin marks an important parallel to his thinking about inoculation. Everything here focuses on the personal, which Mather signals insistently by punctuating his remarks with the first-person singular pronoun:

Be Restless, until the Things that accompany Salvation, and the Evident Tokens of it, be plainly to be found upon thee: Until thou art able to say, My Mind by a New and a strong Biass given from Heaven unto it, is come to make the Serving and Pleasing of the Glorious God, the Chief End of my Life.... I prize Him in all His Offices; I prize Him with All His Benefits; I would fain have Him to fulfil in me all the Good Pleasure of His Goodness.... The Lusts of indwelling Sin, I seek, I Sigh, I Long for a Deliverance from them ... I Love my Neighbour; I am glad, when it goes well with him; I am grieved when it goes Ill with him.[49]

The repetition of "I" in this passage signals, for Mather, the "deepest sense of Self-Abhorrence, and Self-Abasement" that is necessary for the individual to make his way back to the Lord, and as such, provides a sense of how he understood the function of inoculation.[50] In contrast to Douglass's and Grainger's allegations, the focus on individual treatment and salvation is not intended as a selfish act for personal gain, but as a transformative move toward the Lord that must be made on an individual basis, and that will ultimately benefit the entire community.

Many twentieth-century critics have questioned the motives and reasoning behind Mather's advocacy of inoculation, ranging from Miller's uncharitable view that his actions merely reflect an opportunistic attempt to strengthen the ministry by taking advantage of recent developments in medicine, to Otho Beall's and Richard Shryock's far more generous reading that medicine for Mather was "a second vocation," and that even if he had not been trained professionally, he pursued it with rigor and discipline.[51] But Louise Breen has made the most sophisticated attempt to locate Mather's thinking about inoculation at the nexus of his medical writings and his theological beliefs, figuring the procedure as a "natural" analogue to conversion.[52] The religious strictures that Mather calls for are independent of any medical prophylaxis, so his focus on the individual's role in preparing himself for immunity is not incompatible with the jeremiad, and it allows him to conceive of inoculation as a simple extension of this logic of piety. The schema that Breen proposes suggests that inoculation was, for Mather, a method of preparing oneself for future immunity analogous to the preparationist doctrines for receiving grace: the Christian prepared "himself for conversion by relinquishing all to God; in smallpox, the patient could prepare himself for immunity to future epidemics only by taking the deadly virus into his system."[53] In other words, Breen argues that this preparationist framework is critical to understanding Mather's support of inoculation as a logical outgrowth of his ministerial work because it accounts for the apparent disjunction between his Calvinist theology and a procedure that, on the surface, can only tenuously be considered congruent with it. If inoculation falls within Mather's theological apparatus of contagion, it is because he abstracts from the communal rhetoric of the jeremiad to emphasize the role of individual responsibility in preparationist doctrines: humans seek self-abasement and redemption out of their love of God; the community itself can be saved from affliction only when subjects renew themselves individually, because a Christian's personal interest was necessarily mapped on the community's interest. The anti-inoculators, however, did not let Mather off the hook so easily. For them, the union of personal and communal bodies effected in the jeremiad could not be separated at will.

Mather's model of the body's immunological mechanism was medically unorthodox, but this unorthodoxy is central to his early advocacy of inoculation, and it likewise colored his own defense against critics like Douglass. In addition to Breen's insights about the analogical character of Mather's medical and theological ideas, I want to highlight his investment in the rhetorical quality of his writing. Certainly, analogy is rhetorical in and of itself, but beyond this, Mather's focus on the individual's ultimate responsibility for his own treatment manifests itself in a rhetorical shift toward particularity and repetition (of "I") in order to make his point about treatment. If not significant on its own, this attention to language is ironic, when considered in the context of his broader critique of the medical profession, and his wariness that medical knowledge is too often wrapped up in rhetorical affect. For example, Mather asserts his authority by undermining medical practitioners, and he criticizes physicians by outlining what he sees as the fundamental epistemological problem at the heart of the profession itself: "To know the cause" of distemper, he writes, "is half the cure." The statement is not controversial, but Mather goes on to lament "how little Progress is there yett made in that Knowledge." Addressing those physicians who "talk about the Causes of Diseases," he criticizes their ignorance, describing "their talk [as] very Conjectural, very Uncertain, very Ambiguous; and oftentimes a meer Jargon; and in it, they are full of Contradiction to One another."[54] By highlighting the disjunction between knowing and representing the cause of illness, Mather positions medical expertise as a rhetorical affect in which knowledge and jargon stand in opposition to one another, so that medical debate too often becomes illogical or meaningless, and in either case, an impediment to progress. The upshot of such an argument is that *The Angel of Bethesda* promises to be an exemplary medical repository so long as Mather speaks plainly and sidesteps the pitfalls of uncertainty. Mather's gambit here is to ignore Douglass's question about professional qualifications, to reorient the issue by focusing on the representational qualities of medical discourse, and to suggest that physicians do not have a monopoly over the production knowledge. The argument also implies that Mather believed his own writing to be clear enough that audiences ought to be convinced by his pronouncements, and that his lack of formal medical training could be overcome through a combination of reason and careful argument—despite the fact that he is often steeped in ambiguity, jargon, and rhetorical affect himself.

Ironically, the chapter in which Mather criticizes conjecture is titled *Conjecturalities. or, Some Touches upon a New Theory of Many Diseases*, a text that borrows heavily from Benjamin Marten's *A New Theory of Consumptions* (1720), and which therefore lends Mather's work an assertive tone that belies the title's conjectural quality. The chapter itself is as much a commonplace as a synthesis of ideas, with extended passages copied verbatim from Marten's original text. Its broader significance lies in the opportunity it affords Mather to link his model of human health with the latest scientific theories and developments from Europe, as manifested in the work of Marten, Pylarinus, and Timonius. In particular, Mather focuses intently on Marten's proto-germ theory of disease, which was based on the "Microscopical Observations" of "Animalcula or exceeding minute Animals," and on the assumption that "Infinite Numbers" of these animalcula could "insinuate themselves . . . thro' the Pores of our skin; and soon get into the Juices of our Bodies."[55] While Marten hinted that his theory of consumption might eventually be generalized by "some Abler Hand, whose Abilities are more equal to the Task," he nevertheless suggests that animalcula could be responsible for diseases like smallpox, leprosy, venereal disease, measles, and other distempers. Mather elides this uncertainty from his text, leaping at the opportunity to abstract Marten's observation to the general case.[56]

Mather draws further from Marten's observations to posit that these "invisible insects," as he sometimes calls them, could be carried across oceans and deserts by prevailing winds or in the "Bodies or Cloathes or Goods of Travellers," and thus spread diseases throughout the world.[57] In outlining the history of epidemics, Mather (via Marten) recalls Martin Lister's description of the geographic distributions of illness in the world, and his hypothesis that smallpox came to Europe via Africa and the Orient, when the spice trades were opened by the "Princes of Egypt, unto the remoter Parts of the East Indies; from whence it originally came, and where at this day it rages more cruelly than with us," as well as "Dr. [William] Oliver's Opinion, That we received the Small Pox and Measles from Arabia; and that Europe was wholly unacquainted with them, until by frequent Incursions of the Arabians into Africa, and afterwards into Spain, the Venom came to be Spred as now it is"[58] Lister's and Oliver's histories represent Europe as a healthy territory that was originally free from the disease, but became infected as a result of exploration and commerce. And yet, in a remarkable shift from the *Magnalia Christi Americana*, where Mather relied on the mythic explanation that God had cleared Native Americans from New England with miraculous plagues, he includes Marten's observations that Europe, too, had done its share of spreading contagion throughout the world, with a surprisingly frank assessment of the New World's early epidemiological history: "Tis generally Supposed, that *Europe* is Endebted unto America for the Lues Venerea. If so, Europe has paid its debt unto America, by making unto it a Present of the Small Pox, in Lieu of the Great one."[59]

As prescient as this proto-germ theory appears to be, Mather's reliance on current European scientific knowledge went hand in hand with his religious sensibilities, and guided his conjectures about contagion back to theological grounds. His citation of Marten's work is a testimonial to his participation in transatlantic knowledge networks, as are his ongoing reports of *Curiosa Americana* to the Royal Society, and his often mocked decision to identify himself as a Fellow of the Society in his medical and scientific writings. These transatlantic networks are deployed by Mather as evidence of his expertise, but a closer examination of his writings reveals that Marten's animalcular theory was meaningful to him only insofar as it provided an opportunity to use science and medicine as evidentiary frameworks for theological conclusions. Instruments like the microscope were no doubt useful for observing the "invisible world," but they held Mather's attention because they helped him to decipher those observations and draw theological analogues from them. Indeed, as Breen argues, analogical thinking is fundamental to Mather's understanding of disease, and it helps him to close the link between the invisible *physical* world and the invisible *spiritual* world, lending particular significance to his 1716 comments that the cyclical patterns of illness in seventeenth-century Boston were guided by the "peculiar agency of the invisible world."[60] In other words, Douglass's critique of professionalism made little sense to Mather, for whom theology and medicine were two conjoined fields that needed to be understood together in order to properly treat illness.

Mather makes what is perhaps one of his greatest rhetorical leaps when he tries to explain the mechanism of infection. The animalcular theory gives Mather the language through which to bridge the gap between European scientists like Marten, Hooke, and Leewenhoek and the "Sentiments of Piety" that drove his religious writing. Nevertheless, Marten's "microscopical observations" were just as literal to Mather as his theological apparatus was, so analogy provides him with a tool for grounding theology in scientific descriptions of the world around him. And if, as he suspected, diseases were caused by an imbalance in the Nishmath-Chajim, then it was logical to suggest that those imbalances could be caused, in turn, by animalcula, which were but the active agents of God's will. The analogy to the invisible world of spirits was simply too tempting for Mather to ignore, so he constructed his own germ theory that borrowed equally from science and theology, and reinforced traditional Calvinist representations of illness as a sign of divine punishment:

How much does our Life ly at the Mercy of our God! How much do we walk thro' unseen Armies of Numberless Living Things, ready to Seize and Prey upon us! . . . What Unknown Armies had the Holy One, wherewith to Chastise, and Even destroy, the Rebellious Children of Men? Millions of Billions of Trillions of Invisible Velites! Of Sinful

Men they say, Our Father, Shall We Smite them? On His order, they
do it Immediately; they do it Effectually. What a poor Thing is Man;
that a Worm inconceivably less than the Light Dust of the Balance, is
too hard for him.[61]

This fantastical vision in which animalcula literally become God's armies sent
to fight sinners from within their own bodies provides a rich metaphorical
construction, and reflects Mather's own thinking about smallpox, given observations about the swarms of animals observed in the "Pustles of the"
disease.[62] Combined with analogical evidence, such metaphors created ready-
made explanations for Mather to describe how smallpox operates on mankind; invisible velites are not the direct cause of disease, but the effectual
means through which God reduces humans. Indeed, in his chapter on the
disease titled *Variolae trimphatae*, Mather finally makes the link between
smallpox, animalcula, and theology explicit, reporting, "It begins now to be
Vehemently Suspected That the Small-Pox may be more of an Animalculated
Business, than we have been generally aware of. The Millions of — — — —
which the Microscopes discover in the Pustules, have Confirmed the Suspicion," and he continues: "What would a Nieuentyt now say, Reading Job.
VII.5. upon it?"[63]

The reference to Job ("my flesh is clothed with worms and clods of dust")
provides any theologically minded thinker like Mather with the necessary
analogy to locate the generic cure for God's scourge in repentance. And yet,
Mather actively advocated for the physical as well as spiritual treatment of
disease, so his analogical reasoning begs the question of how, other than
through praying, individual patients might protect themselves from God's
armies of invisible velites? Predictably, the answer lies in what Breen has
described as the preparationist analogue of inoculation. But whereas Breen's
investigation of this analogical relationship helps to account for Mather's certainty in advocating inoculation, I remain curious about the intersection of
that analogical thinking with his metaphorical representations of animalcula.
What I'd like to foreground most emphatically are the representational stakes
of Mather's claims, which are never so evident as when he self-consciously
deploys metaphor to account for medical processes. Mather's defense of inoculation proceeds on the assumption that although smallpox is God's scourge,
the procedure is a gift from God as well, and that God has indeed taught man
"how to make himself Sick, in a way that will save his life."[64] Repeating the
metaphor he used to discuss the workings of animalcula in the human body,
Mather describes the difference between taking smallpox through inoculation, and being infected in the common way by imagining the human body as

a citadel under attack from foreign invaders. When an individual is infected in the common way, miasms of the smallpox enter:

> into the Body, in the Way of Inspiration, [and] are immediately taken into the Blood of the Lungs: And, I pray, how many Pulses pass before the very Heart is pierced with them? . . . Behold, the Enemy at once gott into the very Center of the Citadel: And the Invaded Party must be very Strong indeed, if it can struggle with him, and after all Entirely Expel and Conquer him.[65]

In contrast to this, Mather sticks with the metaphor when describing the insertion of animalcula into the body via the arm or leg (as with inoculation). This method, he argues, introduces foreign bodies through the:

> outworks of the Citadel, and at a Considerable Distance from the Center of it. . . . The Vital Powers are kept so clear from his Assaults, that they can manage the Combats bravely and, tho' not without a Surrender of those Humours in the Blood, which the Invader makes a Siezure on, they oblige him to march out the same way that he came in, and are sure of never being troubled with him any more.[66]

Obviously, Mather was neither the first nor the last person to rely on military metaphors to describe the actions of disease in the human body, but the key point here is that in deploying this metaphor, Mather synthesizes his religious and medical thinking, and literalizes it in its application to inoculation. Indeed, while the citadel metaphor is not part of Marten's hypothesis, Mather's explanation is obviously drawn from Marten's text, which describes animalcula "being drove to the Lungs by the Circulation of the Blood . . . or which possibly being carried about by the Air, may be immediately convey'd to the Lungs by that we draw in, and being there deposited."[67]

Mather used the citadel metaphor on more than one occasion, and by all accounts, he was self-conscious about its rhetorical quality—and about the potential for literalizing that metaphor. For example, the citadel first seems to have appeared publicly in print in Mather's anonymously published London pamphlet titled *An Account of the Method and Success of Inoculating the Small-Pox* (1722), where he tests the limits of metaphor against the animalcular hypothesis directly, and offers what is perhaps his most self-conscious acknowledgment of the rhetorical foundation of his understanding of disease in the human body. After describing the citadel, he concludes that "if the Vermicular Hypothesis of the Small-Pox be receiv'd with us, (and it be, as many now think, an animalculated Business) there is less of Metaphor in our Account, than may be at first imagin'd."[68] Here, then, Mather reveals that his medical metaphor operates *both* figurally *and* literally—that which may have started out as word play now carries vexing implications for theories of knowledge as well as for his stance toward medical discourse. Despite his criticism of physicians who conjecture too much, or who remain mired in jargon, Mather's model of the human body is certainly no less grounded in rhetoric, although his way out of the dilemma is to literalize the metaphor. He immediately comes to this realization, and engages in some critical self-reflection, offering the following refrain: "But to what Purpose is all this Jargon? And of what Significancy are most of our Speculations? Experience! Experience! 'tis to Thee that the Matter must be referr'd after all: a few Empericks here, are worth all our Dogmatists."[69] Catching himself on the verge of dogmatism, Mather steps back, deploying the language of empiricism to regain control of his narrative; he spends the next several pages of his pamphlet avoiding sweeping metaphors, providing instead a detailed history of the 1721 smallpox epidemic, of Boston's experiment with inoculation, and finally, of the controversy itself.

It is unclear how much this rhetorical self-control derives from the fact that the pamphlet was published in London, rather than Boston, but the distance between the two certainly helped Mather to imagine a more sedate audience than the one that would throw a grenade through his window in November 1721.[70] Even so, he is unable to contain himself for long. Metaphor and analogy are so central to how Mather understands health and the human body, that they also shade his experience of the inoculation controversy itself. Turning to the public debate over inoculation, Mather falls back on familiar religious language, and his metaphors multiply, taking on added urgency, until his representation of smallpox merges with those of the mob of anti-inoculators that victimizes him. If the metaphor that had bound medical and theological discourse to one another lost currency as the former became more literal, they take on a renewed vigor when aimed at the public arena, where Mather represents his critics as an epidemical threat to the town:

> But never any Patient had so many Pustules of the Small-Pox, as there were Lies now daily told, and spread among our deluded People. . . . [Those] who made the loudest Cry, (who most commonly were what we may not improperly call of *the confluent Sort*, and such also as were past the Dangers of the Small-Pox themselves) had a very Satanic Fury acting them. They were like the possess'd People in the Gospel, exceeding fierce; insomuch that one could scarce pass by the Way

where they were to be met withal. Their *common Way* was to rail and rave, and with Death, or other Mischiefs, to them that practis'd, or favour'd this devilish Invention. To inflame them in their Transports, and harden them in their Violences and Exclamations, they pretended Religion on their Side.[71] (emphasis added)

Terms like "confluent sort" and "common way" are immediately recognizable for their association with smallpox, and the metaphors that substitute lies for pustules mark a rhetorical shift in Mather's representation of this public health debate *from* a focus on health *to* a focus on the public—on incivility itself as a public health hazard. The point is, however, that the transition from one to the other is relatively seamless for Mather, who thinks analogically to map his medical knowledge onto theological frameworks, and vice versa. Contrary to Miller's characterization of the inoculation controversy, the focus on language does not reflect an absurd detour down a blind alley, but is symptomatic of Mather's drive to read all facets of the epidemic—including inoculation—as part of a theological morality play. As far as Mather is concerned, the inoculation controversy was *always* about language and style, but this made him particularly vulnerable to critics like Douglass and Franklin, who publicly drew attention to his rhetorical affect, churning out pamphlet after pamphlet, mimicking his stylistic quirks, satirizing, and exposing them to public view. In retrospect, these satires might seem to fragment the debate over inoculation, but I want to argue that they are inextricably woven into Mather's attempts to reconcile medical and theological discourses, even as Douglass struggled to drive them apart.

The inoculation controversy remains a fairly esoteric object of study because so much of the primary material seems to distract from what modern audiences would identify as the central pragmatic question—whether inoculation was effective in preventing epidemics. The answer to this question is simple: yes, it did. But regardless of the religious and public health issues raised by the specter of inoculation, one cannot help but be impressed by the extraordinary faith Mather that placed in himself and in the procedure. Arguably, he was right to do so. Despite the fact that he didn't know why inoculation worked, and, more ominously, that if practiced in an unregulated manner, it could help to spread the contagion rather than end it, the method proved to be "effectual."[72] Certainly, Mather felt vindicated by the fact that the mortality rate for inoculees was significantly lower than for those who contracted smallpox in the natural way. And once the procedure had been introduced to New England, this practice of preventative medicine would take hold on both sides of the Atlantic. Finally satisfied with is effectiveness, Douglass became an important proponent of inoculation a decade later, and Benjamin Franklin, too, became a major supporter, conveniently eliding the controversy from his *Autobiography* (an attempt, perhaps, at correcting one of the early errata of his life), and came to regret not having inoculated his son, who died of smallpox in 1636.

As early as the winter of 1777, George Washington, facing constant pressure from British forces who tended to be immune to smallpox, ordered mass inoculations for soldiers of the Continental Army—a policy that had a significant impact on the outcome of the revolution.[73] But despite its effectiveness, the truth of the matter is that inoculation remained a dangerous procedure because it involved the live variola virus. Jonathan Edwards was inoculated in February 1758 on the advice of his physician and the College of New Jersey (Princeton) trustees, but soon developed pustules in his mouth and throat. These sores prevented him from swallowing, and his condition deteriorated until he died at the end of March—less than three months after acceding to the presidency of the college.[74] Despite such inherent risks, inoculation became increasingly popular as the century wore on, until it was finally supplanted by vaccination after Edward Jenner's 1796 experiment on James Phipps, and his publication of *An Inquiry into the Causes and Effects of the Variolae Vaccinae* (1798) to detail his method of replacing smallpox with cowpox as the matter to be inoculated into pustules (thus, the name *vaccination*).[75] But even then the vaccine continued to pose some danger: the United States stopped vaccinating children in 1971 because the risk of contracting smallpox naturally was almost zero, while complications from the vaccine killed six to eight children annually.[76] Jenner's scientific advance on a procedure popularized in Boston in 1721 created a monumental shift that led to the most successful eradication program in the history of medicine, and which finally culminated in Somalia in 1977, with the last recorded case of naturally occurring smallpox in the world.[77]

The details of this eradication have long been considered a triumph of modern Western epidemiology. In its final phases, the battle against disease relied on the concept of herd immunity, while containment strategies called for the vaccination of more than 80 percent of susceptible individuals in certain populations. This strategy, however, proved expensive and problematic because it was often difficult to reach all those targeted to receive the vaccine, and because vaccination teams did not always complete their assignments or keep accurate records of their progress.[78] By the late 1960s, a new strategy of "epidemiological surveillance (active case-hunting) and vigorous containment of outbreaks by selective vaccination" was discovered to be more effective than trying to achieve blanket coverage in a community.[79] Physicians from the

World Health Organization found that they could interrupt epidemics by vaccinating only half of susceptible populations if they monitored those populations carefully, and returned to vaccinate susceptible citizens at the first signs of contagion.[80] This combination of surveillance and selective vaccination balanced communal and individual susceptibility in the development of public health policy. As WHO physicians traveled the globe tracing, identifying, and treating susceptible populations, they contained smallpox within ever-shrinking boundaries until the virus disappeared from its natural environment and was left in but a few select laboratories in the United States and the Soviet Union (and later, Russia). This process of treating population clusters through selective vaccination is significantly different from the inoculation program (if one can call it that) advocated by Cotton Mather. Although the jeremiad functioned by considering the national scope of affliction, it was impossible for Mather to understand the immunological significance of conceiving of community as a distinct ecosystem susceptible to contagion. His recommendation involved treating subjects individually, and saving the community one inhabitant at a time, just as one would identify and elect regenerate members of the church one soul at a time. And yet, Mather stands as a central figure in the annals of medicine, having appropriated inoculation as a procedure that would transform public health practices, and eventually eradicate one of the deadliest diseases in human history. But the final question remains: How did this appropriation take place, and how was it invested in the rhetorical stakes of the inoculation controversy?

III

The significance of the "tiff about style" that for Miller characterized the inoculation controversy becomes increasingly apparent as its forms and conventions are understood in the public context in which they were deployed. The controversy, ostensibly about a medical procedure, emerged as a newspaper and pamphlet war at the moment when the press became an increasingly important tool in negotiating liberal ideologies in New England.[81] It gave rise to *The New England Courant*, and to a wealth of other printed materials; it drew Bostonians together by focusing on a shared susceptibility to smallpox and on the issue of public health; and it created micro-communities on either side of the debate that mirrored print circulations within Boston and across the Atlantic. In this manner, the controversy marks what would eventually come to be recognized as a free press, and in doing so, helped to establish what Benedict Anderson has called "imagined communities."[82] All three of

Boston's papers at the time—the *News-Letter*, the *Gazette*, and the *Courant*—obsessively recorded and publicized the details of the controversy, while propagating the very narratives that gave readers an intellectual stake in the issue beyond their physical vulnerability to smallpox. Even as these various papers aligned themselves in different directions, they nevertheless operated together in creating a space for the citizens of Boston to imagine themselves as part of a broader medical and religious debate, and as a community made distinct by its immunological identity—a point best characterized by Priscilla Wald's use of the phrase "imagined immunities" as a framework for articulating national identities, and making transparent the relation between print, community, and immunity.[83] External to the controversy itself, for example, the papers had already been publishing a series of dispatches from Marseilles and Aix-en-Provence, chronicling the devastating effects of plague in southern France immediately prior to the smallpox outbreak in Boston. These stories described the symptoms of the disease in gory detail, but also reported its effects on the various functions of church and government—perhaps as a lesson on how communities ought and ought not to operate during times of epidemic. If Anderson argues that colonial newspapers helped to bring imagined communities into being by providing a forum for the common interests of otherwise faceless strangers to be made public, the *Courant*'s announcement of a total quarantine of French ships in early August 1721 helped Boston to coalesce around its fears of a shared national affliction and around its shared relief at the protective measures enacted against a foreign one.[84] Thus, even as newspapers provided a point of contact for the imaginings of community, the locus of these imaginings in Boston was the narrative trail of contagious diseases that seemed to converge on the town.

The second issue of the *Courant*, published on August 14, further capitalized on the fear of foreign contagion that had been played up in the *Gazette* and the *News-Letter* reports from southern France by suggesting that smallpox inoculation could breed the plague. The anti-inoculators had already made much of the fact that the procedure described by Timonius and Pylarinus was a "Mahometan" one, hoping that suspicion about a foreign religion would lead to apprehensions about inoculation. But the aim of this latest revelation was to insinuate that the actions taken by the Boston selectmen to protect the town from foreign plagues were being undermined by the inoculators. While the story manipulates public fears to rally the community against inoculation, it does so by superimposing geographically and biologically distinct epidemics onto one another—a kind of contagion by analogy, as if anecdotal similarities between symptoms might somehow cause one disease to mutate into the other: "After the Use of that Operation, Abscesses do sometimes break out in the Emunctorys, which is the only place in the Body, where the Plague Boils do break out."[85] Thus, if Bostonians were not convinced by the town's anti-inoculators that the procedure was dangerous, then surely the prospect of the plague—with its dire consequences so clearly spelled out in the recent pages of Boston's papers—was.

A satirical piece (later attributed to Douglass) in the same issue of the *Courant* precedes this warning. Douglass begins with an overview of two stories about inoculation and a proposed expedition to "check the daring Insults and intended Hostilities of the *Eastern Indians*" that appeared in the paper's first issue.[86] He goes on to affirm that the stories had found a way to lodge themselves in his mind—as likely they would have in the paper's community of readers—before combining the two events into what he calls a project for "reducing the Eastern Indians by *Inoculation*."[87] He reasons that because inoculation is a dangerous practice for both individuals and communities, it would best serve New England colonists as a potent offensive weapon against this second, external threat. His plan calls for sending a party of inoculators into battle, armed with incision-lancets, making sure that:

> their Ammunition be of the best Proof, that is, a composition of Negro Yaws, and confluent Small Pox. That the Inoculators, be all Volunteers, who besides their usual Fees, and travelling Charges, may be allowed a Gratuity of 10 l. per Head, of each Indian who survives, conveys and spreads the Infection amongst his Tribe; and of 5 l. per Head for those who blow up too soon (or die) before they reach the Places where Execution is intended.[88]

This passage highlights the cultural work performed through the use of satire during the controversy. If such work is invisible to its participants, it was nevertheless highly charged. As with Mather's historical reconsideration of the channels of contagion between Europe and America, Douglass's plan functions by reminding his readers of the early colonial effects that epidemics had on Native Americans; if Native American populations had been reduced by a miraculous plague a century earlier, colonists could reprise the event by taking advantage of their newfound medical knowledge and their technological superiority; a new form of invisible bullets.

The implication of this proposal is that communities could strengthen themselves and offset multiple threats by redeploying one against the other to the benefit of the body politic (a kind of immunological triangulation). More pointed, however, is the commercial dimension of Douglass's plan, which even as it offers a satire of physicians who accept fees for giving smallpox to patients, is telling in that it unveils the economic motivating force that lies beneath the controversy, and which is far more powerful than any theological one that the anti-inoculators could have pretended to defend in Boston. There is no pretense here of converting or civilizing the Indians. The goal is total annihilation, and its price can be calculated at 5 l. per Native American head unless, of course, the contagion takes hold, in which case numberless invisible victims can be aggregated, and the fee doubled. This is colonialism seen through the twin lenses of epidemiology and economy, and its effects are made legible on the racialized bodies of its intended victims; events like epidemics and inoculation are communal traumas only until they can be reimagined as part of an offensive military strategy. The economic dimension of the plan is readily evident because of the monetary reference, but it takes on added meaning in light of Douglass's reference to the "Negro Yaws," a highly contagious pox-like disease that was unknown in New England until the slave trade brought it there.

My reading of documents related to the inoculation controversy has been deeply invested in excavating the stylistic and formal effects that were deployed as part of the arguments on both sides of the debate, but I remain aware that this attention to the rhetorical and epistemological implications of these texts—to the metaphorical qualities of Mather's writing—risks merely replicating the attention to the New England mind and soul that characterized Miller's work. In this vein, I want to focus on the New England body that emerged from the epidemic and controversy, and on the bodies that underpin any discussion about smallpox and inoculation; to jump from Anderson's notion of "imagined communities" to a more concrete consideration of the embodied communities that were shaped by shared susceptibility to variola, and to the bodies that became objects of this print debate—that became invisible to the history of Western medicine even as the debate exploded onto the pages of Boston's newspapers. I want to think of the status of these bodies in relation to questions about language and "style." I repeat the statistic that 850 of the approximately 6,000 Bostonians who were infected with smallpox died during the 1721 epidemic, and only 6 of the 247 inoculees perished, to remind us that these are physical—and not metaphorical, or figural—bodies. Clearly, these numbers indicate that inoculation was preferable to being infected in the "common way," and yet as is often the case with samples of this size, the ill and the dead tend to become abstractions, receding into the background while personalities like Mather, Douglass, and Franklin—who all actively participated in the controversy—remain in view, and the controversy itself becomes a staging point in the modern analysis of liberalism and print.

I pause now for a moment to ask what is at stake when we abstract from patients' bodies to theories of illness and treatment, and how print is complicit in making these abstractions. This chapter began with the image of a nameless, faceless African sailor falling sick with smallpox as he arrived in Boston in late April 1721, so I would like to come full circle by thinking further about this solitary African figure—this patient zero—who turns out to be an important touchstone in the controversy because Africans like him, both on the margins and at the center of Boston's smallpox epidemic, cast a long shadow over the history of Western medicine. First, this sailor stands in as a figure of circum-Atlantic trade, reminding us that Africans are both objects and agents in the economic networks that bind Europe, Africa, and America; just as important, he reminds us that trading routes inevitably double as conduits for pathogens to circulate from one community to the next, regardless of national and territorial boundaries; that commerce and illness travel along the same by-ways of global trade.[89] Second, two more Africans take center stage during Boston's 1721 epidemic as the subjects of experimentation: when Zabdiel Boylston performed the first inoculations in Boston, he tested the procedure on his six-year-old son, on one of his slaves, and on his slave's son.[90] Thus, a quintessentially modern Western medical procedure began its life in America as an experiment tested on children and Africans— perhaps one of the first, but certainly not the last time medical experiments were performed on Africans and African Americans in the New World. Third— and this is the direction that I'd like to proceed in for the remainder of this chapter—African knowledge represents an important figure in the circulation of medical technology during the controversy, both materially, and in print.

The first reports of inoculation that circulated in the *Transactions* of the Royal Society identified the procedure as emanating from Constantinople, but returning to Mather's 1716 letter to Woodward, where he describes the genesis of his interest, we see him insist on staking his place in history by assuring Woodward that "many months before [he] met with any intimations of treating the smallpox with the method of inoculation anywhere in Europe," he had heard it from an alternate source. He writes:

Inquiring of my Negro-man Onesimus, who is a pretty intelligent fellow, whether he ever had the smallpox, he answered both yes and no; and then told me that he had undergone an operation which had given him something of the smallpox, and would forever preserve him from it, adding that it was often used among the Garamantese, and that whoever had the courage to use it was forever free from the fear of the contagion.[91]

The letter's significance is manifold: it locates Africa as the source of inoculation, representing the transatlantic circulation of knowledge around the entire Atlantic rim, rather than simply bouncing between the two poles of Boston and London (Mather's correspondence, his desire to be recognized as a Fellow of the Royal Society, and his insistence on the wealth of information to be catalogued in the New World for the benefit of mankind, all suggest an investment in representing Boston—and himself, in particular—as a metropolitan counterpoint to London). But I would like to argue that the letter is significant for other reasons as well. Mather's insistence that he knew about inoculation *before* reading it in the *Transactions* of the Royal Society points to the African origins of the procedure, but does so in a way that reemphasizes the primacy of transatlantic exchange on an American/British axis over the African/North American (or indeed the British/Asian axis that informed the *Transactions'* initial reports from Constantinople). Without ever leaving his Boston home, Mather casts himself as the subject of this narrative—an explorer-colonizer who inquires about the world around him, who translates his slave's ambiguous oral assertions ("he answered both yes and no") into writing, gives those assertions meaning, and, in the process, "discovers" a new procedure that will save "hundreds of thousands of lives." Susan Scott Parrish rightly suggests that such stories help Mather to represent "his place in the British periphery as a center of exotic knowledge, surpassing, in this instance, even the Royal Society," although her reading is based on a subsequent iteration of the Onesimus narrative that I discuss below.[92] Even as Mather points to the African source of inoculation, its inclusion in his correspondence with Woodward relegates the narrative to being but one of the many *Curiosa Americana* that he reported to the Royal Society—one might even argue that Mather sees himself as a model of the Society; as such, Onesimus's story is remarkable to Mather insofar as he codifies it within a growing transatlantic network of medical and scientific knowledge, and uses it to appropriate inoculation into a specifically Western—and American—medical tradition.[93]

The point that I am moving toward is that this process of appropriation is bound in the rhetorical qualities of the controversy, and that "style" and metaphor are therefore fundamental to the racialized logic that emerges from Mather's medical writing, and into the public debate about inoculation. If the Woodward letter appears to be a straightforward representation of fact with few, if any, obvious stylistic markers to distinguish this story from any number of events that Mather reported to the Royal Society, it is worth reading the various permutations of Onesimus's narrative as Mather rewrites it and brings it to print over the next decade. Modern critics tend to extrapolate the significance of the Onesimus narrative by reading any one of its multiple iterations, but I'd like to argue for reading them sequentially, and for piecing together what the various changes signify as they are presented to different audiences over time; rather than being a move toward increased accuracy or authentic replication of African language, Mather's revisions indicate a self-conscious engagement with audience, and an attempt to work through the epistemological relations between knowledge and form. Indeed, here is where the story's circulation in print plays an important role in appropriating inoculation into Western medical tradition—appropriating it *as* Western medicine. While it is difficult to establish the exact order in which these versions were composed—especially because a couple of them were written within days of each other—I will examine them in roughly chronological order, and by intended audience. The first variant I'd like to look at—written around September 7, 1721—is probably not the very first iteration of the story after the Woodward letter, but I begin with it because it was published in London (rather than Boston), as part of Mather's 1722 *Account*, and was thus written with an English audience in mind.

The *Account* is, of course, the pamphlet in which Mather mused explicitly on epistemological questions about metaphor and medical language as these applied to his citadel thesis of infection, so it is not insignificant that he represents Onesimus's story here in a relatively straightforward manner, as he had done in the Woodward letter. And given the overall style of the *Account*, Mather seems to have imagined a more genteel, sedate audience than the "Hell-Fire" club that haunted him in New England. Mather provides the following summary report for his English audience, including no obvious stylistic features to mark his slave's speech:

[Mather] successively met with a Number of Africans; who all, in their plain Way, without any Combination or Correspondence, agreed in one Story, viz. that in their Country (where they use to die like Rotten Sheep, when the Small-Pox gets among them) it is now become a common thing to cut a Place or two in their Skin, sometimes one Place, and sometimes another, and put in a little of the Matter of the Small-Pox; after which, they, in a few Days, grow a little Sick, and a few Small-Pox break out, and by and by they dry away; and that no Body ever dy'd of doing this, nor ever had the Small-Pox after it. Which last Point is confirm'd by their constant Attendance on the Sick in our Families, without receiving the Infection; and so considerable is the Number of these in our Neighbourhood, that he had as

evident Proof of the Practice, Safety, and Success of this Operation, as
we have that there are Lions in Africa.[94]

I draw attention to this version of the story because Mather's retelling all but
evacuates Onesimus's speaking voice (pluralized in this case, to include a
"Number of Africans") from the narrative itself. While Mather does make a
self-conscious stylistic judgment by pointing to the Africans' "plain way" of
speaking, the description is muted here in comparison to the iterations that
would be published in Boston, and is subservient to the fact that they speak
independently (i.e., "without any Combination or Correspondence") and with
one voice. Aside from the description of inoculation, Mather sees evidence of
inoculation's effectiveness in the fact that these Africans all appear to be immune to smallpox, even as they attend to the sick in Boston. Thus, even if
their speech could be discounted as testimony, their immunological condition
speaks for itself.

The story first circulated publicly in Boston, in a pamphlet titled *Some
Account of what is said of Innoculating or Transplanting the Small Pox*, published
some time between August 25 and September 4, 1721, under the name of
Zabdiel Boylston, but likely co-written with Mather.[95] By this time—and for
the Boston audience—Onesimus's narrative had changed in important ways.
Again, it had been generalized from the story of one man to the "one story" in
support of inoculation agreed upon by "all" Africans. Indeed, Mather/
Boylston argue that because these Africans are in agreement, their story is all
the more credible:

> That abundance of poor Negro's die of the Small Pox, till they learn
> this Way; that People take the Juice of the Small Pox, and Cut the
> Skin, and put in a drop; then by'nd by a little Sick, then few Small Pox;
> and no body dye of it: no body have Small Pox any more.[96]

As the narrative shifts from its broad focus on the effects of smallpox to a
decidedly unscientific description of the procedure, it takes on stylistic particularities, presumably in an attempt to mimic the language patterns of African
slaves in New England: the definite articles drop out, and the narrative
becomes increasingly diffuse; *thens* and *ands* follow one on top of the other,
suggesting an almost coincidental temporality in which unsophisticated Africans have as little mastery over the procedure as they have over language. It is
as if the ungrammatical syntax mystifies their use of inoculation in this version of the narrative, and as if Boylston and Mather suggest that to master the
technology of inoculation, one must also master language and storytelling—a

mastery that Mather's various histories of the epidemic and controversy are meant to demonstrate.

This effect is even more pronounced in *The Angel of Bethesda*, where definite articles all but disappear, and where the stilted language becomes central to the story itself:

> Grandy-many dy of the Small-Pox: But now they Learn This Way: People take Juice of Small-Pox; and cutty-skin, and putt in a Drop; then by'nd by a little sicky, sicky: then very few little things like Small-Pox; and no body dy of it; and no body have Small-Pox any more.[97]

Here again, the broken syntax goes hand in hand with the story's awkwardness, and because the story had been recast so may times, we can't simply characterize this latest version as a sign of Mather's desire to transcribe African speech accurately. For example, one should note the rhetorical progression in these three versions, beginning with the Woodward letter in which inoculation gives Onesimus "something of the smallpox," to Africans receiving "few Small Pox" in both the London and the Boylston *Account*, to the *Angel of Bethesda*, which describes "very few little things *like* Small-Pox" breaking out after inoculation. This shift from a clear recognition of the disease to Mather's use of simile in the *Angel of Bethesda* narrative displays a progressive movement from certainty toward ambiguity and confusion—a shift that Mather uses to represent the Africans' failure to master inoculation and medical knowledge. If anything, this latest iteration implies that inoculation is guided by an overarching transcendent authority beyond the Africans' grasp. Boylston and Mather make this point explicit when they write in *Some Account* that "in *Africa*, where the Poor Creatures dye of the *Small Pox* in the common way like Rotten Sheep, a Merciful GOD has taught them a *wonderful Preservative*"—a representation that reduces Africans to unwitting beneficiaries of inoculation, rather than sophisticated medical practitioners or compelling advocates.[98]

In her analysis of the inoculation controversy, Margot Minardi argues that Mather's *Angel of Bethesda* transcription of "eighteenth-century African English" is an attempt to "make his retelling as authentic (to his white readers) as possible."[99] While Minardi's argument is persuasive in its attempt to "read the inoculation controversy as part of the ongoing construction of race in the early modern world," I would clarify that more so than Mather's representation of the language itself in any given version of the Onesimus narrative, it is important to examine the various iterations of the story next to each other.[100] Its evolution over a number of iterations—for audiences in England and in Boston—offers striking evidence of Mather's deliberate editorial attention to the form of African speech as part of a public print performance. Whereas the London versions of the story demonstrate Mather's attempt to write a history of inoculation from the perspective of a detached metropolitan observer, with each iteration of the Boston version, Onesimus's narrative becomes increasingly fragmented, drawing attention to its formal properties, which are no longer mere quirks or curiosities, but central to the controversy itself, and deployed as strategic evidence in the service of creating new public health practices in New England. Boylston and Mather push us toward these conclusions with their quick gloss instructing the readers of *Some Account* on how to receive the story of inoculation's origins. Juxtaposing reason and rationality to narrative markers—and subverting Mather's earlier representation of Onesimus as "a pretty intelligent fellow"—they claim that the Africans "can have no Conspiracy or Combination to cheat us . . . the more plainly, brokenly, and blunderingly, and like Ideots, they tell their Story, it will be with reasonable Men, but the much more credible."[101] Again offering an echo of the London pamphlet, Boylston and Mather here replace "combination or correspondence" with "conspiracy or combination"—a change that hints at the charged reception of African testimony in Boston during the controversy, and suggests that Mather's editorial stance was strongly influenced by his experience of events during the epidemic. Their gloss is, of course, absurd, as it empties Onesimus's story of all but its formal significance, offering an important epistemological claim about the relation between form and truth in the process. It also provides a powerful framework for understanding the public circulation of Onesimus's narrative: it is an empty syllogism that compels repetition and circulation. Broken style stands in as the evidence of an assertion's truth, and this truth can be reproduced in print as brokenly and as often as necessary—certainly, Mather demonstrates as much in the iterations he produces between his 1716 letter to Woodward, and his composition of *The Angel of Bethesda* in the wake of the inoculation controversy.[102]

Not surprisingly, the anti-inoculators refused to buy into the argument, and Douglass bluntly rejected Mather's rhetorical gambit by drawing attention to the inherent fallacy of using style as a signifier of truth:

Their second Voucher is an Army of half a Dozen or half a Score Africans, by others call'd Negroe Slaves, who tell us now (tho' never before) that it is practiced in their own Country. The more blundering and Negroish they tell their Story, it is the more credible Says C.M; a paradox in Nature; for all they say true or false is after the same manner. There is not a Race of Men on Earth more False Lyars, &c. Their Accounts of what was done in their Country was never depended

upon till now for Arguments sake. Many Negroes to my knowledge
have assured their Masters that they had the Small Pox in their own
Country or elsewhere, and have now had it in Boston.[103]

As racially charged as these opening lines are, I want to draw attention to the
last sentence of Douglass's argument, which underscores the Africans' failure
to abide by the well-known temporalities of smallpox—namely, that once
infected with the disease, a person cannot contract it a second time. Having
apparently caught this "Army" describing a medical impossibility, Douglass
marshals heavy-handed racialized rhetoric to cast these many Africans as
either deceitful advocates or hopelessly naïve agents who don't understand
the basic mechanism of immunology. Either way, their failure to master a
common narrative echoes Mather's representation of African storytelling
abilities, even as the two work at cross-purposes. Perhaps just as oddly, Douglass's public comments are privately paralleled by Mather, who noted in his
diary entry for June 6, 1721, that Onesimus, who claimed to have been inoculated in Africa, "was afraid how the Small-pox, if it spread, may handle
him."[104] It is difficult to know what to make of such a revelation, given the
fact that Mather had used Onesimus's speech as evidence of his truth-telling,
and further claims to have seen "the Scar of the Wound made for the Operation" on Onesimus's arm.[105] Whether Onesimus was susceptible to smallpox
during this outbreak or not, Mather's report of his fear clearly undermines
the strength of his prior oral testimony, and emphasizes the faulty epidemiological temporality that Douglass would point to. What these comments
demonstrate is that both Mather and Douglass figure Africans as failed narrators, and stand on this representation—more specifically, on their own
ability to decipher African narrative—as the foundation for their arguments.
This moment in the controversy, which alights self-consciously on the formal
properties of African speech, and on the nuances of reading testimonial evidence, reveals the deep entanglements of medical rhetoric, print, and the
racial tropes that enact public health debates. Thus, what Miller bluntly dismissed as a "tiff about style" points us to the central work done by the ideologies of medical and print technology in early America—or what Mulford
calls the "liberalizing tendendencies" of the press and the "free practice of
medical science."[106]
    And yet even as the dominant trope of print and of the free press (and of
Western medicine) has been their liberalizing tendencies, it is worth considering how these tendencies take shape in Boston during the controversy, and
for whom. Whether the liberal subject that emerges from the inoculation controversy is embodied by Mather, Douglass, or either of the Franklins, it is

clear that he neither looks like nor sounds like Onesimus, or any other member of the "army of Africans" who spoke of inoculation.[107] More to the point, the emergence of this highly charged and narrowly defined liberal subject is built on the appropriation of an African medical practice, and the representation of African speech in print; the controversy's "stylistic" squabbles were not a detour, but central to how the liberal subject sees and speaks of himself in 1721 Boston, and to the exclusionary practices he employs in constraining the limits of that subjectivity. To highlight this point in a particularly graphic manner, even as the controversy might have given voice to the liberal subject in eighteenth-century Boston, it did so by simultaneously silencing—and renaming—the subject of liberalism; in his December 10, 1721, diary entry, Mather complained about the "Indignity" done to him by a stranger who mocked him for his faith in African testimony during the controversy by "call[ing] his Negro-Slave by the Name of Cotton Mather."[108] Thus even here, we see how deeply implicated the conventions of African slavery are in the representational practices of the inoculation controversy. Only by recapturing the sense that style circulated as a material practice do we fully come to terms with the relationship between ideology and narrative form in early-eighteenth-century Boston, and appropriate the function of epidemiological analysis for unpacking those relationships.

The public debate over inoculation was integral to transforming this African practice by first exoticizing it textually, and then systematizing and perfecting it as medicine in the Western tradition. Mather's medical and scientific knowledge is built on rhetorical figures such as the trope of the idiotic, blundering African, who becomes a formal and rhetorical affect, rather than through direct observation and experimentation (the language of science), which is what critics like Douglass advocated. While this trope obviously devalues African medical tradition, its function in the narrative is to provide a counterpoint to Mather's status as a scrupulous recorder of facts, and to his authority as a Fellow of the Royal Society. These representational practices rewrite the history of African medicine, translating it from a story in which Africans are active agents in the dissemination of inoculation, to one in which they figure as inarticulate objects of Western medical discourse. Eventually, texts such as Boylston's 1726 *Historical Account of the Small-Pox inoculated in New England* would continue the process of appropriating inoculation into Western traditions, and locating the procedure as an American one by narrating case histories in scrupulous detail, helping to formalize them within developing evidentiary frameworks, and demonstrating mastery over both the procedure and its narration in medical and scientific print communities. If Boston, Boylston, and Mather each have a place in the history of medicine, so too, is this place linked to specific literary productions and those productions formalized in the public discourse that framed the inoculation controversy. Understanding the controversy within the context of epidemiological frameworks effects a significant step toward reorienting the tools of literary criticism as a means of understanding their deployment in the service of national historiography. This is an argument for reconsidering the materials that we read, for reconfiguring our reading practices, and for addressing the relations between the traditions of our field, and the ideological work that we do when we study national literatures.

Ultimately, Miller may not have been entirely mistaken in his assessment of the controversy, although he certainly could not have seen how implicated these debates were in emerging discourses of slavery and colonialism in the eighteenth-century transatlantic world. As a case in point, although Douglass was opposed to inoculating Bostonians in 1721, this does not mean that he saw no benefit in the procedure. On the contrary, in an uncanny echo of his proposal to subjugate Native Americans through inoculation, he argued—with no satire or irony intended this time—that when tied to the economics of the slave trade, the procedure had a very specific value. Because the middle passage was so lethal, and because slave ships themselves were floating pest houses, Douglass calculated the financial benefits of inoculation as follows:

It is then a palliative Prevention of the Small Pox for some time, and not very mortal; and consequently may be of great Use to the Guinea Traders, when the Small Pox gets among their Slaves aboard to inoculate the whole Cargo, and patch them up for a Market; as is already the Practice with them in the other Pox or Yaws, by some slight, palliative Cure to fit them up for a quick Market, tho' to the great Damage of the next Purchasers.[109]

Here, the entire debate about smallpox and the use of inoculation comes into focus with a clarity that was never completely articulated elsewhere during the controversy. Sure, inoculation was a deep concern for public health in Boston, but this was because Boston did not seem to be the proper place for it in 1721. Where the slave trade helped turn Britain into a colonial empire, the movement of bodies across the Atlantic World facilitated the circulation of disease while at the same time being hindered by it.

Despite the irony of turning inoculation against the practitioners who had taught Westerners how to use it, only to see the procedure enhance their value as commodities, Douglass maintained that this technology was best deployed to make the slave trade more efficient. Slaves gained value if they survived smallpox because they would subsequently be immune to the disease. And to be as clear as possible about how widely such narratives circulated during the controversy, despite the ideological and stylistic differences between pro- and anti-inoculators, Mather, too, included a parallel version of this analysis in his London *Account*: "After this, he heard it affirm'd, That it is no unusual Thing for our Ships on the Coast of *Guinea*, when they ship their Slaves, to find out by Enquiry which of the Slaves have not yet had the Small-Pox; and so carry them a-shore, in this Way to give it to them, that the poor Creatures may sell for a better Price; where they are often (inhumanely enough) to be dispos'd of."[110]

Even as Mather and Douglass had widely divergent stances about medical and ministerial authority, and about the appropriate uses of inoculation in Boston, their writings nevertheless converged on a shared racialized ideology made manifest by the relation between smallpox and the slave trade. More specifically, it is the circulation of their writings as part of a public print debate—with its attendant formal and stylistic shifts—that marks the ideological work of the inoculation controversy: burying African knowledge and the agency of African narrators, on the one hand, while testing the boundaries of professional discourses, on the other. Indeed, my own commitments in this project are to demonstrate the inextricability of these trajectories, and to refocus critical attention on the literary qualities that are central—rather than peripheral—to medical histories such as this one. There remain, of course, deep political and cultural implications for this kind of analysis, and these open further avenues for literary critics to follow.

While the genesis of this project comes from my interest in medicine, I want to make the literary stakes of my broader epidemiological claims clear. Only by recapturing the sense that style circulated as a material practice, do we fully come to terms with the relationship between ideology and narrative form in early-eighteenth-century Boston. For a sense of what I mean by material practices, I point in two directions: first, as both Douglass and Mather attest, prior exposure to smallpox added an intrinsic value to slaves, whose owners did not have to worry about losing them to epidemics; advertisements for slave auctions would specify the fact that Africans being sold were immune to smallpox, and pockmarks—on the face, or like those Onesimus showed Mather on his arm—would come to have value, and become familiar features of the slave trade. Second, I turn to the August 22, 1722, issue of the *New England Courant*, published a year after James Franklin had founded the paper, and barely six months before his brother Benjamin would take over publication under an illicit compact famously recounted in the younger Franklin's *Autobiography*. This very issue opens with letter 11 from Silence Dogood—the fictive identity through which we imagine the origins of Benjamin Franklin as the representative eighteenth-century liberal man of letters, an identity that is, nevertheless, only realized when it is projected backward, abstracted, and read in the context of Franklin's later career as thinker, writer, and statesman. But read in the actual pages of the *Courant*—a text that represented Boston's literate classes to themselves—the Dogood letters must be considered next to the material that framed them, and understood in relation to the ongoing critique of print and liberalism that an epidemiological analysis of seventeenth- and eighteenth-century New England narratives makes available to us. The final words in this issue—an advertisement—draw us back to the smallpox epidemic and to the inoculation controversy of 1721, calling attention to a seemingly innocuous description that nevertheless marked the value of yet another nameless, silenced slave who would now circulate as an object of print culture, alongside Franklin's voice: "A Negro Man about Twenty Years of Age, fit for Town or Country Work, and has had the Small Pox, to be sold by Mr. Edward Pell, in Bennet Street at the North end of Boston."[111]

Afterword

The master's house must be dismantled. Only Allmuseri was to
be spoken by the crew when in contact with the newly empow-
ered bondmen. Cringle was to use maps Ghofan was preparing;
he did not trust the ones Falcon had left. In addition to this, he
forbade us to sing songs in English, his oppressor's tongue, whilst
we worked. He said we must learn their stories. Nurture their god.
Allmuseri medicine was to be used to treat sickness and injuries.

—Charles Johnson, *Middle Passage*[1]

As I outlined in the introduction to this book, *Miraculous Plagues* is bookended
by two major epidemics: the 1616–19 outbreaks that devastated Native populations in New England, and the smallpox epidemic that infected more than
half of the people living in Boston in 1721. I have argued that by considering
these epidemics as part of a common immunological trajectory rather than as
independent historical events, we can better understand the role of epidemiology in shaping colonial narrative practices. In the analytic model that I have
proposed, New England's literary history is embedded in local population densities, migration patterns, and shared immunities, which, considered in the
aggregate, complicate narratives of how and where settlers understood their
place in the world, and how they came to terms with their experiences of illness and health; colonial responses to early epidemics set in motion a discursive trajectory that guided the forms and assumptions deployed by later
generations of settlers who sought to explain the epidemical patterns they
witnessed and lived through. As I have shown, these communal assumptions
are visible in the formal and thematic properties of epidemiological texts, so
my aim in this afterword is to reflect on how such seventeenth-century

properties speak to an analysis of modern epidemiology. Throughout the book, I have insisted on supplementing spatial mappings of epidemics with a temporal analysis of epidemiology in order to account for the cross-generational dynamics that inflected the history of illness in New England. It is this temporal analysis that connects the 1616–19 epidemics to Boston's 1721 smallpox outbreak by highlighting the cyclical operation of herd immunity, and, just as significantly, that structures colonial encounters between English settlers, Native Americans, and Africans throughout the seventeenth and early eighteenth centuries. As a case in point, I call attention to a set of parallels between the narratives of Tisquantum and Onesimus—or, to be more accurate, between the various English iterations of those narratives. The first and most obvious similarity is that both stories were obsessively edited and rewritten by English settlers until the principal actors (Tisquantum and Onesimus) literally disappeared from the texts, to be replaced by a nameless "salvage" when Thomas Morton repeated Tisquantum's narrative, and an "Army of Africans" when Cotton Mather finally abstracted Onesimus's during the inoculation controversy.[2] While this abstraction erases individual Native American and African agency from the texts, I want to argue that the process reveals how self-conscious the representations are. This erasure underscores the colonialist ends of epidemiology, and it helps to appropriate the experience of English settlers as a function of their health and their mastery of narrative practices.

     As powerful as this mechanism is for structuring colonial encounters, I now focus on a second parallel that exists between the narratives—this one having to do specifically with the temporal function of epidemiology. In the case of Tisquantum's description of epidemics, we will recall that his etiology of the plague inverted the basic temporality of English justification narratives: instead of diseases preceding the migration, as in the traditional trope of these epidemiological narratives, Tisquantum's story implied that epidemics arrived in the wake of early colonial encounters—that Europeans were responsible for the epidemics, and had it under their control. Though this counter-epidemiology is at odds with English justifications, the fact of the matter is that by abstracting, generalizing, and ventriloquizing Tisquantum's words, settlers represented his temporal framework as a sign of Native American superstition, and a fundamental inability to master the basic genre of epidemiology. It further becomes clear by reading their commentaries on Tisquantum's narrative that the English were more interested in what they saw as his awkward attempt to manipulate epidemiological rhetoric for his own political and economic ends, than in his actual etiology of the "miraculous plague," which, in their version of events, was absurd. In short, though Tisquantum's counter-epidemiology might seem to disrupt or undermine

English etiologies, the representation of Tisquantum's apparently self-serving goal helps to paper over the settlers' use of epidemiology for the same political and economic ends—a move that is thus integral to the narrative role that Native Americans play in early colonial epidemiology.

Onesimus's narrative likewise functions in an inverted temporal space— manifested both in the syntactical confusion that arises when Mather ventril- oquized African explanations for the mechanism of inoculation, and, more potently, in William Douglass's assertion that African narratives failed to abide by the well-known temporalities of smallpox. When Douglass points to slaves who claim to have had smallpox in Africa only to be infected by it in New England, he does so with an eye to undermining their credibility as witnesses, and to label them as a "Race of . . . False Lyars."[3] By the same token, Mather's report that Onesimus was afraid of succumbing to smallpox even after having been inoculated in Africa (a claim that if made public would undermine his advocacy of the procedure) highlights his slave's failure to verbalize the well- known temporalities of smallpox immunity.[4] Such admissions certainly reflect Mather's broader ambivalence about the particular significance of Onesimus's speech, which, as he translates it into its various print editions, comes to sig- nify formally rather than for its specific content. Thus, what becomes clear in the print circulation of Onesimus's narrative is how quickly the content of his speech is subsumed to its formal and stylistic features in order to enact colo- nial relations between Anglo-Americans and Africans in New England.

Through the multiple iterations of their respective narratives, Tisquantum and Onesimus are both transformed into rhetorical figures, and appropriated by English epidemiologies in the service of colonialism. What I want to emphasize here is that this appropriation is structured by the temporalities that define colonial spaces: the inverted temporalities make Onesimus and Tisquantum interesting to colonial audiences, but these inversions, by virtue of the fact that they appear to be so absurd to seventeenth- and eighteenth- century readers, come to stand as evidence in support of English colonial epi- demiologies—that is, as epidemiological evidence in support of the colonial project. The temporality of colonial subjects like Tisquantum and Onesimus serves as the backdrop against which English settlers structure their epidemi- ologies, and narrate their immunological reactions to the environment. It is this structuring—or mapping—that I have argued is central to the work of colonial epidemiology, and which, if traced further, reveals a critical frame- work for rethinking the relation between place, history, and identity. Indeed, my interest in the temporal schema of epidemiology is meant to draw attention to the way that local and regional experiences of disease work at cross-purposes with teleological models of historiography by disrupting the role of nation as a coherent organizing principle. This is an aim that resonates with the work of historians such as Thomas Bender, who, in his commitment to rethinking American history in a global age, questions the primacy of nationhood as "the principle of organization for history departments and graduate training."[5] In Bender's model, nation and temporality form a matrix for historiographic analysis, but, he adds, an overreliance on national paradigms leads to an uneasy circular argument in which the discipline promises to examine the very political entities that it is invested in reproducing:

> To the degree that European and American historians (and the public) were committed to evolutionary theories (and the commitment was considerable), place in time distinguished historical from nonhistorical societies. One could even say that this temporal difference was spatialized. Those peoples not organized in nations—referring mainly to colonies of European powers—were not only outside of the system of nations, they were outside of its understanding of "normal" time, or put differently, they were "backward," even though they were contemporary and entangled with the imperial powers.[6]

Bender's critique identifies the determinant quality of national historiography as a framework that collapses spatiality and temporality into the normative unit of political analysis, and he recognizes that this process is legitimized through academic and popular tellings and retellings of stories. As I understand it, the task Bender proposes is to seek out entanglements rather than smooth them over, and to locate reading practices that abide by the ongoing ideological work of community and nation building in order to defamiliarize what he later calls "the American historical experience."[7] This is not the same thing as displacing one narrative for another in an effort to construct increasingly accurate national histories, but it compels us to consider the critical tools at our disposal, as well as the grammars of reading that these tools introduce to us—grammars that organize literary practices and traditions into national frameworks, and that help us to reimagine the commitment we make when we test the boundaries of our field.

As I have argued throughout *Miraculous Plagues*, a close attention to epidemiology offers critical and analytic strategies that display the entanglements Bender points to. In particular, my elaboration of Tisquantum's and Onesimus's narratives demonstrates that these counter-epidemiologies speak directly to the work that colonial powers do in representing colonial subjects as "nonhistorical" entities, and that these representations become starkly visible in the obsessive rewriting and editing of their stories. Thus, what looks at first to be an odd, but coincidental series of temporal inversions that crop up at different moments in New England's history, reveals instead the way that epidemiology structures colonial hierarchies, and gives voice to specific historiographic traditions. With this in mind, the epidemiology of narrative that I have undertaken here has been calibrated to expose the role of immunity and susceptibility in making geographic landscapes and nationalist historiographies transparent as the strategic effects of colonial rhetoric. As I project these epidemiological functions into the late twentieth and early twenty-first centuries, I am most interested in reflecting on how modern Western epidemiology continues to map non-Western spaces in relation to the boundaries between health and illness. Insofar as this book is an Early American studies monograph, I take an unorthodox approach by focusing the remainder of my energies on late-twentieth- and early-twenty-first-century HIV/AIDS epidemiology with a specific emphasis on Africa. Unusual as this trajectory may seem, my analysis suggests that Western epidemiologies of HIV/AIDS in Africa call on a long tradition of colonial tropes, and bring pressure to bear on national and territorial boundaries by translating modern political geographies onto nineteenth-century images of the continent. HIV/AIDS epidemiology is a useful subject because of the way that the virus and disease have confounded medical and public health communities by disrupting categories of health, behavior, and pathogens even as geopolitical boundaries have continued to fragment themselves in the wake of the Cold War.

The significance of a virus like HIV and of a disease like AIDS at the beginning of the twenty-first century lies in the power of each to reconfigure apparently stable categories of identity, and to alienate national, medical, and critical boundaries from their territorial contexts. Their significance to the field of Early American studies is perhaps less clear at first glance, but I mean my reading of HIV/AIDS epidemiology to reflect on the intertwined medical, theological, and juridical landscapes of colonial New England, as these engage increasingly vexed notions of territoriality. To draw out the point further, I contend that positioning HIV/AIDS epidemiology in Africa as a model for approaching Early American studies is not, in fact, as counterintuitive as appears on the surface. Indeed, the inspiration for this approach comes from a rereading of Perry Miller's notoriously epiphanic moment on the banks of the Congo, when "the mission of expounding what [he] took to be the innermost propulsion of the United States" was "thrust" upon him in the vision of a singular, monolithic narrative New England history.[8] Early Americanists have revisited Miller's scene time and again, usually to point out that its deeply imperialist world view has important implications for the way that his work unfolded, and for the monolithic vision of New England that he represented—often at the expense of marginalized voices, and of what Janice Knight has called the plural *orthodoxies* that were integral to the early colonial experience in Puritan New England.[9] My reading of HIV/AIDS epidemiology is thus a deliberate return to the scene of Miller's epiphany, where our alternate visions of African geography reflect on our relationship to the field in important ways. If Miller's stance toward the people and scenery before him on the banks of the Congo shaped his understanding of a New England "mind," my reading of Africa is also guided with an eye to framing a vision of Early American studies that is steeped in biological and cultural heterogeneity rather than homogeneity, that is fractured rather than monolithic, and for which a history of epidemics focuses attention on colonial bodies as well as minds.

To illustrate these claims, I consider how epidemiologies of the African HIV/AIDS pandemic reify representations of the continent in the popular historical imagination, and how these representations are bound in a broader discourse about the identity of HIV, as well as the search for a vaccine against the disease. On January 6, 2002, for example, the *San Francisco Chronicle* published an article by Rian Malan under the title "Megadeath and Megahype."[10] Ignoring, for a moment, the ironic self-reflexivity of the headline, Malan describes the difficulties of tracking AIDS statistics in Africa, and the impact of these problems on what he calls the transformation of "the destiny of AIDS." Simply speaking, this is a lay-epidemiological account of the relationship between medical practices and history, and, as it turns out, the geographies of the third world. A passage from the middle of the article illustrates the kinds of representations that I examine:

> In 1985, the WHO people asked experts to hammer out a simple description of AIDS that would enable bush doctors to recognize the symptoms and start counting cases. It was a fiasco—mostly because African governments were too disorganized to collect the numbers and send them in. Hence, when it's announced that 14 million Africans have succumbed to AIDS, it does not mean that 14 million infected bodies have been counted. It means that 14 million people have theoretically died, some of them unseen in Africa's swamps, shantytowns and vast swaths of terra incognita.[11]

Malan's sweeping characterization of African governments as being too disorganized to keep accurate statistical records of AIDS cases and fatalities provides a striking counterpoint to his own reorganization of African geography around Western taxonomies of the epidemic. His reference to 14 million deaths—theoretical or otherwise—draws a metonymic relation between an amorphous, ill-defined population of provisionally dead subjects, and what he calls "Africa's swamps, shantytowns and vast swaths of terra incognita," where individual susceptibility to an immuno-suppressant retrovirus becomes symbolic of the medical deficiencies of an entire continent.

Such representations of HIV/AIDS transform the political history of Africa into the history of a continent's failures to treat disease—as if bush doctors were incapable of recognizing a mysterious new illness until Western doctors had discovered it within their own well-defined borders and named it themselves, or as if Western medical and economic models were not at least complicit in producing the African pandemic. It is Malan's implied thesis about the taxonomies and treatments of HIV/AIDS that frame his conception of Africa as a "terra incognita"—a move that clearly represents differences in medical technology between Africa and modern Western nations spatially. By highlighting African failures to contain HIV/AIDS as an endemic function of governmental disorganization, Malan's narrative implicitly suggests the power of Western medicine to do so—a tall claim indeed. And by transforming African geographies into a series of illegible spaces where geopolitical borders are washed away by waves of disease, Malan further implies that Western nations are themselves healthy, coherent, and stable. Although this transformation of colonial history by Western medicine appears to be seamless, the elision of geopolitical boundaries is rarely so neat, and medical discourses are rarely so transparent. In the contemporary African case, these discourses operate in a prior colonial context, reformulating rather than replacing it, and revealing the power of epidemiological narratives to simultaneously cover over and reappropriate geographical spaces while reimagining national, cultural, and ideological matrices.

Where the history of African colonization once structured national borders according to economic and geopolitical interests, these borders were destabilized at the end of the Cold War when the two global superpowers began to renegotiate their own boundaries in relation to the world. This is not to say that African nation-states have disappeared during the last twenty years (although some have, while others have undergone major political reorganizations and name changes, and yet others have come into being), but that the continent has been dramatically reconceptualized in relation to the West. Among the various paradigms that have reoriented geopolitical borders are the polarization of religious difference (especially of Islam in relation to the American "global" war on terror), ethnic cleansing and genocide (in the Sudan and Rwanda), national programs of land redistribution (in Zimbabwe), and the epidemiological mappings of disease (like malaria, Ebola, and HIV/AIDS). If the visual representation of Africa in the modern Western imagination has historically relied on the trope of a dark continent, or been given as a relation between charted and uncharted territory (representations still produced in association with hemorrhagic fevers like Ebola), the imaginary reconstruction of its post–Cold War geography is most apparent in HIV/AIDS clade maps that trace the spatial distribution of HIV's distinct genetic subtypes. As with Malan's description, nations tend to lose their individual autonomies and are recast according to regional immunological sensitivities and transmission networks in these maps.[12] But because HIV/AIDS itself is not constrained by national boundaries, these clade maps tend to organize information in ways that bypass geopolitical structures of governance, reconfiguring them according to regional circulations of HIV, and highlighting the notion that African lands themselves are unhealthy. While these maps do not represent Africa as "terra incognita," they do suggest a continent whose turbulent political boundaries reflect heterogeneous populations of sick subjects.

It is exactly this transformative power to map land that I argue is fundamental to the ideological work done by epidemiology. And while I have briefly charted this power on a geopolitical axis with respect to representing African geographies, these mappings are, in fact, contiguous with representations of pathogens. In the case of HIV/AIDS, the clade maps that trace the related but diverging genetic histories of the virus reveal that the Western industrialized world is predominantly affected by one major strain of HIV (Clade B), while Africa is by at least three (including Clades A, C, and D). The multiple African strains of HIV demonstrate that the virus—or viruses, depending on how we want to categorize identity—has spread across the continent at an alarming pace, offering a striking counterpoint to the relative homogeneity of HIV/AIDS distribution in industrialized nations. Unlike Francis Black's analysis of "New World" immune systems, homogeneity in this case is neither a bad sign nor necessarily imprinted genetically on humans.[13] Indeed, if homogeneity is a rhetorical concept that can be applied to HIV/AIDS in the West, it might best describe the economic and ideological apparatus that characterizes current medical approaches to the treatment of HIV and AIDS—a philosophy of treatment based on policing personal behaviors, on tracking viral loads, and on treating individual immune systems, rather than on reorganizing social and economic networks. The heterogeneity of Africa's HIV/AIDS pandemic suggests the failure of these policing techniques, and implies that solutions might best be drawn from an array of medical as well as nonmedical strategies. African HIV/AIDS clade maps may therefore not describe the unfitness of African bodies or cultures to resist the epidemic, but reveal deep fissures in the application of Western medical and infrastructural strategies on the African continent. Although more "official" than Malan's representations, such maps reconfigure geopolitical borders, suggesting that these are as mutable as the virus, and they raise fundamental questions about the very notion of boundary itself. Not to draw too fine a point on the matter, these representations imply a deeply embedded relation between the conception of identity on national and viral scales.

While the development of HIV/AIDS medicines will necessarily take place in laboratories, treatments themselves must consider the historical, geographic, legal, and economic stages on which the disease operates to be successful in a timely fashion and on a global scale. Such considerations, I argue, are available through a narrative analysis of epidemiology, and through an understanding of the way that HIV/AIDS epidemiology shapes medical practices and spatial organizations of the world. Indeed, the virus's mutability is central to the question of HIV/AIDS treatments, and hangs over the continuing efforts to develop an AIDS vaccine. In a claim that privileges the primary importance of identifying pathogenic agents in order to treat illness successfully, Margaret Heckler, the Secretary of Health and Human Services under Ronald Reagan, projected in 1984 that a vaccine would be completed in little more than two years after the discovery of HIV as the causative agent of AIDS. Nearly twenty years after this claim, Carol Ezzell revisited Heckler's pronouncement, and addressed the major roadblocks that continued to hinder the development of an HIV/AIDS vaccine in a way that makes the representational issues of this seemingly biological question remarkably clear for literary critics: "Retroviruses also reproduce rapidly and sloppily, providing ample opportunity for the emergence of mutations that allow HIV to shift its identity and thereby give the immune system or antiretroviral drugs the slip."[14] For HIV to be defined by its ability to "shift its identity" suggests a deeper question about the nature of identity in relation to illness and epidemic. HIV's success at giving immune systems "the slip" disrupts seemingly stable ontological categories, and positions the identity of HIV as a function of its mutability, rather than as a quality that rests in any fixed essential or physical characteristic. In other words, the identity of HIV in the context of medical research and vaccination programs—that which makes it so difficult to treat—inheres in its ability to disrupt stable categories of identity.

This ontological problem manifests itself microscopically in the behaviors of HIV just outlined, and macroscopically in the way that AIDS repositions international and geopolitical boundaries in official maps as well as in lay epidemiologies such as Malan's. Here, I am arguing for reading practices that recognize the fundamental tension between health and nation in an ontological framework over and against a representational one. What HIV/AIDS (or more appropriately, HIV/AIDS epidemiology) reveals are the ways in which epidemics and their treatments cannot easily be separated from the

representational practices that describe them. But these effects describe neither HIV nor AIDS. They are symptomatic of the cultural and the medical discourses that help us to imagine HIV/AIDS and its treatments in the Western
world. Where national myths reveal ontological assumptions about cultural
and territorial boundaries, these assumptions reflect a similar ontological understanding of bodies and human health. Since Western epidemiologists first
became aware that a loose set of physical symptoms could be grouped under
the umbrella of AIDS in the early 1980s, the disease has gone from epidemic
to pandemic in Africa, obviating the nineteenth- and twentieth-century borders drawn by European colonial powers to organize the continent into national and colonial economies. As these borders collapse on one another and
reconfigure African geographies, they bear a haunting reminder that the problem is not just a foreign one; despite the United States' struggles to contain
HIV/AIDS within clearly defined communal spaces, its failures to do so point
to the porousness of the same borders that it is so determined to protect.

Even as I focus on HIV/AIDS in Africa, I remain aware that in doing so, I
risk replicating the very representational stance that I seek to dismantle, by
projecting illness onto the developing world over and against a national imaginary that assumes a standard of healthfulness within America's borders;
indeed, such an imaginary is dependent on these very projections in order to
represent itself as fundamentally healthy. I would like to trouble this imaginary by closing with a brief word on the 2004 debate between Vice President
Dick Cheney and the Democratic nominee John Edwards. During the debate,
moderator Gwen Ifill asked the candidates about the HIV/AIDS epidemic in
America. "In particular," she said, "I want to talk to you . . . not about AIDS in
China or Africa, but AIDS right here in this country, where black women
between the ages of twenty-five and forty-four are thirteen times more likely
to die of the disease than their counterparts. What should the government's
role be in helping to end the growth of this epidemic?"[15] Appearing as it did in
a debate on national security, Ifill's question turned the discussion inward at a
crucial moment—not with an eye to protecting a nebulously defined homeland, but to define the spaces within America that continue to remain unseen
and unprotected as Americans look outward to identify potential threats to
the nation. Answering first, Cheney focused immediately on the very topic
that Ifill had asked him not to address, and pointed to the Bush administration's $15 billion package to "help in the international effort" against HIV/
AIDS, and touted the "significant progress" that the United States had made
in treating the disease on the domestic front. Nevertheless, he ended with the
strikingly candid admission that "I have not heard those numbers with respect
to African American women. I was not aware that it was—that they're in

epidemic there, because we have made progress in terms of the overall rate of AIDS infection . . . . Obviously we need to do more." Not to be outdone, Edwards responded to the same question by pledging that a Kerry administration would double Bush's international investment in HIV/AIDS programs, before he moved on to speak about genocide in Sudan, and about what he called the "bigger question" of health-care coverage in America.

Ifill was visibly frustrated with these responses. Both candidates addressed issues that she had specifically asked them not to discuss, and both ignored the effects of HIV/AIDS on black women in America. Indeed, though Cheney at least acknowledged Ifill's question, his admission that he was "not aware" AIDS was still epidemic in this country—and both his and Edwards's instinct to shift the site of HIV/AIDS infection from America to Africa—is symptomatic of a model of nationhood that doesn't quite know what to do with unhealthy American bodies. Moreover, Cheney's use of the phrase "they're in epidemic there" severs the community of 25- to 44-year-old African American women from the broader conceptual notion of America, figuring this population as a "they," rather than part of the collective national "we," but just as significantly, representing these women as a location—a "there"—distinct from the "here" of the healthy American body politic. While one is tempted to suggest that it would be easier to ignore these women by exiling them to a foreign space, the debate's great irony is that the candidates were more than willing to talk about HIV/AIDS in Africa, where its presence across the Atlantic acts as an ideological counterpoint to America's imagined healthfulness, and its "progress" against the disease on the home front. Indeed, Cheney's "there" isolates African American women with HIV/AIDS in an indeterminate space that is neither foreign nor domestic, where they become a rhetorical affect, relegated to the margins of public discourse, and where their HIV status does not contradict images of the nation's mythically robust health.

Whether the subject is the war on terror, homeland security, or illegal immigration, the default rhetorical strategy of America's political discourse assumes that the nation is, at its core, composed of a united, coherent citizenry, and clearly defined borders. As I have argued, these rhetorical strategies are intimately bound to representations of health, and we can certainly turn to colonial New England to examine the process that gives weight to these strategies by imagining the West in relation to Africa. If the seventeenth century doesn't teach us how to treat disease in the twenty-first century, attention to the reading practices at the heart of justification narratives, the Antinomian controversy, the halfway covenant, the jeremiad, and public health debates like Boston's 1721 inoculation controversy does defamiliarize our understanding of what epidemiology is, and of how medical rhetoric functions; the figures of

Tisquantum and Onesimus teach us about the history of epidemics and their treatments in New England, about the interlinked histories of colonialism and Western medicine, and about how to read the ideological fields of medical rhetoric—whether professional or circulating openly in the public sphere. These reading practices teach us about the ways in which health and nation constitute one another in terms of a geopolitics of medicine. Indeed, as the United States is forced to confront the health of its own citizens, and as geopolitical boundaries around the world collapse on and reconfigure one another, they provide an uncanny reminder that the problem is not just a foreign one.

I end with the Cheney–Edwards vice-presidential debate because this is where the enduring legacy of epidemiology's discursive practices comes to the forefront. If providing aid to African nations is laudable in and of itself, Ifill's question—and both Cheney's and Edwards's inability to address, let alone answer it—suggests that acknowledging Africa's systemic problems in treating HIV/AIDS has a significant effect on the terms through which we imagine American health and national identity. Like it had for Mather and Malan, Africa functions in the vice-presidential debate as a rhetorical figure that, because it is in the midst of a pandemic, projects the Western world—and the U.S. in particular—as a model of health. These figures imply that America has been successful at treating HIV/AIDS within its own borders, that its treatment programs are effective, and that they can be exported to the world as a model of humanitarianism, if only developing nations could replicate Western medical and governmental infrastructures. Ifill's alarming statistic about the incidence of HIV/AIDS among 25- to 44-year-old African American women puts the lie to this image, and reveals that the virus remains entrenched within America's borders, that those very treatments we are exporting are themselves suspect on local, regional, and geopolitical scales, and that the stable national identities implied by Malan's rhetoric are anything but. So what are the stakes of Ifill's desire to shift attention from African to African *American* HIV/AIDS in the middle of a debate about national security? Deliberate or not, Cheney's—and Edwards's—language is particularly meaningful in the context of the 2004 general election, which made protecting America *the* central overarching issue of the new millennium. If both campaigns cast the election as a referendum on who could best protect the nation's borders, we should note that since September 2001, few have addressed these seemingly simple questions in a comprehensive fashion: *Where* are those borders located? *How* are they constituted? And *what* is the homeland? The vice-presidential candidates' inability to talk about HIV/AIDS and African American women suggests that the concept of nationhood—and therefore of national borders—is more tangled than we would like to imagine at the beginning of the twenty-first century.

NOTES

Introduction

1. John Edgar Wideman, *Fever* (New York: Penguin, 1989), 145.
2. For histories of the biological conquest of North America, see Sherburne F. Cook, "The Significance of Disease in the Extinction of the New England Indians," *Human Biology* 45 (1973): 485–508; William Cronon, *Changes in the Land: Indians, Colonists, and the Ecology of New England* (New York: Hill and Wang, 1989); Alfred W. Crosby, "Virgin Soil Epidemics as a Factor in the Aboriginal Depopulation in America," *William and Mary Quarterly*, 33 (1976): 289–99, and *The Columbian Exchange: Biological and Cultural Consequences of 1492*, 30th ann. ed. (Westport, CT: Praeger, 2003); John Duffy, *Epidemics in Colonial America* (Baton Rouge: Louisiana State University Press, 1953); Donald R. Hopkins, *Princes and Peasants* (Chicago: University of Chicago Press, 1983); Francis Jennings, *The Invasion of America: Indians, Colonialism and the Cant of Conquest* (New York: Norton, 1975); David S. Jones, *Rationalizing Epidemics: Meanings and Uses of American Indian Mortality since 1600* (Cambridge, MA: Harvard University Press, 2004), and "Virgin Soils Revisited," *William and Mary Quarterly*, 60 (2003): 703–42; William McNeill, *Plagues and Peoples* (New York: Anchor, 1998); Roy Harvey Pearce, *Savagism and Civilization* (Berkeley: University of California Press, 1988); E. Wagner Stearn and Allen E. Stearn, *The Effects of Small-Pox on the Destiny of the Amerindian* (Boston: Humphries, 1945); Sheldon Watts, *Epidemics and History: Disease, Power and Imperialism* (New Haven, CT: Yale University Press, 1997); and Noah Webster, *A Brief History of Epidemic and Pestilential Diseases*, 2 vols. (Hartford, CT, 1799).
3. Thomas C. Timmreck, *An Introduction to Epidemiology*, 3rd ed. (Boston: Jones, 2002), 4.
4. For more on the work of epidemiologists, see Timmreck; Abraham M. Lilienfeld and David E. Lilienfeld, *Foundations of Epidemiology*, 2nd ed. (New York: Oxford University Press, 1980); and Judith S. Mausner and Anita K. Bahn, *Epidemiology: An Introductory Text* (Philadelphia: Saunders, 1974).
5. John Snow, *On the Mode of Communication of Cholera* (1855), repr. in *Snow on Cholera* (London: Oxford University Press, 1936). See also Steven Johnson, *The Ghost Map: The Story of London's Most Terrifying Epidemic—and How It Changed Science, Cities, and the Modern World* (New York: Penguin 2006).
6. Robert Koch was recognized as the first to isolate the *vibrio cholerae* bacillus in 1883, though it was later acknowledged that Filippo Pacini had done so in 1854, the same year as the London epidemic (Johnson, 213).
7. See Cindy Patton's critique of tropical medicine and the mapping of HIV/AIDS in urban environments: *Globalizing AIDS* (Minneapolis: University of Minnesota Press, 2002), esp. chap. 4, "A Dying Epidemiology," 114–32, and "Performativity and Spatial Distinction:

The End of AIDS Epidemiology," *Performativity and Performance*, eds. Andrew Parker and Eve Kosofsky Sedgwick (New York: Routledge, 1995), 173–96.

8. See Patton, *Globalizing AIDS* and "Performativity and Spatial Distinction"; and Priscilla Wald, *Contagious: Cultures, Carriers, and the Outbreak Narrative* (Durham, NC: Duke University Press, 2008), and "Imagined Immunities," *Cultural Studies and Political Theory*, ed. Jodi Dean (Ithaca, NY: Cornell University Press, 2000), 189–208.

9. Patton, *Globalizing AIDS*, xxvi. See also Wald, *Contagious*, 3.

10. Patton, *Globalizing AIDS*, 33.

11. Patton, *Globalizing AIDS*, 40.

12. Wald, *Contagious*, 3.

13. Wald, *Contagious*, 33. See also Benedict Anderson, *Imagined Communities: Reflections on the Origin and Spread of Nationalism*, rev. ed. (New York: Verso, 1991).

14. Wald, *Contagious*, 54.

15. Wald, *Contagious*, 53, 49.

16. For more on virgin soil, see Crosby, "Virgin Soil Epidemics"; and Jones, "Virgin Soils Revisited," and *Rationalizing Epidemics*.

17. Letter from Cotton Mather to John Woodward, July 12, 1716, *Selected Letters of Cotton Mather*, ed. Kenneth Silverman (Baton Rouge: Louisiana State University Press, 1971), 213.

18. John Winthrop, *Generall Considerations for the Plantation in New England, with an Answer to Several Objections* (1629), repr. in *The Winthrop Papers*, vol. 2, ed. Stewart Mitchell (Boston: Massachusetts Historical Society, 1931), 120.

19. John Winthrop, *A Short Story of the Rise, reign, and ruine of the Antinomians, Familists & Libertines, that infected the Churches of New-England* (1644), repr. in David Hall, ed., *The Antinomian Controversy 1636–1638: A Documentary History*, 2nd ed. (Durham, NC: Duke University Press, 1990), 199–310, 218.

20. Winthrop, *Short Story*, 263.

21. Winthrop, *Short Story*, 262, 310; and *A Report of the Trial of Anne Hutchinson* in Hall, ed., 349–88, 383.

22. Patton, *Globalizing AIDS*, 118. See also Patton, "Performativity and Spatial Distinction."

23. For more on herd immunity, see Lilienfeld and Lilienfeld, 61; Timmreck, 49–51; and Wald, *Contagious*, 48–53.

24. See Duffy, 19–23, 106.

25. Perry Miller, *The New England Mind: From Colony to Province* (Cambridge, MA: Harvard University Press, 1953), 316.

26. See Anderson; and Wald, "Imagined Immunities," and *Contagious*.

27. Letter from Cotton Mather to John Woodward, July 12, 1716, repr. in *Selected Letters of Cotton Mather*, ed. Kenneth Silverman (Baton Rouge: Louisiana State University Press, 1971), 214.

28. William Douglas, *Inoculation of the Small Pox as practiced in Boston, Consider'd in a Letter to A__S__M.D. & F.R.S. in London* (Boston, 1722), 7.

Chapter 1

1. Ishmael Reed, *Mumbo Jumbo* (New York: MacMillan, 1972), 6.

2. Samuel de Champlain, *The Voyages of Sieur de Champlain* (1613), trans. Charles Pomeroy Otis, repr. in *Publications of the Prince Society* (1878; repr., New York: Burt Franklin, 1966), 12:64–65, 72–73.

3. John Smith, *A Description of New England: Or The Observations, and discoveries, of Captain John Smith (Admirall of that Country) in the North of America, in the year of our Lord 1614* (London, 1616), 26. This description is also repeated in Smith, *The Generall Historie of Virginia, New-England, and the Summer Isles with the names of the Adventurers, Planters, and Governours from their first Beginning Anno 1584 to this present 1624* (London, 1624), 215.

4. Robert Cushman, *Reasons and Considerations touching the lawfulness of removing out of England into the parts of America,* in *A Journal of the Pilgrims at Plymouth* [*Mourt's Relation*], ed. Dwight Heath (1622; repr., Cambridge, MA: Applewood Books, 1986), 88–96, 93.

5. Prime examples of such narratives include Cushman, *Reasons and Considerations;* John Winthrop, *Generall Considerations for the Plantation in New England, with an Answer to Several Objections* (1629), repr. in *The Winthrop Papers,* vol. 2, ed. Stewart Mitchell (Boston: Massachusetts Historical Society, 1931); [John White], *The Planters Plea. Or The Grounds of Plantations Examined, and Usuall Objections Answered* (London, 1630); Francis Higginson, *New Englands Plantation. Or, A Short and True Description of the Commodities and Discommodities of that Countrey* (London, 1630); and Smith, *Advertisements for the Unexperienced Planters of New-England, or any where. Or, the Pathway to experience to erect a Plantation* (London, 1631). Long after the initial migrations themselves, justification narratives maintained their ideological hold on New England's mythologized past in histories such as Edward Johnson, *A History of New-England* [*Wonder-Working Providence of Sions Saviour*] (London, 1654).

6. Thomas Dermer, "To his Worshipfull Friend M. Samuel Purchas, Preacher of the Word, at the Church a little within Ludgate, London," (1619) in Samuel Purchas, *Hakluytus Posthumus or Purchas His Pilgrimes* (1625; repr., Glasgow: James MacLehose, 1906), 19:129.

7. The characterization of these events as a "series" of epidemics is problematic in and of itself, and I use the plural because the range of years covered suggests that in spite of seventeenth-century English accounts that the epidemic was a singular event, it is far more likely that several diseases recurred periodically; Smith, for example, noted that "they had three plagues in three years successively neere two hundred miles along the Sea coast" (*Advertisements,* 9). The lack of extant concrete eyewitness accounts of these epidemics means that the range of years during which they occurred is itself in question, with most references placing its beginning around 1616; some see its end as early as 1617, and others as late as 1620. Estimates for pre-contact populations are notoriously difficult to calculate—as are, by extension, estimates of mortality rates for epidemics, which in this case range from 30 to 95 percent. In addition to these uncertainties, modern epidemiologists and historians have not pinpointed the exact identity of these epidemics. Although Dermer and several others referred to it as "the Plague," this was a catch-all term, and the debate has raged since then, including in early histories such as John Josselyn, *An Account of two Voyages to New-England* 2nd ed. (London, 1675); and Daniel Gookin, *Historical Collections of the Indians in New England* (Boston, 1792). Modern hypotheses range from influenza to smallpox, chicken pox, trichinosis, and yellow fever, although none of these seems to fit exactly with period accounts. For a more detailed discussion of the identity and effects of these epidemics, see Charles Francis Adams, *Three Episodes of Massachusetts History,* vol. 1 (Cambridge, MA: Riverside, 1903); Timothy L. Bratton, "The Identity of the New England Indian Epidemic of 1616–1619," *Bulletin of the History of Medicine* 62 (1988): 351–83; Noble David Cook, *Born to Die: Disease and New World Conquests, 1492–1650* (Cambridge, UK: Cambridge University Press, 1998); Sherburne F. Cook, "The Significance of Disease in the Extinction of the New England Indians," *Human Biology* 45 (1973): 485–508; William Cronon, *Changes in the Land: Indians, Colonists, and the Ecology of New England* (New York: Hill and Wang, 1989); Alfred W. Crosby, *The Columbian Exchange: Biological and Cultural Consequences of 1492,* 30th ann. ed. (Westport, CT: Praeger, 2003) and "Virgin Soil Epidemics as a Factor in the Aboriginal Depopulation in America," *William and Mary Quarterly* 33 (1976): 289–99; Henry F. Dobyns, *Their Numbers Become Thinned* (Knoxville: University of Tennessee Press, 1983) and "Disease Transfer at Contact," *Annual Review of Anthropology* 22 (1993): 273–91; John Duffy, *Epidemics in Colonial America* (Baton Rouge: Louisiana State University Press, 1953); Francis Jennings, *The Invasion of America: Indians, Colonialism and the Cant of Conquest* (New York: Norton, 1975); David S. Jones, *Rationalizing Epidemics: Meanings and Uses of American Indian Mortality since 1600* (Cambridge, MA: Harvard University Press,

2004), and "Virgin Soils Revisited," *William and Mary Quarterly* 60 (2003): 703–42; William McNeill, *Plagues and Peoples* (New York: Anchor, 1998); Dean R. Snow and Kim M. Lanphear, "European Contact and Indian Depopulation in the Northeast: The Timing of the First Epidemics," *Ethnohistory* 35 (Winter 1988): 15–33; Arthur J. Spiess and Bruce D. Spiess, "The New England Pandemic of 1616–1622: Cause and Archaeological Implication," *Man in the Northeast* 34 (1987): 71–83; E. Wagner Stearn and Allen E. Stearn, *The Effect of Smallpox on the Destiny of the Amerindian* (Boston: Humphries, 1945); and Russell Thornton, "Aboriginal North American Population and Rates of Decline, ca. A.D. 1500–1900," *Current Anthropology* 38, no. 2 (April 1997): 310–15.

8. Smith, *New Englands Trials*, 2nd ed. (London, 1622), 9. See also Smith, *Generall History*, 229; and *Advertisements*, 9.

9. William Bradford, *Of Plymouth Plantation 1620–1647*, ed. Samuel Eliot Morison (New York: Knopf, 1952), 87. These narratives were increasingly repeated over the following century. For other roughly contemporaneous accounts of these epidemics, see note 5, as well as Edward Winslow, *Good Newes From New England. A True Relation of Things Very Remarkable at the Plantation of Plimoth in New England* (1624; repr., Bedford, MA: Applewood Books, 1996) and *Mourt's Relation*; and William Wood, *New England's Prospect*, ed. Alden T. Vaughan (1634; repr., Amherst: University of Massachusetts Press, 1977). For later descriptions in the seventeenth and eighteenth centuries, see Josselyn, Gookin, and Cotton Mather, *Magnalia Christi Americana*, ed. Kenneth B. Murdock (1702; repr., Cambridge, MA: Harvard University Press, 1977).

10. Thomas Morton, *New English Canaan* (Amsterdam, 1637), 23.

11. Morton, 24.

12. The parallel between Bradford and Morton's rhetoric is startling, given the political and religious tensions between them. Even as Morton does not revel in providential rhetoric in quite the same way that his Separatist and Puritan counterparts do, his reliance on this language to describe epidemics underscores the shared cultural ideologies that shaped the first-generation experience of settlers in New England. For more on the broad rhetorical appeal of epidemics in justification narratives, see Jim Egan, *Authorizing Experience: Refigurations of the Body Politic in Seventeenth-Century New England Writing* (Princeton, NJ: Princeton University Press, 1999), esp. 25.

13. Johnson, 16–17.

14. Jorge Cañizares-Esguerra, *Puritan Conquistadors: Iberianizing the Atlantic, 1550–1700* (Stanford, CA: Stanford University Press, 2006), 12. Cañizares-Esguerra's reading of Spanish and English narratives aims to recuperate "demonology" to Christians' "ongoing epic struggle" in the New World (5). For more on the Spanish influence on English colonial discourses, see also Gesa Mackenthun, *Metaphors of Dispossession: American Beginnings and the Translation of Empire 1492–1637* (Norman: University of Oklahoma Press, 1997).

15. Cañizares-Esguerra, 207.

16. Cañizares-Esguerra, 69.

17. These twin concerns about the legitimacy and safety of migration to New England drove the rhetoric of many early justification narratives. Indeed, the New England colonists were so concerned with avoiding the ongoing problems faced by the colonists in Jamestown, Virginia, and with distancing themselves from the "black legend" of Spanish colonialism, that they looked everywhere for signs to justify their efforts even as they borrowed language from these very same colonial traditions. For more on the language of colonial expansion, especially as it relates to Virginia and Spain, see Cañizares-Esguerra; Mackenthun; Joyce E. Chaplin, *Subject Matter: Technology, the Body, and Science on the Anglo-American Frontier, 1500–1676* (Cambridge, MA: Harvard University Press, 2001); Eric Cheyfitz, *The Poetics of Imperialism: Translation and Colonization from "The Tempest" to "Tarzan"* (New York: Oxford University Press, 1991); and Peter Hulme, *Colonial Encounters: Europe and the Native Caribbean 1492–1797* (New York: Methuen, 1986).

18. For more on the doctrine of *vacuum domicilium*, on civil and natural law in the North American context, and on the influences of these colonial discourses on John Locke's theories of property, see Barbara Arneil, *John Locke and America: The Defence of English Colonialism* (Oxford: Clarendon Press, 1996); Stuart Banner, *How the Indians Lost Their Land: Law and Power on the Frontier* (Cambridge, MA: Harvard University Press, 2005); C. B. Macpherson, *The Political Theory of Possessive Individualism: Hobbes to Locke* (New York: Oxford University Press, 1962); Mackenthun; Cronon; Cheyfitz; Hulme; and, of course, John Locke, *Two Treatises of Government*, ed. Peter Laslett (1690; repr., Cambridge, UK: Cambridge University Press, 2005). Early-seventeenth-century justification narratives that address the doctrines of civil and natural law explicitly include Winthrop, *Generall Considerations*; and Cushman, *Reasons and Considerations*.

19. Cañizares-Esguerra, 14.

20. White, 25. White is one of those writers whom Cañizares-Esguerra situates explicitly in the epic tradition (68–69), especially as he calls on his countrymen to join the "glorious" conquest. It strikes me that his identification of Johnson and White within such a tradition draws attention to the direct influence of Spanish writings on the English colonial experience, as well as to English attempts to appropriate those traditions within locally specific experiences as well. For more on the construction of and appeal to "experience" as an epistemological category, see Egan.

21. Winslow also makes the relation between epidemics and the appropriation of land explicit in *Mourt's Relation*, writing that "about four years ago all the inhabitants [of Patuxet] died of an extraordinary plague, and there is neither man, woman, nor child remaining, as indeed we have found none, so as there is none to hinder our possession, or lay claim unto it" (51).

22. Cushman, *A Sermon Preached at Plimmoth in New-England December 9, 1621. In an assemblie of his Majesties faithfull Subjects, there inhabiting. Wherein is shewed the danger of selfe-love, and the sweetnesse of true Friendship. Together, with a Preface, Shewing the state of the Country, and Condition of the Savages* [*The Sin and Danger of Self-Love*] (London, 1622), A3.

23. Cushman, *Reasons and Considerations*, 92.

24. Winthrop, *Generall Considerations*, 120. He revised and circulated this document numerous times, and several variants exist, all collected in *The Winthrop Papers*. I cite the "Higginson copy" that is taken from Thomas Hutchinson's *Collection of Original Papers* (1769) because it is the most fully fleshed out. For more on the pamphlet's history, see *The Winthrop Papers*, 2:106–49.

25. To the extent that seventeenth-century justification narratives recognize Native Americans as part of the colonial migration project, this recognition is marked by an inherent absence or void: while civil law is projected onto New England with the effect that the Native Americans *could* establish property rights if they were to actively cultivate land, narratives such as William Wood's *New England's Prospect* make this seem unlikely, as Wood describes Natives who are "fettered in the chaines of idleness; so as that they had rather starve than work" (96). Ironically, just as with Cushman's use of the word "waste," Wood's "idleness" also has a dual connotation, relating both to vacant (idle) land and poor work habits. As if to belabor the point, Wood explicitly describes the "lazy" (35) nature of Native Americans in relation to their unwillingness to fertilize the ground, so that dispossession is figured as inherent in their inability to labor properly as required by civil law. Like these other writers, Winthrop's justifications internalize the failure to cultivate land as a characteristic that disqualifies the Native Americans from ownership of property, and thus from adequate protection under civil law.

26. Before going on to argue that Native Americans were unfit to own property in New England, Winthrop asks, "Why may not christians have liberty to go and dwell amongst them in their waste lands and woods (leaving them such places as they have manured for their corne) as lawfully as Abraham did among the Sodomites?" (*Generall Considerations*, 120). Although this comment acknowledges Native American agriculture explicitly (and thus

provides evidence of a right to property), its parenthetical nature buries the evidence in the midst of his broader argument, and effectively hides its presence from the text. Wood likewise acknowledges that Native Americans had "very good crops," although this is used as evidence for how rich the New England soil was, as he notes that they were "too lazy" to fertilize their fields (35).

27. In the early years of New England's history, this threat was often felt as an extension of violence in Virginia. Matthew Craddock of the Massachusetts Company warned John Endicott in a February 1629 letter "not to be too confident of the fidelity of the salvages. It is [a proverb trite] as true, 'the burnt child dreads the fire.' Our countrymen have suffered by their too much confidence in Virginia" (Letter from Matthew Craddock to John Endicott, February 16, 1628, repr. in *Chronicles of the First Planters of the Colony of Massachusetts Bay, from 1623 to 1636*, ed. Alexander Young [Boston, 1846], 131–38, 136). While one is first struck by Craddock's conflation of Virginia and Massachusetts tribes, this wariness reflects an insistence that the Massachusetts Company appropriate land legally in order to remain on good terms with the Native Americans. For more on the colonists' fear of Native American aggression, see note 17, and Cañizares-Esguerra, who argues that the so-called 1622 Virginia massacre "dramatically changed English perceptions of the Amerindians" (28).

28. Winthrop, *Generall Considerations*, 120.

29. The parallel between Winthrop and White is hardly surprising, given that a copy of Winthrop's *Generall Considerations* was confiscated from White by government agents in 1635 (*Winthrop Papers* 2:109).

30. Letter from John Winthrop to Sir Simonds D'Ewes, July 21, 1634, repr. in *The Winthrop Papers*, ed. Allyn Bailey Forbes (Boston: Massachusetts Historical Society, 1943), 3:171–72. While this letter references a new wave of smallpox epidemics that struck New England's Native American populations in the mid-1630s, it is worth noting that five years after his earlier work, Winthrop refers to Native Americans here as "natives," rather than "savages," but also that he explicitly maintains a line between the ongoing epidemics and the "title" that settlers now have to land in New England.

31. Where modern epidemiologists consider the 1616–19 epidemics to have been Old World diseases spread to susceptible New World populations, this is not an etiology that had much traction in early-seventeenth-century justification narratives, although in the years prior to the Pilgrim landing at Plymouth, there had been ample opportunity for Old World pathogens to infect Native Americans (by explorers such as Smith, or by European fishing boats that made periodic landfall in the Massachusetts region). By the early eighteenth century, theories about the European origins of Native American epidemics circulated widely, and Cotton Mather, citing Benjamin Marten, includes the following in his medical writings: "Tis generally Supposed, that *Europe* is Endebted unto America for the Lues Venerea. If so, Europe has paid its debt unto America, by making unto it a Present of the Small Pox, in Lieu of the Great one" (*The Angel of Bethesda*, ed. Gordon W. Jones [Barre, MA: American Antiquarian Society, 1972], 44). For the source of Mather's comment, see Marten, *A New Theory of Consumptions: More Especially of a Phthisis, or Consumption of the Lungs* (London, 1720), 64.

32. These English readings of disease are static insofar as they fail to account for the possibility that Native Americans could have amplified the effects of the epidemics by spreading infection as they traveled from one location to the next—a scenario that likely played a significant role in the spread of disease in the New World. In 1640, Jesuits in New France would report that during an epidemic, the Hurons typically lived among the sick, "in the same indifference, and community of all things, as if they were in perfect health . . . [and] the evil spread from house to house, from village to village, and finally became scattered throughout the country" (Crosby, "Virgin Soil Epidemics," 297). An added factor that may have worsened the impact of disease on Native American communities during this period is that although epidemics were devastating in and of themselves,

high rates of adult mortality would lead to broader social collapses, such as when Bradford reports that sick individuals could not look after one another. In particular, when adults succumbed to disease, parents left orphaned children to die of famine and exposure; see Chaplin, 158.

33. Cronon, 164.
34. Arneil, 38.
35. Cheyfitz, 48.
36. Cheyfitz, 59.
37. Arneil, 49.
38. William Brigham, ed. *The Compact with the Charter and Laws of the Colony of New Plymouth* (Boston, 1836), 3.
39. For more on the historiographic project to date, see note 7.
40. For more on the notion of shaping conceptual "frames" and frameworks for disease, see Charles E. Rosenberg and Janet Golden, *Framing Disease: Studies in Cultural History* (New Brunswick, NJ: Rutgers University Press, 1992), esp. xiii–xxvi; and Priscilla Wald, *Contagious: Cultures, Carriers, and the Outbreak Narrative* (Durham, NC: Duke University Press, 2008).
41. Thomas C. Timmreck, *An Introduction to Epidemiology*, 3rd ed. (Boston: Jones, 2002), 21.
42. I use the term "modern" to distinguish what we commonly think of as epidemiology from this collection of seventeenth-century texts. Strictly speaking, its use is redundant because epidemiology is, by definition, a modern statistical science. My work of displacing epidemiology into the seventeenth and eighteenth centuries is an attempt to recuperate and analyze the narrative effects of this medical practice. I contend that this anachronistic displacement reveals the transparent relation between narrative and epidemiology, thus freeing the term for a critique of current medical practices, as well as an analysis of the historical and literary developments that I examine here.
43. Abraham M. Lilienfeld and David E. Lilienfeld, *Foundations of Epidemiology*, 2nd ed. (New York: Oxford University Press, 1980), 4. An example of such philosophical models in modern medicine—that of objective scientific detachment—would be used to identify certain predetermined signs to make accurate diagnoses; would chart the prescription of medicines according to age, weight, gender, and possible drug interactions; and would conduct controlled drug trials that go through rigorous stages of testing by adhering to strict predetermined programs. While these modes of practice have become highly efficient, if not indispensable in the modern industrialized world, we ought to bear in mind that any reliance on statistical analysis, by its very nature, produces case histories that will deviate from, or fail to conform to normal distribution patterns. We might call these *diagnostic failures*. Such diagnostic failures are treated as anomalous events because they do not conform to projected patterns; but even as they diverge from standard models, these failures can be used to draw more accurate predictive formulas in the future, thus reinforcing precision and specialization as the primary modes of modern medicine. But as the potential accuracy of projections increases, as Old World diseases become increasingly rare in industrialized countries, and as medicine, technology, and agriculture become more specialized, so, too, does the risk of hazards from unforeseen sources, such as cross-species infections like the Avian bird flu, SARS, H1N1, BSE (mad-cow disease), and its human counterpart, new-variant Creutzfeldt-Jakob disease, and drug-resistant strains of illnesses like tuberculosis, MRSA, and HIV, as well as the evolution of iatrogenic diseases, increase. This is a thorny public health issue because as the perception of these hazards increases, so too does skepticism about the effectiveness and danger of medical practices, which has led some parents to opt their children out of basic medical services like vaccination. In its most problematic form, diagnostic failure has the capacity to exacerbate public health crises when communities are not fully equipped to make sense of broad anomalies in data sets. A full generation after the emergence of HIV/AIDS in America, we can begin to understand how a reliance on the medical world to provide a quick

and full analysis of this epidemic at a time when it was incapable of doing so left communities unable to combat the disease effectively, and implicated them, even if unwittingly,
in its spread. The model critiques for such histories are Randy Shilts, *And the Band Played
On: Politics, People, and the AIDS Epidemic* (New York: St. Martin's, 1987); and Cindy Patton, "Performativity and Spatial Distinction: The End of AIDS Epidemiology," *Performativity and Performance*, eds. Andrew Parker and Eve Kosofsky Sedgwick (New York:
Routledge, 1995): 173–96, and *Globalizing AIDS* (Minneapolis: University of Minnesota
Press, 2002).

44. Similarly, we can take a second look at modern epidemiology and medical practice to dis-
cern their narrative elements. Indeed, modern medical practices have seen a shift in
recent years from a deep reliance on hierarchical models of the doctor–patient relationship, toward incorporating a more conscious awareness of the stories that patients tell
with and about their bodies. This trend is most conspicuous in the development of narrative medicine programs, palliative care units, nurse-practitioner clinics, and the self-
management of morphine and other pain medications, as well as in ongoing discussions
about euthanasia. The clearest example of the inextricable nature of epidemiology and
narrative in contemporary epidemics is revealed in the developing analyses of HIV/AIDS
in relation to public policy—both on domestic and international fronts. Finally, the Internet, with its burgeoning communities and ready store of information about new medicines and potential treatments, has put additional pressure on doctors and hospitals to
shift their attentions in order to cope with and manage patients who now have highly
specialized, if incomplete, medical knowledge.

45. Although the word "discrimination" appears odd in this context, it properly ascribes a
special (divine) agency to disease that modern epidemiologies would not. Where modern
epidemiologists might eventually agree on a series of events that would locate the biological source and identity of the epidemics of 1616–19, Puritan writers traced this source
providentially.

46. Chapter 3 of this book engages just this dilemma, as epidemiological patterns shifted in
unforeseen ways, and forced New England colonists to rethink and revise their epidemiological assumptions in relation to their migration project midway through the seventeenth century.

47. Cushman, *Sin and Danger*, A3.

48. White, 25. Similarly, Smith recounted that "it seems God hath provided this Country for
our Nation, destroying the natives by the plague, it not touching one Englishman, though
many traded and were conversant amongst them" (*Advertisements*, 9).

49. White, 23–24. Immediately following this passage, White also notes that "Neyther are
the Natives at any time troubled with paine of teeth, sorenesse of eyes, or ache in their
limbes," so that in this narrow point at least, the environment looks to be healthy for all
humans. The upshot is that if New England is healthful for Native Americans as well, then
the epidemics signify even more meaningfully as divinely ordained plagues. Johnson also
notes that "naturally the Country is very healthy" (17), and Wood, that "the common
diseases of England, they be strangers to the English now in that strange land. To my
knowledge I never knew any that had the pox, measles, green-sickness, headaches, stone,
or consumptions, etc. Many that have come infirm out of England retain their old griev-
ances still, and some that were long troubled with lingering diseases, as coughs of the
lungs, consumptions, etc., have been restored by that medicinable climate to their former
strength and health" (32).

50. Higginson, [14].

51. Higginson, [9]. Ironically, Higginson died in the summer of 1630, within a year of his
arrival in New England. Wood also used himself as an example, noting that "the last
argument to confirm the healthfulness of the country shall be from mine own experience,
who although in England I was brought up tenderly under the careful hatching of my
dearest friends, yet scarce could I be acquainted with health . . . but being planted in that

new soil and healthful air, which was more correspondent to my nature . . . yet scarce did I know what belonged to a day's sickness" (33).

52. Egan, 20.

53. Egan, 28.

54. Egan, 25. See note 18 and Arneil for more on the influence of America's colonial history on Locke. It is no great coincidence that Locke's *Second Treatise* would rely so heavily on the figure of the Native American to ground his reading of property and natural law, although by the time he would write that "in the beginning all the World was America" (301), the justification narrative's epidemiological rhetoric had essentially fallen to the wayside—perhaps, in part, because its arbitrariness was by then too problematic to maintain. It nevertheless speaks to the power of epidemiological rhetoric that Winthrop's, Cushman's, Johnson's, and White's narratives relied on the scene of epidemic to help shape this important political tradition that would come to have a critical impact in the eighteenth century.

55. Henry Nash Smith, *Virgin Land: The American West as Symbol and Myth* (Cambridge, MA: Harvard University Press, 1970).

56. Jennings, 15–31. See also Dobyns, "Brief Perspective on a Scholarly Transformation: Widowing the 'Virgin Land,'" *Ethnohistory* 23, no. 2 (Spring 1976): 95–104.

57. Jones, "Virgin Soils Revisited," 714. The metonymy has become so pervasive that it continues to finds its way into surprising places, such as Chaplin's nuanced study of the history of science during the early period of the British Atlantic empire, and of the influence played by encounters with Native Americans and Africans. Chaplin highlights the fact that "the historiography on post-Columbian epidemic disease in America has taken care to explain that Indian mortality was *not* a racial characteristic" (158, emphasis added), and yet much of that historiography—including her own overview of those epidemics—falls back on the land/body metonymy as an explanatory model. Chaplin herself uses the concept of virgin soil epidemics in her analysis, and notes that "the population is then virgin soil for the disease's firm root and rapid spread" (158). My focus on her words here does some injustice to the complexity of her argument, but I merely wish to demonstrate how far-ranging this colonialist trope is.

58. Cindy Patton, "Performativity and Spatial Distinction," 188. See also *Globalizing AIDS*.

59. Bradford, 87. For more on the Narragansett and the disparate effect of epidemics, see Winslow, *Good Newes*, 75n1; and Jones, *Rationalizing Epidemics*, 34.

60. Jones, "Virgin Soils Revisited," 707–8. For more on the relationship between immunological determinism and literary criticism, see Wald, "Future Perfect: Grammar, Genes, and Geography," *New Literary History* 31 (2000): 681–708.

61. Francis L. Black, "An Explanation of High Death Rates among New World Peoples When in Contact with Old World Diseases," *Perspectives in Biology and Medicine* 37 (1994): 292–307, 299.

62. Black, 299.

63. This is a framework that has a close affinity to the question of cultural homogeneity in early Puritan New England, and is one that I explore more fully in Chapter 3, while engaging Wald's study of *imagined immunities* (*Contagious*, and "Imagined Immunities," *Cultural Studies and Political Theory*, ed. Jodi Dean [Ithaca, NY: Cornell University Press, 2000]: 189–208).

64. Black, 301.

65. For a study that attempts to correlate the evolution of religious diversity with epidemics in geographic terms, see Corey L. Fincher and Randy Thornhill, "Assortative Sociality, Limited Dispersal, Infectious Disease and the Genesis of the Global Pattern of Religion Diversity," *Proceedings of the Royal Society B* 275 (July 2008): 2587–94.

66. Jones, *Rationalizing Epidemics*, 19.

67. There were, of course, those justification narratives that made exactly this claim. Cushman's *Reasons and Considerations*, for example, described Native Americans and their land

as "spacious and void, and there are few and do but run over the grass, as do the foxes and wild beasts. They are not industrious, neither have art, science, skill or faculty to use either the land or the commodities of it, but all spoils, rots, and is marred for want of manuring, gathering, ordering, etc" (91–92).

68. Adams, 9.

69. Wood, 38. Likewise, recall that White had remarked that there was "much cleared ground for tillage . . . which came to pass by the desolation hapning through a three yeeres Plague" (25).

70. Young, ed., *Chronicles of the Pilgrim Fathers of the Colony of Plymouth from 1602 to 1625* (Boston, 1844), 184.

71. Cronon, 90.

72. Wood, 74.

73. Bradford, 85.

74. Morton, 23.

75. Smith, *Advertisements*, 9.

76. A century later, Cotton Mather told the story in his *Magnalia Christi Americana*. Writing that these events occurred "not long before" the epidemics, Mather goes on to say that a Frenchman told "those *Tawny Pagans, that God being angry with them for their Wickedness, would not only destroy them all, but also People the place with another Nation, which would not live after their Brutish Manners.* Those Infidels then Blasphemously reply'd, *God could not kill them;* which Blasphemous mistake was confuted by an horrible and unusual *Plague"* (129). Such narratives were, of course, not new to New England, having been recounted, for example, by Thomas Harriot in the late sixteenth century (*A Briefe and True Report of the New Found Land of Virginia* [1588/1590; repr., New York: Dover, 1972]).

77. Chaplin, 34.

78. For more on Tisquantum's history, see Bradford, 81; and Smith, *Generall Historie*, 233. See also Frank Shuffelton, "Indian Devils and Pilgrim Fathers: Squanto, Hobomok, and the English Conception of Indian Religion," *The New England Quarterly* 49, no. 1 (March 1976): 108–16; John H. Humins, "Squanto and Massasoit: A Struggle for Power," *The New England Quarterly* 60, no. 1 (March 1987): 54–70; and Leonard A. Wolf, "Squanto's Role in Pilgrim Diplomacy," *Ethnohistory* 11, no. 3 (Summer 1964): 247–61.

79. Winslow, *Good Newes*, 16.

80. Smith, *Generall Historie*, 229.

81. Bradford, 99. See also Smith's *Generall Historie* for the following version of the account: "divers Salvages also [Tisquantum] had caused to believe we would destroy them, but he would doe his best to appease us; this he did onely to make his Country-men believe what great power hee had with us to get bribes on both sides, to make peace or warre when he would, and the more to possesse them with feare, he perswaded many we had buried the plague in our store house, which wee could send when we listed whither wee would" (235). Finally, Mather would also repeat the scene in his *Magnalia*, writing that Tisquantum "went on to terrifie them with a ridiculous *Rhodomantado*, which they Believed, that this People kept the *Plague* in a Cellar (where they kept their *Powder*) and could at their pleasure let it loose to make such Havock among them, as the Distemper had already made among them a few Years before. Thus was the *Tongue of a Dog* made useful to a feeble and sickly *Lazarus!"* (135).

82. Shuffelton, 115.

83. Morton, 104–5.

84. Harriot, 28.

85. For more on this ambiguity, see Mackenthun, who argues that "it is not at all clear whether Wingina's persuasion was based on his independent judgment or was the result of an explanatory dialogue with the colonists. The scene in fact recalls the one between Columbus and his Arawak interpreters, who 'are always assured' of his divine origin by their frequent 'intercourse [*conversación*]' with him" (148). The key to this interpretation (and to the relationship between the Harriot and New England narratives) is that

regardless of the ambiguity, the story itself circulates as a tropic convention of colonial exploration narratives.

86. Harriot, 29.
87. See Smith, *Generall Historie*, 12.
88. Chaplin, 29. For more on the invisible bullets, see also Mackenthun and Stephen Greenblatt, *Shakespearean Negotiations: The Circulation of Social Energy in Renaissance England* (Berkeley: University of California Press, 1988).
89. Chaplin, 26, 27.
90. Letter from Roger Williams to Governor Henry Vane and Deputy Governor John Winthrop, May 1, 1637, repr. in *The Correspondence of Roger Williams, 1629–1653*, ed. Glenn W. LaFantasie (Providence, RI: Brown University Press, 1988), 1:72.
91. According to Bradford, Tisquantum "fell sick of an Indian fever, bleeding much at the nose (which the Indians take for a symptom of death) and within a few days he died there; desiring the Governor to pray for him that he might go the Englishmen's God in Heaven" (114).
92. John Winthrop, *A Short Story of the Rise, reign, and ruine of the Antinomians, Familists & Libertines, that infected the Churches of New-England*, in David D. Hall, ed., *The Antinomian Controversy, 1636–1638: A Documentary History*, 2nd ed. (Durham, NC: Duke University Press, 1990), 218.

Chapter 2

1. Maryse, Condé, *I, Tituba, Black Witch of Salem*, trans. Richard Philcox (New York: Ballantine, 1992), 150.
2. John Stetson Barry, *History of Massachusetts: The Colonial Period*, 4th ed., vol. 1 (Boston, 1856), 162.
3. Letter from Matthew Craddock to John Endicott, February 16, 1628, repr. in *Chronicles of the First Planters of the Colony of Massachusetts Bay, from 1623 to 1636*, ed. Alexander Young (Boston, 1846), 131–38, 133.
4. One such competing claim was made by John Oldham, who argued that much of the land granted to the Company by the Plymouth council in 1628 actually belonged to him by a prior grant from John Gorges ("Records of the Governor and Company of the Massachusetts Bay in New-England," repr. in Young, ed., 39–128, 51). Although the Company was "well satisfied by good counsel" that Oldham's grant was "void in law," it felt compelled to hold hearings into the matter, and pressed Endicott to "send forty or fifty persons . . . whereby the better to strengthen our possession there against all or any that shall intrude upon us, which we would not have you by any means to give way unto" (The Company's First General Letter of Instructions to Endicott and His Council, April 17, 1629, repr. in Young, ed., 141–71, 148, 150).
5. The Company's First General Letter to Endicott, 167.
6. The Company's First General Letter to Endicott, 167.
7. The Company's Second General Letter of Instructions to Endicott and His Council, May 28, 1629, repr. in Young, ed., 172–91, 177.
8. The Company's Second General Letter to Endicott, 177.
9. The Company's First General Letter to Endicott, 163, 162; and Letter from Matthew Craddock to John Endicott, 133.
10. Letter from Matthew Craddock to John Endicott, 133.
11. Letter from Matthew Craddock to John Endicott, 133.
12. Barry, 169.
13. William Bradford, *Of Plymouth Plantation 1620–1647*, ed. Samuel Eliot Morison (New York: Knopf, 1952), 223.
14. The "old planters" at Naumkeag (those who had arrived with the Dorchester Company) had previously been ministered by John Lyford, who himself had left Plymouth because

he was disenchanted with its rigid Separatism. Lyford stayed briefly in Naumkeag, before going to Virginia, leaving the settlement "without [a minister], till Mr. Higginson and Mr. Skelton came over" (William Hubbard, *A General History of New England, from the Discovery to 1680*, Massachusetts Historical Society Collection, 2nd ser., vol. 5 [ca. 1682; repr., Boston,1848], 116).

15. Two of the most notable physician-ministers in early-seventeenth-century New England were John Eliot and Michael Wigglesworth. In an odd twist to be explored in Chapter 4, Cotton Mather positioned himself as a minister who was knowledgeable in matters of medicine, and attempted to serve his community on two fronts. By this time, however, a process of professionalization and specialization was beginning to take hold in New England, and his medical expertise (or lack of it) would be roundly criticized.

16. Thomas Morton, who perhaps ought not to be taken as the last word in these matters, wrote this satirical description of Fuller: "How hee went to worke with his gifts is a question; yet hee did a great cure for Captaine [Endicott], hee cured him of a disease called a wife . . . [he was] made Phisition generall of Salem: where hee exercised his gifts so well, that of full 42. that there hee tooke to cure, there is not one has more cause to complaine, or can say black's his eie." Morton then went on to write "in mine opinion, hee deserves to be set upon a palfrey and lead up and downe in triumph throw new Canaan . . . that men might know where to finde a Quacksalver" (*New English Canaan* [Amsterdam, 1637], 152–53).

17. Bradford, *Plymouth Plantation*, 224.

18. Williston Walker, *A History of the Congregational Churches in the United States*, (New York, 1894), 101.

19. Walker, 65.

20. Perry Miller, *Orthodoxy in Massachusetts 1630–1650: A Genetic Study* (Cambridge, MA: Harvard University Press, 1933), 128. In evidence for this assertion, Miller declares that Hugh Peter was a friend of Endicott's, and became a patentee of the New England Company in 1628, attending at least two council meetings. According to Miller, "Peter's devotion to the Congregational polity was well known at this time, and his affiliation with the Company may very possibly have been the entering wedge of the Congregationalists' control" (124). Craddock's February 1629 letter to Endicott suggests that the Company had intended to send Peter to New England as minister, but that he was in Holland at that time, "whence his return . . . [was] uncertain" (Letter from Matthew Craddock to John Endicott, 135).

21. Miller, *Orthodoxy*, 134, 131.

22. The Company's First General Letter to Endicott, 144.

23. Miller, *Orthodoxy*, 130.

24. Bradford, *Plymouth Plantation*, 225.

25. Bradford, *Plymouth Plantation*, 224; Walker, 106.

26. Nathaniel Morton, *New Englands Memoriall* (Cambridge, 1669), 76.

27. "The Form of Government for the Colony," repr. in Young, ed., 192–96.

28. In its September 28th council, the Company decided that some of the Brownes's "letters should be opened and publicly read" in case they "defamed the country of New-England, and the Governor and government there" ("Records of the Governor and Company of the Massachusetts," 91). This type of oversight was not unusual (Winthrop keeps track of similar events in his journal), and simply reinforces the colonial government's reliance on maintaining transparency within New England communities. Coincidently, the Company had far more pressing matters to attend to at that meeting, forming a committee to study the question of whether the government and patent could be transferred to New England.

29. Letter from the Massachusetts Bay Company to the Ministers, October 16, 1629, repr. in Young, ed., 287–89, 288.

30. Nathaniel B. Shurtleff, ed., *Records of the Governor and Company of the Massachusetts Bay in New England*, vol. 1 (Boston, 1853), 37.

31. Letter from the Massachusetts Bay Company to the Ministers, 289.

32. Letter from the Massachusetts Bay Company to John Endicott, October 16, 1629, repr. in Young, ed., 290–92, 291.

33. Robert Baillie, *A Dissuassive From the Errours Of the Time* (London, 1645), 54–55.

34. Letter from John Dudley to the Countess of Lincoln, March 28, 1631, repr. in Young, ed., 303–41, 311.

35. Letter from Samuel Fuller to William Bradford, June 28, 1630, repr. in *Governor William Bradford's Letter Book* (Bedford, MA: Applewood Books, 2001), 56.

36. Walker, 108. News of the Salem congregation's refusal to baptize Coddington's child traveled back to England quickly, and John Cotton replied with alarm to admonish Skelton on October 2nd. Cotton found two primary errors in Skelton's actions: first, that no one could be admitted to the sacrament if not also a member of "some particular reformed church," and second, that "none of our congregacions in England are particular reformed churches, but Mr. Lathrops & such as his" (*The Correspondence of John Cotton*, ed. Sargent Bush, Jr. [Chapel Hill: University of North Carolina Press, 2001], 144). The first of these complaints would become the cornerstone of Congregationalist doctrine (later to be espoused by Cotton himself), and the second was a direct affront to the Church of England. John Lathrop's church in England had been built on John Robinson's model of Separation, and his acceptance into the Salem congregation points to the influence of Plymouth. Indeed, Cotton wrote that this error required "a booke rather than a letter to answere it: you went hence of another judgment, & I am afraid your chaunge hath sprung from new-Plymouth-men, whom though I much esteeme as godly and loving Christians, yet their grounds which they received for this tenent from Mr Robinson, do not satsfye mee" (144). This letter, to which Larzer Ziff argues Miller did not have access, reveals the anxiety that the Massachusetts Bay Company felt with respect to the power of Plymouth's influence over its settlers ("The Salem Puritans in the "Free Aire of a New World," *The Huntington Library Quarterly*, 20 [1956]: 373–84).

37. Letter from Samuel Fuller and Edward Winslow to William Bradford, July 26, 1630, *Bradford's Letter Book*, 57.

38. Letter from Samuel Fuller to William Bradford, August 2, 1630, *Bradford Letter Book*, 58. The aggregate London Bills of Mortality collected by John Graunt do indeed show that 1630, with 1,317 fatalities, was a year in which the plague was significant (as opposed to 0 deaths in 1629, 247 in 1631, and 9 in 1632). Nevertheless, despite this spike in mortality, Graunt does not list 1630 as a major plague year (*Natural and Political Observations Mentioned in a Following Index and Made Upon the Bills of Mortality 1662* [New York: Arno Press, 1975]).

39. Fuller to Bradford, August 2, 1630, *Bradford's Letter Book*, 58.

40. Fuller to Bradford, August 2, 1630, *Bradford's Letter Book*, 58.

41. Shurtleff, 87.

42. Slayden Yarbrough, "The Influence of Plymouth Colony Separatism on Salem: An Interpretation of John Cotton's Letter of 1630 to Samuel Skelton," *Church History*, 51 (1982): 290–303, 302. See also Ziff, "The Salem Puritans."

43. Perhaps an early example of exceptionalist rhetoric, Robert Baillie published his criticism of New England Congregationalism in *A Dissuasive from the Errours of the Time* (to which John Cotton responded with *The Way of Congregational Churches Cleared* in 1648), advancing the idea that the "free aire of a new world" might have been contagious, and led to the Puritans' unorthodox practices. Of course, Miller takes issue with this notion, and with historians who "take refuge in citing the mystical declaration of Scotch Baillie" (xiii).

44. Hubbard, 117.

45. Edward Winslow, *Hypocrisie Unmasked* (London, 1646), 92. The process Winslow describes is grounded in the "written word onely. . . . So that here also thou maist see they set not the Church at Plimouth before them for example, but the Primitive Churches were and are their and our mutuall patterns and examples, which are onely worthy to be followed" (92).

46. Miller, xiii.

47. John Dudley to the Countess of Lincoln, 319, 325.

48. John Dudley to the Countess of Lincoln, 325.

49. John Dudley to the Countess of Lincoln, 326.

50. Shurtleff, 83.

51. After Knopp paid part of the fine, the remaining 3 pounds were remitted in August 1634 (Shurtleff, 99), and the fine was definitively discharged in September 1638 (243).

52. The *Short Story* (1644) is Weld's quick repackaging of John Winthrop's *Antinomians and Familists Condemned By the Synod of Elders in New England* (1644). Except where the words are specifically Weld's (such as in the title and preface), I will generally refer to the text as Winthrop's—a convenient shorthand used in David Hall's edition of the controversy's primary documents (*The Antinomian Controversy 1636–1638: A Documentary History*, 2nd ed. [Durham, NC: Duke University Press, 1990], 199–310).

53. I use the term "Orthodoxy" with full knowledge that it describes a cultural coherence that was far from settled by the time the controversy erupted. It is my contention that a crisis like this one (and ongoing epidemics that I will explore in Chapter 3) helps to engender cultural coherence retroactively by positing a corporate body around which the community could rally, and by framing dissent as the work of pathological agents who could be expelled from the community. In this temporal inversion, "Orthodoxy" does not so much represent the state of affairs in Massachusetts Bay 1636–38, as it describes the representation of those affairs after the fact. Even as Orthodoxy becomes a representational term, it assumes an ontological coherence on the model of healthy bodies confronted with foreign pathogens. See Janice Knight for more on the question of New England's multiple Orthodoxies (*Orthodoxies in Massachusetts: Rereading American Puritanism* [Cambridge, MA: Harvard University Press, 1994]).

54. Patricia Caldwell, "The Antinomian Language Controversy," *Harvard Theological Review* 69, no. 3–4 (1976): 345–67, 346.

55. See Michael P. Winship, *Making Heretics: Militant Protestantism and Free Grace in Massachusetts, 1636–1641* (Princeton, NJ: Princeton University Press, 2002); Phillip Round, *By Nature and by Custom Cursed: Transatlantic Civil Discourse and New England Cultural Production, 1620–1660* (Hanover, NH: University Press of New England, 1999); Elizabeth Maddock Dillon, *The Gender of Freedom: Fictions of Liberalism and the Literary Public Sphere* (Stanford, CA: Stanford University Press, 2004); and Jim Egan, *Authorizing Experience: Refigurations of the Body Politic in Seventeenth-Century New England Writing* (Princeton, NJ: Princeton University Press, 1999). For more on the controversy, see also Emery Battis, *Saints and Sectaries: Anne Hutchinson and the Antinomian Controversy in the Massachusetts Bay Colony* (Chapel Hill: University of North Carolina Press, 1962); Michelle Burnham, "Anne Hutchinson and the Economics of Antinomian Selfhood in Colonial New England," *Criticism*, 39:3 (1997): 337–58; Andrew Delbanco, *The Puritan Ordeal* (Cambridge, MA: Harvard University Press, 1989); Lisa M. Gordis, *Opening Scripture: Bible Reading and Interpretive Authority in Puritan New England* (Chicago: University of Chicago Press, 2003); Philip F. Gura, *A Glimpse of Sion's Glory: Puritan Radicalism in New England, 1620–1660* (Middletown, CT: Wesleyan University Press, 1984); Jane Kamensky, *Governing the Tongue: The Politics of Speech in Early New England* (New York: Oxford University Press, 1997); Ann Kibbey, *The Interpretation of Material Shapes in Puritanism: A Study of Rhetoric, Prejudice, and Violence* (New York: Cambridge University Press, 1986); Amy Schrager Lang, *Prophetic Woman: Anne Hutchinson and the Problem of Dissent in the Literature of New England* (Berkeley: University of California Press, 1987); Perry Miller, *The New England Mind: The Seventeenth Century* (Cambridge, MA: Harvard University Press, 1939); Lad Tobin, "A Radically Different Voice: Gender and Language in the Trials of Anne Hutchinson" *Early American Literature* 25 (1990): 253–70; and Ziff, *Puritanism in America: New Culture in a New World* (New York: Viking Compass, 1973).

56. Jonathan Beecher Field, "The Antinomian Controversy Did Not Take Place," *Early American Studies: An Interdisciplinary Journal* 6, no. 2 (2008): 448–63.
57. Field, 449. See also Jean Baudrillard, *The Gulf War Did Not Take Place*, trans. Paul Patton (Bloomington: Indiana University Press, 1995).
58. Dillon, 76.
59. Field, 448.
60. Dillon, 72.
61. This observation has almost become commonplace in contemporary parlance, with what we might call an epidemic of epidemics that focus on social and political behavior. The most famous such representations in twentieth-century America may well have been that of Communism at the height of McCarthyism and the Red Scare, while the end of the Cold War marked a renewed interest in societal ills such as crime, drugs, and illiteracy; since 2001, representations of terrorism and terrorist cells have likewise relied on epidemiological tropes of contagion and containment. Because of epidemiological successes in treating biological diseases, the implicit subtext of such representations of figural epidemics is that these problems are not natural to the community's healthy state, and can therefore be cured.
62. See Tobin; Margaret V. Richardson and Arthur T. Hertig, "New England's First Recorded Hydatidiform Mole," *New England Journal of Medicine* 207, no. 11 (March 1959): 544–45; Anne Jacobson Schutte, "'Such Monstrous Births': A Neglected Aspect of the Antinomian Controversy," *Renaissance Quarterly* 38, no. 1 (1985): 85–106; and Bryce Traister, "Anne Hutchinson's 'Monstrous Birth' and the Feminization of Antinomianism," *Canadian Review of American Studies/Revue canadienne d'études américaines* 27, no. 2 (1997): 133–58.
63. Winthrop, *Short Story*, 201.
64. Winthrop, "A Model of Christian Charity" in *The Norton Anthology of American Literature*, eds. Nina Baym et al., 7th ed., vol. A (New York: Norton, 2007), 147–58, 153.
65. Winthrop, *Model*, 156.
66. Louise Breen maintains that while the Court's decision helped to maintain a disciplinary grip over the colony, it also meant that "the 'visible' saint necessarily became the spiritual reflection of the good citizen, and diversity in the means of reaching salvation had to be curtailed" (*Transgressing the Bounds: Subversive Enterprises among the Puritan Elite in Massachusetts, 1630–1692* [New York: Oxford University Press, 2001], 20). This curtailment describes a process of formalization in which admission to the church is revealed as an artificial arbiter of good citizenship. It is little wonder that such a move would raise the ire of fundamentalist Calvinists. In effect, this formalization collapses the space between secular and sacred acts for visible saints, while the gap between citizens and noncitizens (church members and nonmembers) widens. The political fallout from such a strategy would become the locus of the Antinomian controversy.
67. Breen, 6.
68. Breen, 6.
69. Winthrop, *Short Story*, 203.
70. Lang, 19.
71. Winthrop, *Short Story*, 221, 203.
72. Winthrop, *Short Story*, 284.
73. See Dillon for more on how she argues that "the miscarriages . . . function as publicity or evidence of heresy rather than as punishment for heresy" (90).
74. John Wheelwright, "A Fast Day Sermon," in Hall, ed., *The Antinomian Controversy*, 152–72, 154.
75. Wheelwright, 158.
76. Winthrop, *The Journal of John Winthrop 1630–1649*, eds. Richard S. Dunn, James Savage, and Laetitia Yeandle (Cambridge, MA: Harvard University Press, 1996), 196.
77. Winthrop, *Journal*, 197.

78. For an exploration of the significant differences between the language of the Orthodoxy and the Antinomians, see Ross J. Pudaloff, "Sign and Subject: Antinomianism in Massachusetts Bay," *Semiotica* 54 (1985): 147–63. Pudaloff's argument arises from an analysis of Foucault's work on Renaissance and Classical epistemes. For Pudaloff, although both factions were conversant in each language, the Puritan elders tended to rely on the language of "Classical contractualism," while the Antinomians primarily invoked "Renaissance organicism" (152). He argues that the Antinomian controversy marks the Puritan confrontation of the "conflict between the two *epistemes* as it imputes to the [subject] a particular concept of subjectivity" (158).

79. Winthrop, *Short Story*, 253.

80. Lang, 10.

81. Winthrop, *Short Story*, 214.

82. Winthrop, *Short Story*, 249.

83. "Acknowledgment of Samuel Cole and Others," repr. in *The Winthrop Papers*, vol. 3, ed. Allyn Bailey Forbes (Boston: Massachusetts Historical Society, 1943), 513.

84. "Acknowledgment of Thomas Savage," repr. in Forbes, ed., 3:515–16.

85. The focus on Hutchinson has increasingly been problematized since Knight's study of Orthodoxies in Massachusetts, which all but sidelines her role in the theological debates that raged in early New England colonies. Likewise, Egan is interested in the way that Winthrop would "exaggerate her role in the controversy to the extent of naming her the principal cause of [the colony's] trouble even though any number of influential male leaders, including the ministers John Cotton and John Wheelwright, lectured on Antinomian doctrine to larger groups on a more regular basis in an unambiguously acceptable context for religious teaching" (73).

86. See Cotton Mather, *Magnalia Christi Americana*, ed. Kenneth B. Murdock (1702; repr., Cambridge, MA: Harvard University Press, 1977); and Edward Johnson, *A History of New-England [Wonder-Working Providence of Sions Saviour]* (London, 1654).

87. Mary Beth Norton, *Founding Mothers & Fathers: Gendered Power and the Forming of American Society* (New York: Knopf, 1996), 375.

88. Although I point out that scholars often refer to Hutchinson's prosecution for sedition, the mistake itself is usually not central to their arguments. Breen explains that Hutchinson did not have the political status to sign the petition (and thus did not commit the same crime that her male counterparts did). Winthrop accuses her of having "countenanced" the petitioners (*Short Story*, 266; and "The Examination of Mrs. Anne Hutchinson at the Court at Newtown," in Hall, ed., 311–48, 313), but her trial is nonetheless marked by a confusion of *what* exactly she had been charged with; thus, until the latter part of her trial, the crisis she represented to the Court is reflected in the problem of *how* to identify her crime.

89. Pudaloff, 149.

90. Dillon, 52.

91. "The Examination of Anne Hutchinson," 312.

92. "The Examination of Anne Hutchinson," 312.

93. Dillon, 58.

94. "The Examination of Anne Hutchinson," 312.

95. "The Examination of Anne Hutchinson," 313.

96. Winthrop, *Short Story*, 267.

97. "The Examination of Anne Hutchinson," 314.

98. "The Examination of Anne Hutchinson," 315.

99. "The Examination of Anne Hutchinson," 315, 316.

100. "The Examination of Anne Hutchinson," 314.

101. "The Examination of Anne Hutchinson," 312.

102. From the time he arrived in Massachusetts Bay in September 1633, John Cotton was concerned with issues surrounding a woman's place in public. He argued that his wife

should be allowed to forego the habitual public conversion testimony, requesting "that she might not be putt to make open Confession &c: which he said was against the Apostles Rule & not fitt for women's modestye, but that the Elders might examine her in private" (Winthrop, *Journal*, 96).

103. Dillon, 67.
104. "The Examination of Anne Hutchinson," 343.
105. "The Examination of Anne Hutchinson," 337.
106. "The Examination of Anne Hutchinson," 341.
107. Winthrop, *Short Story*, 310.
108. The opportunity to recant and reenter the fold was an important function of prosecutions in New England, as it allowed for the community to represent itself as contiguous and whole, rather than fractured or vengeful.
109. "A Report of the Trial of Mrs. Anne Hutchinson before the Church in Boston," in Hall, ed., 349–88, 361.
110. "A Report of the Trial," 383.
111. "A Report of the Trial," 372.
112. Winthrop, *Short Story*, 236. In an interesting parallel, Winthrop remarked in December 1638 that a woman by the name of Mary Oliver had recently begun to cause trouble in Salem. As evidence that Hutchinson's prosecution served to model the behavior of women, here are Winthrop's words: "She was," he says "(for ability of speech, and appearance of zeal and devotion) far before Mrs. Hutchinson, and so the fitter instrument to have done hurt, but that she was poor and had little acquaintance" (*Journal*, 275). While this description disparages Hutchinson, it also points to the social gap that could hinder or facilitate dissent—and infection—within the colony.
113. Winthrop, *Short Story*, 263.
114. Norton, 222.
115. Norton, 227.
116. Cotton, 412.
117. Hubbard, 283.
118. Egan, 75.
119. Egan, 75.
120. Egan, 69.
121. Cindy Patton, "Performativity and Spatial Distinction: The End of AIDS Epidemiology," *Performativity and Performance*, eds. Andrew Parker and Eve Kosofsky Sedgwick (New York: Routledge, 1995): 173–96, 174. See also Patton, *Globalizing AIDS* (Minneapolis: University of Minnesota Press, 2002), 119.
122. Lang, 8.
123. I am indebted to Karen O. Kupperman and the Atlantic History Workshop at NYU for this particular insight into the trajectory of Dyer's life. It is worth recollecting that the title of Winthrop's history of the controversy (*Antinomians and Familists Condemned*) as well as the longer title of Weld's narrative (*the Rise, reign, and ruine of the Antinomians, Familists & Libertines*) juxtapose Quakerism with Antinomianism, so the threat that Massachusetts Bay saw Dyer as representing was not at all far-fetched.
124. Shurtleff, 224. See Traister for this useful observation regarding Winthrop's suspicions about Hawkins, and the fact that "she practiced obstetrical homeopathy suggests that the Puritans were predisposed to fear Hutchinson's theological power on the basis of her gendered lay activities" (140).
125. Winthrop, *Short Story*, 218.
126. "Report of the Trial," 373. One is left to marvel at the irony of Cotton's representation, as it is he, after all, whose opinions most influenced the Antinomians, and who inspired Hutchinson to migrate to New England.
127. Pudaloff, 155.
128. Shurtleff, 196.

129. Winthrop, *Journal,* 240.
130. Johnson, 99.

Chapter 3

1. Toni Morrison, *Song of Solomon* (New York: Penguin, 1977), 157.
2. For more on "virgin soil," see my discussion in Chapter 1, and Alfred W. Crosby, *The Columbian Exchange: Biological and Cultural Consequences of 1492,* 30th ann. ed.(Westport, CT: Praeger, 2003), and "Virgin Soil Epidemics as a Factor in the Aboriginal Depopulation in America," *William and Mary Quarterly* 33 (1976): 289–99; and David S. Jones, *Rationalizing Epidemics: Meanings and Uses of American Indian Mortality since 1600* (Cambridge, MA: Harvard University Press, 2004), and "Virgin Soils Revisited," *William and Mary Quarterly* 60 (2003): 703–42. John Duffy traces the history of colonial epidemics, offering compelling arguments about the causes of specific epidemical patterns (*Epidemics in Colonial America* [Baton Rouge: Louisiana State University Press, 1953]). Likewise, Elizabeth Fenn has given a detailed and nuanced history of smallpox during the Revolutionary War (*Pox Americana: the Great Smallpox Epidemic of 1775–82* [New York: Hill and Wang, 2001]).
3. Joyce Chaplin argues that "scholarship on American exceptionalism has usually focused on the cultural dimension of colonial history without paying equal attention to the way English settlers constructed a corporeal identity for themselves" (*Subject Matter: Technology, the Body, and Science on the Anglo-American Frontier, 1500–1676* [Cambridge, MA: Harvard University Press, 2001], 21). While I am not making a claim for the Puritan body as exceptional, the immunological and epidemiological histories that I outline in this chapter helped to inform the exceptionalist rhetoric that emerged from the colonists' seemingly unique experience of disease in New England.
4. See Jones, *Rationalizing Epidemics* for further descriptions of the 1633–34 smallpox epidemics. Jones explains that "in contrast to the epidemic of 1616, the [later] outbreak did not remain confined to the coast. Instead, it spread quickly throughout New England and into New York and Quebec. The epidemic, apparently the northeast Algonquin's first experience with smallpox, became the greatest epidemic ever to strike the New England Indians. Overall mortality approached 86 percent" (31).
5. Winthrop writes: "For the natives in these parts, Gods hand hath so pursued them, as for 300 miles space, the greatest parte of them are swept away by the small poxe, which still continues among them: So as God hathe hereby cleered our title to this place." (Letter from John Winthrop to Sir Simonds D'Ewes, July 21, 1634, *The Winthrop Papers,* ed. Allyn Bailey Forbes [Boston: Massachusetts Historical Society, 1943], 3:171–72). For more on the ways that the English sense of body and self was influenced by interaction with and observations of Native Americans and Africans, see Chaplin; and Karen Ordahl Kupperman, *Indians and English: Facing Off in Early America* (Ithaca, NY: Cornell University Press, 2000).
6. William Bradford, *Of Plymouth Plantation 1620–1647,* ed. Samuel Eliot Morison (New York: Knopf, 1952), 270–71. Referring back to the epidemics of 1616–19, John White made a similar observation about English immunity to the diseases that were decimating Native Americans (*The Planter's Plea* [London, 1630], 25).
7. William Wood, *New England's Prospect,* ed. Alden T. Vaughan (1634; repr., Amherst: University of Massachusetts Press, 1977), 32.
8. Bradford, 260 and 445.
9. The letter is most often cited because of Mather's early reference to inoculation, a process that he claims to have learned from his slave Onesimus before reading about it in the *Transactions* of the Royal Society. While the history of inoculation has long made for a compelling story, Mather's reference to the cyclical recurrence of smallpox provides equally crucial information about the early history of New England (Letter from

Cotton Mather to John Woodward, July 12, 1716, repr. in *Selected Letters of Cotton Mather*, ed. Kenneth Silverman [Baton Rouge: Louisiana State University Press, 1971], 213). Mather's reference to the "invisible world" offers an interesting counterpoint to the latter half of my analysis, which I will take up in Chapter 4. See Louise Breen for more on this phrase and on Mather's role in the 1721 inoculation controversy ("Cotton Mather, the 'Angelical Ministry,' and Inoculation," *Journal of the History of Medicine and Allied Sciences* 46 [July 1991]: 333–57).

10. Ola Elizabeth Winslow, *A Destroying Angel: The Conquest of Smallpox in Colonial Boston* (Boston: Houghton Mifflin, 1974), 26–27; and Duffy, 44–45. Smallpox is the primary focus of my analysis here, but it is one of several viral diseases—including the measles—that would have behaved in this cyclical pattern in New England, as I describe below.

11. For further discussions of smallpox and variola, see Derrick Baxby, *Jenner's Smallpox Vaccine: The Riddle of the Vaccinia Virus and Its Origin* (London: Heinemann, 1981); and Abbas M. Behbehani, *The Smallpox Story in Words and Pictures* (Kansas City, MO: Kansas Medical Center, 1988).

12. For a further discussion of this demographic effect, see Duffy, 19–23, 106; Fenn, 28; Donald R. Hopkins, *Princes and Peasants* (Chicago: University of Chicago Press, 1983), 238; and Priscilla Wald, "Imagined Immunities," *Cultural Studies and Political Theory*, ed. Jodi Dean (Ithaca, NY: Cornell University Press, 2000): 189–208, 194, and *Contagious: Cultures, Carriers, and the Outbreak Narrative* (Durham, NC: Duke University Press, 2008).

13. S. R. Duncan, Susan Scott, and C. J. Duncan, "The Dynamics of Smallpox Epidemics in Britain, 1550–1800," *Demography* 30, no. 3 (August 1993): 405–23, 406; and S. R. Duncan, Susan Scott, and C. J. Duncan, "Smallpox Epidemics in Cities in Britain," *Journal of Interdisciplinary History* 25, no. 2 (Autumn 1994): 255–71, 256.

14. Duncan, Scott, and Duncan, 259. The mean age of death from smallpox in larger cities was often between 2.5 and 5 years of age (259). And, in a point that will become central to my argument, this number was often fairly similar in smaller English towns as well. Likewise, immigrants to the city, if they were not already immune to smallpox, would more likely than not be infected relatively soon after their arrival.

15. Duncan, Scott, and Duncan, 407; and 266.

16. Duncan, Scott, and Duncan, 406; and 256.

17. The most isolated English villages likely experienced longer intervals between epidemics (Duncan, Scott, and Duncan, 411, 406).

18. For more on this, see Ola Elizabeth Winslow, who also argues that "most adults among the earliest passengers on these seventeen ships to arrive in New England [in 1630] had already acquired immunity from smallpox infection in an earlier attack, probably in childhood. Throughout the seventeenth century smallpox was still regarded as a childhood disease" (24). Francis Higginson gives brief insight into this dynamic in the description of his 1629 voyage to New England ("Higginson's Journal of His Voyage," repr. in *Chronicles of the First Planters of the Colony of Massachusetts Bay, from 1623 to 1636*, ed. Alexander Young [Boston, 1846], 215–38). The voyage began on April 25 from Gravesend, and Higginson, his wife, and his daughter Mary disembarked at Cowcastle on May 5 (219), before rejoining the ship at Yarmouth on the 11th (220). On May 17, Higginson relates that his "two children, Samuel and Mary, began to be sick of the small pox and purples together, which was brought into the ship by one Mr. Brown, which was sick of the same at Gravesend" (222). Mary died on May 19, and Higginson reports that her death "was a grief to us her parents, and a terror to all the rest, as being the beginning of a contagious disease and mortality" (223). Without being too specific, he concludes that "some of our men fell sick of the scurvy, and others of the small pox, which more and more increased; yet, thanks be to God, none died of it but my own child mentioned" (226). While light on the specifics, Higginson's journal certainly suggests a heightened susceptibility and mortality among children without denying that adults could be susceptible as well.

19. Wald, *Contagious*, 48.

20. See Lilienfeld and Lilienfeld, 61; Timmreck, 49–51; and Wald, *Contagious*, 48–53.
21. See Behbehani, 118–19, for more on the importance of herd immunity in developing modern immunization programs.
22. Duncan, Scott, and Duncan, 265; and 409.
23. William McNeill, *Plagues and Peoples* (New York: Anchor, 1998), 143.
24. Duffy, 22. Duffy posits that population density may not be the sole factor involved in this development because smallpox was often endemic (rather than epidemic) in smaller English towns (with a population ranging from 10,000 to 15,000) as well as large cities, a fact that can be addressed by the differences in local, regional, and national densities (106). He argues that by the eighteenth century, higher living standards in America meant that more people had access to procedures such as inoculation, which therefore regulated epidemics more effectively than in Europe. Although this economic premise is undoubtedly significant in contemporary health-care systems, Fenn's work seems to undermine Duffy's hypothesis—particularly as it relates to the British and American armies during the Revolutionary War.
25. Duffy, 109. Duffy also observes that American susceptibility to smallpox had a deep cultural impact throughout the seventeenth and eighteenth centuries, leading colonists to establish American schools and colleges, at least in part to minimize the dangers of traveling to Europe. My argument parallels Duffy's claim insofar as I link epidemiological patterns to the evolution of religious practices and narrative genres.
26. Wald, *Contagious*, 49.
27. For more on the concept of immunological determinism, see Chapter 1, as well as Jones, "Virgin Soils"; and Wald, "Future Perfect: Grammar, Genes, and Geography," *New Literary History* 31 (2000): 681–708.
28. Wald, "Imagined Immunities," 191, 208, and *Contagious*, 67. Although Wald's analysis describes a twentieth-century phenomenon where bacteriology, microbiology, sociology, and the "language of contagion" ("Imagined Immunities," 192) helped to reimagine the bonds of community and to break down national boundaries, I am describing much the same effects in the seventeenth century, when these boundaries were being constituted in New England. The tendency to visualize epidemics geographically (which Wald points to) leads me to believe that what we often term *national* ought to be recast as *territorial* in order to undo the pervasive metonymy of nation and territory. In this manner, the effects of a disease like HIV/AIDS, which does indeed know no territorial boundaries, manifest themselves quite differently within regional—or cultural—boundaries, depending on such factors as economic, transportation, and public health infrastructures. See also Benedict Anderson, *Imagined Communities: Reflections on the Origin and Spread of Nationalism* rev. ed. (New York: Verso, 1991).
29. Williston Walker, *A History of the Congregational Churches in the United States,* (New York, 1894), 115. For the decision to limit the franchise, see Nathaniel B. Shurtleff, ed., *Records of the Governor and Company of the Massachusetts Bay in New England,* vol. 1 (Boston, 1853), 87.
30. Edmund S. Morgan, *Visible Saints: The History of a Puritan Idea* (New York: New York University Press, 1963), 114.
31. Walker, *The Creeds and Platforms of Congregationalism* (Boston [1893]: Pilgrim, 1960), 107.
32. Walker, *Creeds,* 165. The relation between church membership and the franchise was not applied universally in New England. Unlike Massachusetts and New Haven, Plymouth and Connecticut did not limit the franchise to church members (160).
33. The debate was wide-ranging, but two responses to the Antinomian controversy—John Winthrop's *Short Story* (1644), and John Cotton's *Way of the Congregational Churches Cleared* (1648)—were published in England as a defense of the New England Congregationalist system.

34. Walker, *Creeds*, 159.
35. Walker, *Creeds*, 144.
36. The earliest covenants were exceedingly simple, as is evident from Salem's 1629 document: "We Covenant with the Lord and one with an other; and doe bynd our selves in the presence of God, to walke together in all his waies, according as he is pleased to reveale himself unto us in his Blessed word of truth" (Walker, *Creeds*, 116). Local distinctions between these covenants were to have a significant impact on the tensions between church members and nonmembers very soon after settlement. The 1648 *Cambridge Platform* was an attempt to bridge these differences and offer a consensus vision of Puritanism in New England. For more on the Covenant systems, see Morgan; Walker, *Creeds*, and *Congregational Churches;* Perry Miller, *The New England Mind: From Colony to Province* (Cambridge, MA: Harvard University Press, 1953); Norman Pettit, *The Heart Prepared: Grace and Conversion in Puritan Spiritual Life*, 2nd ed. (Middletown, CT: Wesleyan University Press, 1989); Sacvan Bercovitch, *The American Jeremiad* (Madison: University of Wisconsin Press, 1978); Janice Knight, *Orthodoxies in Massachusetts: Rereading American Puritanism* (Cambridge, MA: Harvard University Press, 1994); David Hall, *The Faithful Shepherd: A History of the New England Ministry in the Seventeenth Century* (Chapel Hill: University of North Carolina Press, 1972); Robert G. Pope, *The Half-Way Covenant: Church Membership in Puritan New England* (Princeton, NJ: Princeton University Press, 1969); and Michael P. Winship, *Making Heretics: Militant Protestants and Free Grace in Massachusetts, 1636–1641* (Princeton, NJ: Princeton University Press, 2002).
37. See, John T. Waters, "Hingham, Massachusetts, 1631–1661: An East Anglian Oligarchy in the New World," *Journal of Social History* 1, no. 4 (1968): 351–70.
38. The petition appeared in England under the title of *New-England's Jonas Cast up at London* (London, 1647), and Edward Winslow's rebuttal, *New-Englands Salamander* (London, 1647), was published shortly thereafter, giving the Court's version of events. In addition to Child, the signers of the petition were Thomas Fowle, Samuel Maverick, Thomas Burton, David Yale, John Smith, and John Dand. This group was anything but tolerant, and it was by no means homogeneous or bound by ideological beliefs beyond a fortuitous convergence of disparate complaints that focused on the goal of overturning the Massachusetts Government, and establishing the Presbyterian Church in New England. George Lyman Kittredge's characterization puts it best: "A moment's reflection shows that [their diversity of views] is equally disconcerting to *any* theory that would strive to explain the united action of this ill-assorted group" ("Dr. Robert Child the Remonstrant," *Transactions of the Colonial Society of Massachusetts* 21 [Boston, 1920]: 1–146, 28, original emphasis). See also Waters; and Margaret E. Newell, "Robert Child and the Entrepreneurial Vision: Economy and Ideology in Early New England," *The New England Quarterly* 68, no. 2 (1995): 223–56.
39. John Winthrop, "A Model of Christian Charity," in *The Norton Anthology of American Literature*, 7th ed., Vol. A, eds. Nina Baym, et al. (New York: Norton, 2007): 147–58, 147.
40. John Child, *New Englands Jonas Cast up at London* (London, 1647), 6.
41. Child, 7.
42. Winthrop, *The Journal of John Winthrop 1630–1649*, eds. Richard S. Dunn, James Savage, and Laetitia Yeandle (Cambridge, MA: Harvard University Press, 1996), 620.
43. Winthrop, *Journal*, 620.
44. Kittredge, 2.
45. Kittredge, 7–8. Kittredge also reports that Child was the subject of correspondence between Hugh Peter and the elder Winthrop in which his Presbyterianism was noted explicitly as a cause for concern (16).
46. Winthrop, *Journal*, 657.
47. Winthrop, *Journal*, 657.
48. Child, 10, 11–12.

49. Pettit, 158.
50. Walker, *Creeds*, 246.
51. Morgan, 126.
52. Miller, *Colony*, 88.
53. Miller, *Colony*, 89.
54. Walker, *Creeds*, 169. While the question was left unsettled until 1662, the Cambridge Synod of 1646–48 was explicitly charged with answering this question.
55. Winthrop, *Journal*, 690.
56. Winthrop, *Journal*, 691.
57. Walker, *Creeds*, 224.
58. Bercovitch, 27.
59. Bercovitch, 65; and Morgan, 137.
60. Morgan, 125, 128.
61. Although this commitment moves from a local to a nationalist project through the process of negotiation that is the function of a synod, David Hall notes that individual congregations did not apply the halfway covenant consistently throughout New England (the freedom to adhere to doctrinal decisions being a special feature of New England Congregationalist synods or "councils"). Instead, Hall cites Pope's study that "documented patterns of response to the halfway covenant so various as to defy interpretation," so that even the analysis that I give here reflects an attempt to describe a deeply contested and dynamic evolution, rather than a cultural model that was universally accepted ("On Common Ground: The Coherence of American Puritan Studies," *William and Mary Quarterly* 44, no. 2 [1987]: 193–229, 224).
62. Bercovitch, 64.
63. Bercovitch, 65.
64. Miller, *Orthodoxy in Massachusetts 1630–1650: A Genetic Study* (Cambridge, MA: Harvard University Press, 1933).
65. Bercovitch, 65.
66. Bercovitch, 33.
67. Bercovitch, 62.
68. Michael Wigglesworth, "God's Controversy with New England," *Electronic Texts in American Studies*, ed. Reiner Smolinski (Lincoln: University of Nebraska Press, 2007). Line citations will be given parenthetically in the text.
69. Miller, *Colony*, 30.
70. My reference to orthodoxy in this context is not meant to suggest the existence of a singular, capital "O" Puritan Orthodoxy in Massachusetts, but to an internal debate aimed at giving voice to a set of core theological tenets that could be described as orthodox in and of themselves. Part of my broader argument is that the immunological syntax of epidemiological rhetoric helps to articulate cultural consensus and orthodoxy by pathologizing certain behaviors believed to produce illness (literal or figurative), and creating regulatory mechanisms to protect communities by policing these behaviors.
71. This rhetorical move is quite similar to Edward Johnson's representation of dead Native Americas as failed crops in the wake of the 1616–19 epidemics (*A History of New-England* [*Wonder-Working Providence of Sions Saviour*] [London, 1654]). See Chapter 1 for a more extensive discussion of this trope.
72. Wigglesworth was born in England in 1631, but immigrated to New England in 1638, so I am representing him as a voice of the second generation. He was educated at Harvard, and became a minister, although his life-long interest in medicine led him to become a practicing physician later in life. See Richard Crowder, *No Featherbed to Heaven* (East Lansing: Michigan State University Press, 1962).
73. Wigglesworth, *The Diary of Michael Wigglesworth, 1653–1657*, ed. Morgan (New York: Harper & Row, 1965), 64.

Chapter 4

1. William Wells Brown, *Clotel; or, The President's Daughter* (New York: Modern Library, 2000), 100.
2. *The Boston Gazette*, no. 71, April 17–24, 1721. See also Ola Elizabeth Winslow, *A Destroying Angel: The Conquest of Smallpox in Colonial Boston* (Boston: Houghton Mifflin, 1974), 44.
3. Both *The Boston Gazette* and *The Boston News-Letter* reported that as of May 27th, "there are now Eight Persons Sick of the Small-Pox in the Town, and no more, according to the best Information" (*BNL*, no. 899, May 22–29, 1721; see also *BG*, no. 77, May 22–29, 1721).
4. *BNL*, no. 898, May 15–22, 1721.
5. *BNL*, no. 900, May 29–June 5, 1721.
6. Winslow, 58. Although the Boston selectmen ordered a report of the number of cases in 1721, it is difficult to say with certainty what the final figures for this epidemic were. Using the selectmen's records, John Duffy reports a population of 10,670 with 5,980 cases and 844 deaths, while he says that William Douglass's estimate put the number of deaths at 899 (*Epidemics in Colonial America* [Baton Rouge: Louisiana State University Press, 1953], 51); John Blake reports 5,759 cases with 842 fatalities (*Public Health in the Town of Boston 1630–1822* [Cambridge, MA: Harvard University Press, 1959], 61); Otho T. Beall and Richard Shryock report 5,889 cases with 844 fatalities (*Cotton Mather: First Significant Figure in American Medicine* [Baltimore: Johns Hopkins University Press, 1954], 107); and Oscar Reiss records 5,759 cases with 844 fatalities (*Medicine in Colonial America* [Lanham, MD: University Press of America, 2000], 302). The epidemic began in late May, and peaked in the fall of 1721, before receding early in 1722. Elsewhere, Blake breaks down the epidemic's progress as follows: "One person died in May, eight in June, eleven in July, and twenty-six in August," 101 in September, 411 in October, 249 in November, and by late February 1722, "there were no more known cases in the town ("The Inoculation Controversy in Boston, 1721–1722," *The New England Quarterly* 25, no. 4 [December 1952]: 489–506, 495, 496, repr. in I. Bernard Cohen, ed., *Cotton Mather and American Science and Medicine*, vol. 1 [New York: Arno Press, 1980]).
7. Carla Mulford, "Pox and 'Hell-Fire': Boston's Smallpox Controversy, the New Science, and Early Modern Liberalism," *Periodical Literature in Eighteenth-Century America*, eds. Mark L. Kamrath and Sharon M. Harris (Knoxville: University of Tennessee Press, 2005): 7–27, 7.
8. Timonius's letter was printed in *Transactions*, no. 339 (1714), while Pylarinus's appeared in No. 347 (1716), and both were collected in vol. 29 (1717). See George Lyman Kittredge, "Some Lost Works of Cotton Mather," *Proceedings of the Massachusetts Historical Society*, vol. 45 (Boston, 1912): 418–79, 419. For Lady Mary Wortley Montagu's role in advocating inoculation, see Abbas M. Behbehani, *The Smallpox Story in Words and Pictures* (Kansas, MO: Kansas Medical Center, 1988), 17. Arnold C. Klebs offers a slightly more detailed history, reporting that while the Montagus and the 1721 Boston inoculators represent the most widely publicized experiments with the procedure, European physicians did have knowledge of it going back at least to 1670, when practitioners in Leipzig referred to it cryptically as "buying the smallpox" ("The Historic Evolution of Variolation," *Bulletin of the Johns Hopkins Hospital* 24, no. 265 [1913]: 69–83, 70, repr. in Cohen, vol. 1). See also Maxine Van De Wetering, "A Reconsideration of the Inoculation Controversy," *The New England Quarterly* 58, no. 1 (1985): 46–67.
9. Winslow, 77. This figure reflects the inoculations performed in Boston by Zabdiel Boylston (six of the patients in his care died). According to Reiss, thirty-nine more people were inoculated in towns such as Roxbury and Cambridge, for a grand total of 286 (302); Blake's aggregate total is 287, also with six deaths (*Public Health*, 61).
10. See Letter from Cotton Mather to John Woodward, July 12, 1716, *Selected Letters of Cotton Mather*, ed. Kenneth Silverman (Baton Rouge: Louisiana State University Press,

1971): 213–14 (this is the same letter in which Mather mentions the twelve-year cyclical pattern of smallpox epidemics in Boston discussed in Chapter 3). William Douglass was a Scottish-born doctor who was educated in Edinburgh, Leyden, and Paris (Raymond P. Stearns, *Science in the British Colonies of America* [Urbana: University of Illinois Press, 1970]: 477–84).

11. Cotton Mather, *Selected Letters,* 214. See also *Diary of Cotton Mather,* 2 vols. (New York: Ungar, 1957), 2:662, and *The Angel of Bethesda,* ed. Gordon W. Jones (Barre, MA: American Antiquarian Society, 1972), 107.

12. Boston experienced another smallpox epidemic in 1730, but this time Douglass supported inoculation. See Blake, *Public Health,* 75 and 84; and Douglass, *A Dissertation Concerning Inoculation of the Small-Pox* (Boston, 1730).

13. The ministers who signed this letter were Cotton and Increase Mather, Benjamin Colman, Thomas Prince, John Webb, and William Cooper (*BG,* no. 88, July 27–31, 1721). Anti-inoculators included James Franklin, Samuel Grainger, John Checkly, and John Williams.

14. See, for example, *The New England Courant,* no. 18, November 27–December 4, 1721. See also Mulford, "Pox and 'Hell-Fire,'" 11. James Franklin, of course, was assisted by his younger brother and apprentice Benjamin, who would go on to publish the *New England Courant* when James was forbidden to do so in 1723.

15. Examples of such minister–physicians in the seventeenth century include John Eliot, Michael Wigglesworth, and Thomas Thacher. See Patricia A. Watson, *The Angelical Conjunction: The Preacher-Physicians of Colonial New England* (Knoxville: University of Tennessee Press, 1991).

16. Douglass, *The Abuses and Scandals of some late Pamphlets in Favour of Inoculation of the Smallpox, Modestly obviated, and Inoculation further consider'd in a Letter to A___S___M.D. & F.R.S. in London* (Boston, 1722), 8.

17. Douglass, *Abuses and Scandals,* 8. See also Van De Wetering, 53.

18. Douglass, *Abuses and Scandals,* 6. The anti-inoculators derived endless amusement from mocking Mather. They joked that he had discovered methods for solving unsolvable mathematical problems such as "squaring a circle," and for calculating a ship's longitudinal position with ease (6). Among the most ridiculed of his observations was his "particular Fancy, that the *wild* Pidgeons, when they leave New-England at certain Seasons, repair to some undiscover'd Satellite, accompanying the Earth at a near Distance" (6). The fact that Mather's name did not appear on the Royal Society's rolls seems to have been a clerical oversight, rather than fraud on his part. See Kittredge, "Cotton Mather's Election into the Royal Society," *Transactions of the Colonial Society of Massachusetts, 1911–1913* (Boston, 1913), 14:81–114, repr. in Cohen, vol. 1, and "Further Notes on Cotton Mather and the Royal Society," *Transactions of the Colonial Society of Massachusetts, 1911–1913* (Boston, 1913), 14:281–92, repr. in Cohen, vol. 1.

19. See Cotton Mather to John Woodward, 213–14.

20. Douglass, *Inoculation of the Small Pox as practiced in Boston, Consider'd in a Letter to A___S___M.D. & F.R.S. in London* (Boston, 1722), A2. Although the introduction to Douglass's pamphlet is unsigned, Perry Miller attributes it to James Franklin (*The New England Mind: From Colony to Province* [Cambridge, MA: Harvard University Press, 1953], 357).

21. *NEC,* no. 1, August 7, 1721.

22. This was a common point of attack against the pro-inoculation forces, and Samuel Grainger took up the charge by framing the issue in terms of the Sixth Commandment, because inoculation was potential fatal to inoculees: "I think it very Evident that the Voluntary Transplanting upon my self an Infectious and Pestilential Distemper, is the encouraging and producing of a Moral Cause, which has a Tendency to take away my own Life, and the Life of my Neighbour unjustly, if Pestilential distempers have a Tendency to take away Life, which I hope you will allow" (*The Imposition of Inoculation as a Duty Religiously Considered in a Leter to a Gentleman in the Country Inclin'd to Admit it* [Boston, 1721], 16). See also Edmund Massey, who took up the anti-inoculation argument in

England (*A Sermon against the Dangerous and sinful Practice of Inoculation*, 3rd ed. [London 1722, rpt. Boston, 1730], esp. 21–22). While this logic is straightforward, Increase Mather argued the exact opposite stance with equal conviction. He claimed that because humans were commanded to take whatever means necessary to protect themselves from harm (and inoculation protected them from harm), they were obliged to submit themselves to it: "It is then a wonderful Providence of GOD, that all that were Inoculated should have their Lives preserved.... I confess I am afraid, that the Discouraging of this Practice, may cause many a Life to be lost, which for my own part, I should be loth to have any hand in, because of the Sixth Commandment" (*Several Reasons Proving that Inoculating or Transplanting the Small Pox, is a Lawful Practice, and that it has been Blessed by GOD for the Saving of many a Life* [Boston, 1721], 1). The fact that these arguments were so easily transposed from one side to the other inevitably led to rhetorical posturing in which equally empty logical forms became the object of ridicule; the syllogisms offered one day became fodder for satire the next.
23. Douglass, *Inoculation of the Small Pox*, 12.
24. Grainger, 19.
25. Grainger, 4.
26. Grainger, 5.
27. Grainger, 9.
28. Grainger, 4–5.
29. Grainger, 8.
30. Perry Miller, 358.
31. Grainger, 11.
32. Massey, 24. This notion of using a treatment to put oneself in harm's way is by no means new. Mitchell Breitwieser briefly explores the relation between inoculation and Derrida's analysis of Plato's pharmakon (*Cotton Mather and Benjamin Franklin: The Price of Representative Personality* [Cambridge, UK: Cambridge University Press, 1984], 120–23).
33. Grainger, 12.
34. Increase Mather, 1.
35. *NEC*, no. 1, August 7, 1721, and *NEC*, no. 17, November 21–27, 1721. This particular line of attack appeared to be one of the anti-inoculators' favorites. In mid-August, they wrote that "'twas hop'd ... those Gentlemen of Piety and Learning who pleaded for the Practice, would have brought some other Arguments upon the Stage than the *naked Merits* of their *Character* (which Sort of Argument, if insisted upon, they were told, might possibly be inquir'd into) and we leave the World to judge, whether any Man's *Ipse dixit* without any proof, ought to be sufficient to weigh down the Scale against *Sufficient Evidence, right Reason* and the *Safety* and *Welfare* of a People" (*NEC*, no. 3, August 14–21, 1721).
36. See Perry Miller; Beall and Shryock; Stearns; Duffy; Winslow; Mulford, "Pox and 'Hell-Fire'" and "New Science and the Question of Identity in Eighteenth-Century British America," *Finding Colonial Americas Essays Honoring J. A. Leo Lemay*, ed. Carla Mulford and David S. Shields (Newark: University of Delaware Press, 2001): 79–103; Robert Middlekauff; *The Mathers: Three Generations of Puritan Intellectuals, 1596–1728* (New York: Oxford University Press, 1971); Louise Breen, "Cotton Mather, the 'Angelical Ministry,' and Inoculation," *Journal of the History of Medicine and Allied Sciences* 46 (1991): 333–57; Genevieve Miller, *The Adoption of Inoculation for Smallpox in England and France* (Philadelphia: University of Pennsylvania Press, 1957); Margot Minardi, "The Inoculation Controversy of 1721–1722: An Incident in the History of Race," *The William and Mary Quarterly* 61, no. 1 (2004): 47–76; Eugenia W. Herbert, "Smallpox Inoculation in Africa," *Journal of African History* 16, no. 4 (1975): 539–59; Thomas H. Brown, "The African Connection: Cotton Mather and the Boston Smallpox Epidemic of 1721–1722," *The Journal of the American Medical Association* 260, no. 15 (October 12, 1988): 2247–49; and Margaret Humphreys Warner, "Vindicating the Minister's Medical Role: Cotton Mather's Concept

of the *Nishmath-Chajim* and the Spiritualization of Medicine," *Journal of the History of Medicine and Allied Sciences* 36, no. 3 (1981): 278–95.

37. Perry Miller, 361.

38. The debate did quite literally make its way onto the streets of Boston when an anonymous anti-inoculator hurled a homemade bomb through Cotton Mather's window under cover of darkness in the early morning of November 14th. The next day Mather wrote in his diary that "when the Granado was taken up, there was found a Paper so tied with String about the Fuse, that it might out-Live the breaking of the Shell, which had these words in it; COTTON MATHER, You Dog, Dam you: I'l inoculate you with this, with a Pox to you" (2:658). Far from discouraging him, Mather wrote that this event "filled [me] with unutterable Joy at the Prospect of my approaching Martyrdom . . . when I think on my suffering Death for saving the Lives of dying People, it even ravishes me with a Joy unspeakable and full of Glory" (2:659).

39. Although Mather intended to publish *The Angel of Bethesda*, it did not appear in print during his lifetime; in the February 20, 1724, entry of his diary, he notes that "my large Work, entituled *The Angel of Bethesda*, is now finished. If my glorious Lord will please to accept of it, it may prove on of the most useful Books, that have been written in the World" (2:698–99).

40. Breen, 340.

41. Cotton Mather, *Angel of Bethesda*, 28.

42. Cotton Mather, *Angel of Bethesda*, 30, 33. For more on Mather's understanding of the *Nishamath-Chajim*, see Breen, and Warner, who identifies it as an explicit attempt on Mather's part to create "a rationale for the minister to enter the sick room, even though the increasingly well educated physician was busily attempting to usher him out" (294).

43. Cotton Mather, *Angel of Bethesda*, 31.

44. Cotton Mather, *Angel of Bethesda*, 33.

45. Cotton Mather, *Angel of Bethesda*, 35. See also Mulford, "New Science," 89.

46. Cotton Mather, *Angel of Bethesda*, 37.

47. Cotton Mather, *Angel of Bethesda*, 94.

48. Cotton Mather, *Angel of Bethesda*, 94.

49. Cotton Mather, *Angel of Bethesda*, 95.

50. Cotton Mather, *Angel of Bethesda*, 96.

51. Beall and Shryock, 6.

52. Breen, 338.

53. Breen, 356.

54. Cotton Mather, *Angel of Bethesda*, 43.

55. Benjamin Marten, *A New Theory of Consumptions: More Especially of a Phthisis, or Consumption of the Lungs* (London, 1720), 50, 52. See also Cotton Mather, *Angel of Bethesda*, 43.

56. Marten, v. Interestingly, Gordon Jones, the modern editor of *The Angel of Bethesda*, suggests that Mather's reading and adoption of Marten's ideas made him unique in America: "No other American, according to Doctor Shryock, discussed the germ theory until John Crawford did so in 1807" (333n2).

57. Cotton Mather, *Angel of Bethesda*, 44.

58. Cotton Mather, *Angel of Bethesda*, 45. See also Marten, 64–65.

59. Cotton Mather, *Angel of Bethesda*, 44. See also Marten, 64.

60. See Breen, 354.

61. Cotton Mather, *Angel of Bethesda*, 47.

62. Cotton Mather, *Angel of Bethesda*, 45.

63. Cotton Mather, *Angel of Bethesda*, 94.

64. [Cotton Mather], *Sentiments on the Small Pox Inoculated* (Boston, 1721), 2.

65. Cotton Mather, *Angel of Bethesda*, 112.

66. Cotton Mather, *Angel of Bethesda*, 112.

67. Marten, 51. See also Cotton Mather, *The Angel of Bethesda*, 45–46.

68. [Cotton Mather], *An Account of the Method and Success of Inoculating the Small-Pox in Boston, in New-England* (London, 1722), 8. For an attribution of this pamphlet to Mather, see Kittredge, "Some Lost Works."

69. [Cotton Mather], *An Account,* 8.

70. See Cotton Mather, *Diary* 2:657.

71. [Cotton Mather], *An Account,* 17.

72. Zabdiel Boylston, *Some Account of what is said of Innoculating or Transplanting the Small Pox* (Boston, 1721), 21.

73. Elizabeth A. Fenn, *Pox Americana: The Great Smallpox Epidemic of 1775–82* (New York: Hill and Wang, 2001), 93.

74. See Philip F. Gura, *Jonathan Edwards: America's Evangelical* (New York: Hill and Wang, 2005), 218; and Iain H. Murray, *Jonathan Edwards: A New Biography* (Carlisle, PA: Banner of Truth Trust, 1987), 441.

75. Derrick Baxby, *Jenner's Smallpox Vaccine: The Riddle of the Vaccinia Virus and Its Origin* (London: Heinemann, 1981). 53. See also Edward, Jenner, *An Inquiry into the Causes and Effects of the Variolae Vaccinae* (London, 1798).

76. Behbehani, 109.

77. Behbehani, 122.

78. Behbehani, 118.

79. Behbehani, 119.

80. Behbehani, 118.

81. See Mulford, "Pox and 'Hell-Fire.'"

82. Benedict Anderson, *Imagined Communities: Reflections on the Origin and Spread of Nationalism* rev. ed. (New York: Verso, 1991). See also Mulford, "Pox and 'Hell-Fire.'"

83. See Priscilla Wald, "Imagined Immunities," *Cultural Studies and Political Theory,* ed. Jodi Dean (Ithaca, NY: Cornell University Press, 2000), 189–208, and *Contagious: Cultures, Carriers, and the Outbreak Narrative* (Durham, NC: Duke University Press, 2008).

84. *NEC,* no. 1, August 7, 1721.

85. *NEC,* no. 2, August 7–14, 1721.

86. *NEC,* no. 1, August 7, 1721.

87. *NEC,* no. 2, August 7–14, 1721.

88. *NEC,* no. 2, August 7–14, 1721. Although intended satirically, a similar plan would be discussed during the Seven Years' War, when Sir Jeffrey Amherst, the commander of the British forces in North America, suggested that Native American alliances might be broken if they were "inoculated" with smallpox-infested blankets (Behbehani, 7).

89. A contemporary reminder of this fact has been on the front pages of international newspapers since early in the new millennium, as public health officials worldwide have struggled with the threat of SARS, Avian influenza (H5N1), H1N1, and multiple-drug-resistant tuberculosis, each of which has caused disruptions in trade and travel routes.

90. Zabdiel Boylston, *An Historical Account of the Small Pox Inoculated in New England, Upon all Sorts of Persons, Whites, Blacks, and of all Ages and Constitutions,* 2nd ed. corr. (London, 1726; Boston 1730), 2.

91. Cotton Mather to John Woodward, 214. Practiced as he was in gathering medical knowledge from Pagan as well as Christian sources, Mather did not seem deeply concerned with Onesimus's trustworthiness—although it turns out that many Bostonians were. Certainly, the fact that Onesimus's testimony was corroborated in the *Transactions* of the Royal Society must have influenced Mather's later decision to advocate the procedure publicly.

92. Susan Scott Parrish, *American Curiosity: Cultures of Natural History in the Colonial British Atlantic World* (Chapel Hill: University of North Carolina Press, 2006), 286.

93. For more on Cotton Mather's correspondence with the Royal Society, see Kittredge, "Cotton Mather's Scientific Communications with the Royal Society" *Proceedings of the American Antiquarian Society* (Worcester, 1916): 3–42, repr. in Cohen, vol. 1.

94. [Cotton Mather], *An Account*, 1–2.
95. See Boylston, *Some Account*. There is some controversy about the exact authorship of this pamphlet, although it seems clear that Mather had at least a hand in it, writing in his August 25 diary entry, that "I will assist my Physician, in giving to the Public, some Accounts about releeving the Small-Pox in the way of Transplantation; which may be of great consequence!" (2:639). For a primary attribution of the pamphlet to Mather, see Kittredge, "Some Lost Works," esp. 428–29. For an argument about attribution to Boylston, see Jennifer Lee Carrell, who nonetheless acknowledges Mather's likely contribution (*The Speckled Monster: A Historical Tale of Battling the Smallpox* [New York: Dutton, 2003], 474). I tend to agree with Kittredge on this point, especially considering the close parallels between the passage of the Boylston tract that I examine here, and the other versions provided by Mather, including in *The Angel of Bethesda*.
96. Boylston, *Some Account*, 9.
97. Cotton Mather, *Angel of Bethesda*, 107.
98. Boylston, *Some Account*, 9.
99. Minardi, 63.
100. Minardi, 48.
101. Boylston, *Some Account*, 9.
102. Likewise, Minardi critiques these awkward epistemological claims, writing that "stripped of its paternalist platitudes, the inoculation advocates' argument for the truthfulness of slave testimony rested on this staggering logic: African knowledge was trustworthy precisely because African people had no knowledge. In one stroke, those who used this explanation inverted the traditional relationship between status and knowledge and then set that linkage aright again by filtering the words of the base and simple Africans through the Englishmen's own authoritative prose" (65).
103. Douglass, *Inoculation of the Small Pox*, 7.
104. Cotton Mather, *Diary*, 2:624.
105. Cotton Mather, *Angel of Bethesda*, 107
106. Mulford, "Pox and 'Hell-Fire,'" 12.
107. [Cotton Mather], *Sentiments*, 2.
108. Cotton Mather, *Diary*, 2:663.
109. Douglass, *Inoculation of the Small Pox*, 20.
110. [Cotton Mather], *An Account*, 2.
111. *NEC*, no. 55, August 13–20, 1722.

Afterword

1. Charles Johnson, *Middle Passage* (New York: Atheneum, 1990), 154–55.
2. Thomas Morton, *New English Canaan* (Amsterdam, 1637), 104–5; and [Cotton Mather], *Sentiments on the Small Pox Inoculated* (Boston, 1721), 2.
3. William, Douglass, *Inoculation of the Small Pox as practiced in Boston, Consider'd in a Letter to A__S__M.D. & F.R.S. in London* (Boston, 1722), 7.
4. Mather, *Diary of Cotton Mather*, 2 vols. (New York: Ungar, 1957), 2: 624.
5. Thomas Bender, "Introduction: Historians, the Nation, and the Plenitude of Narratives," in *Rethinking American History in a Global Age*, ed. Bender (Berkeley: University of California Press, 2002), 1–21, 3.
6. Bender, 7.
7. Bender, 11.
8. Perry Miller, *Errand into the Wilderness* (Cambridge, MA: Harvard University Press, 1956), viii.
9. See, for example, Janice Knight, *Orthodoxies in Massachusetts: Rereading American Puritanism* (Cambridge, MA: Harvard University Press, 1994) and Gesa Mackenthun,

Metaphors of Dispossession: American Beginnings and the Translation of Empire 1492–1637 (Norman: University of Oklahoma Press, 1997).

10. Rian Malan, "Megadeath and Megahype" *San Francisco Chronicle,* January 6, 2002: D1+. A longer, epistolary version of this article first appeared as Malan, "AIDS in Africa: In Search of the Truth" *Rolling Stone,* November 22, 2001: 70+.

11. Malan, "Megadeath and Megahype," D1.

12. Carol Ezzell, "Hope in a Vial," *Scientific American,* June 2002: 37–45. In particular, see the map titled "World AIDS Snapshot," 41.

13. Francis L. Black, "An Explanation of High Death Rates among New World Peoples When in Contact with Old World Diseases," *Perspectives in Biology and Medicine* 37 (1994): 292–307.

14. Ezzell, 40.

15. Commission on Presidential Debates, "The Cheney-Edwards Vice Presidential Debate," October 5, 2004, http://www.debates.org/index.php?page=october-5-2004-transcript.

WORKS CITED

Adams, Charles Francis. *Three Episodes of Massachusetts History*. vol. 1. Cambridge, MA: Riverside, 1903.

Anderson, Benedict. *Imagined Communities: Reflections on the Origin and Spread of Nationalism*. Rev. ed. New York: Verso, 1991.

Arneil, Barbara. *John Locke and America: The Defence of English Colonialism*. Oxford: Clarendon Press, 1996.

Baillie, Robert. *A Dissuassive From the Errours Of the Time*. London: Printed for Samuel Gellibrand, 1645.

Banner, Stuart. *How the Indians Lost Their Land: Law and Power on the Frontier*. Cambridge, MA: Harvard University Press, 2005.

Barry, John Stetson. *History of Massachusetts: The Colonial Period*. 4th ed., vol. 1. Boston: Phillips, Sampson, 1856.

Battis, Emery. *Saints and Sectaries: Anne Hutchinson and the Antinomian Controversy in the Massachusetts Bay Colony*. Chapel Hill: University of North Carolina Press, 1962.

Baudrillard, Jean. *The Gulf War Did Not Take Place*. Trans. Paul Patton. Bloomington: Indiana University Press, 1995.

Baxby, Derrick. *Jenner's Smallpox Vaccine: The Riddle of the Vaccinia Virus and Its Origin*. London: Heinemann, 1981.

Beall, Otho T., and Richard Shryock. *Cotton Mather: First Significant Figure in American Medicine*. Baltimore: Johns Hopkins, 1954.

Behbehani, Abbas M. *The Smallpox Story in Words and Pictures*. Kansas City, MO: Kansas Medical Center, 1988.

Bender, Thomas. "Introduction: Historians, the Nation, and the Plenitude of Narratives." In *Rethinking American History in a Global Age*. Ed. Bender, 1–21. Berkeley: University of California Press, 2002.

Bercovitch, Sacvan. *The American Jeremiad*. Madison: University of Wisconsin Press, 1978.

Black, Francis L. "An Explanation of High Death Rates among New World Peoples When in Contact with Old World Diseases." *Perspectives in Biology and Medicine* 37 (1994): 292–307.

Blake, John. "The Inoculation Controversy in Boston, 1721–1722." *The New England Quarterly* 25, no. 4 (December 1952): 489–506.

———. *Public Health in the Town of Boston 1630–1822*. Cambridge, MA: Harvard University Press, 1959.

Boylston, Zabdiel. *An Historical Account of the Small Pox Inoculated in New England, Upon all Sorts of Persons, Whites, Blacks, and of all Ages and Constitutions*. 2nd ed. corr. London, 1726. Boston: Printed for S. Gerrish and T. Hancock, 1730.

————. *Some Account of what is said of Innoculating or Transplanting the Small Pox by the Learned Dr. Emanuel Timonius, and Jacob Pylarinus. With some Remarks thereon.* Boston: Printed for S. Gerrish, 1721.

Bradford, William. *Governor William Bradford's Letter Book.* Bedford, MA: Applewood Books, 2001.

————. *Of Plymouth Plantation 1620–1647.* Ed. Samuel Eliot Morison. New York: Knopf, 1952.

Bratton, Timothy L. "The Identity of the New England Indian Epidemic of 1616–1619." *Bulletin of the History of Medicine* 62 (1988): 351–83.

Breen, Louise. "Cotton Mather, the 'Angelical Ministry,' and Inoculation." *Journal of the History of Medicine and Allied Sciences* 46 (July 1991): 333–57.

————. *Transgressing the Bounds: Subversive Enterprises among the Puritan Elite in Massachusetts, 1630–1692.* New York: Oxford University Press, 2001.

Breitwieser, Mitchell. *Cotton Mather and Benjamin Franklin: The Price of Representative Personality.* Cambridge, UK: Cambridge University Press, 1984.

Brigham, William, ed. *The Compact with the Charter and Laws of the Colony of New Plymouth.* Boston: Dutton and Wentworth, 1836.

Brown, Thomas H. "The African Connection: Cotton Mather and the Boston Smallpox Epidemic of 1721–1722." *The Journal of the American Medical Association* 260, no. 15 (October 12, 1988): 2247–49.

Brown, William Wells. *Clotel; or, The President's Daughter.* New York: Modern Library, 2000.

Burnham, Michelle. "Anne Hutchinson and the Economics of Antinomian Selfhood in Colonial New England." *Criticism* 39 no. 3 (1997): 337–58.

Caldwell, Patricia. "The Antinomian Language Controversy." *Harvard Theological Review* 69, no. 3–4 (1976): 345–67.

Cañizares-Esguerra, Jorge. *Puritan Conquistadors: Iberianizing the Atlantic, 1550–1700.* Stanford, CA: Stanford University Press, 2006.

Carrell, Jennifer Lee. *The Speckled Monster: A Historical Tale of Battling the Smallpox.* New York: Dutton, 2003.

Chaplin, Joyce E. *Subject Matter: Technology, the Body, and Science on the Anglo-American Frontier, 1500–1676.* Cambridge, MA: Harvard University Press, 2001.

Cheyfitz, Eric. *The Poetics of Imperialism: Translation and Colonization from "The Tempest" to "Tarzan."* New York: Oxford University Press, 1991.

Child, John. *New-England's Jonas Cast up at London.* London: Printed for T.R. and E.M., 1647.

Cohen, I. Bernard, ed. *Cotton Mather and American Science and Medicine.* 2 vols. New York: Arno Press, 1980.

Commission on Presidential Debates. "The Cheney-Edwards Vice Presidential Debate." October 5, 2004. http://www.debates.org/index.php?page=october-5-2004-transcript.

Condé, Maryse. *I, Tituba, Black Witch of Salem.* Trans. Richard Philcox. New York: Ballantine Books, 1992.

Cook, Noble David. *Born to Die: Disease and New World Conquests, 1492–1650.* Cambridge, UK: Cambridge University Press, 1998.

Cook, Sherburne F. "The Significance of Disease in the Extinction of the New England Indians." *Human Biology* 45 (1973): 485–508.

Cotton, John. *The Correspondence of John Cotton.* Ed. Sargent Bush, Jr. Chapel Hill: University of North Carolina Press, 2001.

————. *The Way of Congregational Churches Cleared* (1648). Repr. in Hall, ed., *The Antinomian Controversy,* 396–437.

Cronon, William. *Changes in the Land: Indians, Colonists, and the Ecology of New England.* New York: Hill and Wang, 1989.

Crosby, Alfred W. *The Columbian Exchange: Biological and Cultural Consequences of 1492.* 30th ann. ed. Westport, CT: Praeger, 2003.

————. "Virgin Soil Epidemics as a Factor in the Aboriginal Depopulation in America." *William and Mary Quarterly* 33 (1976): 289–99.

Crowder, Richard. *No Featherbed to Heaven*. East Lansing: Michigan State University Press, 1962.

Cushman, Robert. *Reasons and Considerations touching the lawfulness of removing out of England into the parts of America* (1622). Repr. in *A Journal of the Pilgrims at Plymouth [Mourt's Relation]*. Ed. Dwight Heath, 88–96. Cambridge, MA: Applewood Books, 1986.

———. *A Sermon Preached at Plimmoth in New-England December 9, 1621. In an assemblie of his Majesties faithfull Subjects, there inhabiting. Wherein is shewed the danger of selfe-love, and the sweetnesse of true Friendship. Together, with a Preface, Shewing the state of the Country, and Condition of the Savages [The Sin and Danger of Self-Love]*. London: Printed by I.D. for John Bellamie, 1622.

de Champlain, Samuel. *The Voyages of Sieur de Champlain* (1613). Trans. Charles Pomeroy Otis. Repr. in *Publications of the Prince Society*. New York: Burt Franklin (1878) 1966.

Delbanco, Andrew. *The Puritan Ordeal*. Cambridge, MA: Harvard University Press, 1989.

Dermer, Thomas. "To his Worshipfull Friend M. Samuel Purchas, Preacher of the Word, at the Church a little within Ludgate, London." In Samuel Purchas, *Hakluytus Posthumus or Purchas His Pilgrimes* (1625). Repr. Glasgow: James MacLehose, 1906.

Dillon, Elizabeth Maddock. *The Gender of Freedom: Fictions of Liberalism and the Literary Public Sphere*. Stanford, CA: Stanford University Press, 2004.

Dobyns, Henry F. "Brief Perspective on a Scholarly Transformation: Widowing the 'Virgin Land.'" *Ethnohistory* 23, no. 2 (Spring 1976): 95–104.

———. "Disease Transfer at Contact." *Annual Review of Anthropology* 22 (1993): 273–91.

———. *Their Numbers Become Thinned*. Knoxville: University of Tennessee Press, 1983.

Douglass, William. *The Abuses and Scandals of some late Pamphlets in Favour of Inoculation of the Smallpox, Modestly obviated, and Inoculation further consider'd in a Letter to A___S___M.D. & F.R.S. in London*. Boston: Printed by James Franklin, 1722.

———. *A Dissertation Concerning Inoculation of the Small-Pox*. Boston: Printed for D. Henchman and T. Hancock, 1730.

———. *Inoculation of the Small Pox as practiced in Boston, Consider'd in a Letter to A__S__M.D. & F.R.S. in London*. Boston: Printed by James Franklin, 1722.

Duffy, John. *Epidemics in Colonial America*. Baton Rouge: Louisiana State University Press, 1953.

Duncan, S. R., Susan Scott, and C. J. Duncan. "The Dynamics of Smallpox Epidemics in Britain, 1550–1800." *Demography* 30, no. 3 (August 1993): 405–23.

———. "Smallpox Epidemics in Cities in Britain." *Journal of Interdisciplinary History* 25, no. 2 (Autumn 1994): 255–71.

Egan, Jim. *Authorizing Experience: Refigurations of the Body Politic in Seventeenth-Century New England Writing*. Princeton, NJ: Princeton University Press, 1999.

Ezzell, Carol. "Hope in a Vial." *Scientific American*, June 2002: 37–45.

Fenn, Elizabeth. *Pox Americana: The Great Smallpox Epidemic of 1775–82*. New York: Hill and Wang, 2001.

Field, Jonathan Beecher. "The Antinomian Controversy Did Not Take Place." *Early American Studies: An Interdisciplinary Journal* 6, no. 2 (2008): 448–63.

Fincher, Corey L., and Randy Thornhill. "Assortative Sociality, Limited Dispersal, Infectious Disease and the Genesis of the Global Pattern of Religion Diversity." *Proceedings of the Royal Society B* 275 (July 2008): 2587–94.

Gookin, Daniel. *Historical Collections of the Indians in New England*. Boston: Apollo Press, 1792.

Gordis, Lisa M. *Opening Scripture: Bible Reading and Interpretive Authority in Puritan New England*. Chicago: University of Chicago Press, 2003.

Grainger, Samuel. *The Imposition of Inoculation as a Duty Religiously Considered in a Leter to a Gentleman in the Country Inclin'd to Admit it*. Boston: Printed for Nicholas Boone and John Edwards, 1721.

Graunt, John. *Natural and Political Observations Mentioned in a Following Index and Made Upon the Bills of Mortality* (1662). Repr. New York: Arno Press, 1975.

Greenblatt, Stephen. *Shakespearean Negotiations: The Circulation of Social Energy in Renaissance England*. Berkeley: University of California Press, 1988.

Gura, Philip F. *A Glimpse of Sion's Glory: Puritan Radicalism in New England, 1620–1660*. Middletown, CT: Wesleyan University Press, 1984.

———. *Jonathan Edwards: America's Evangelical*. New York: Hill and Wang, 2005.

Hall, David D., ed. *The Antinomian Controversy, 1636–1638: A Documentary History*. 2nd ed. Durham, NC: Duke University Press, 1990.

———. "On Common Ground: The Coherence of American Puritan Studies." *William and Mary Quarterly* 44, no. 2 (1987): 193–229.

———. *The Faithful Shepherd: A History of the New England Ministry in the Seventeenth Century*. Chapel Hill: University of North Carolina Press, 1972.

Harriot, Thomas. *A Briefe and True Report of the New Found Land of Virginia* (1588/1590). Repr. New York: Dover, 1972.

Heath, Dwight, ed. *A Journal of the Pilgrims at Plymouth [Mourt's Relation]* (1622). Cambridge, MA: Applewood Books, 1986.

Herbert, Eugenia W. "Smallpox Inoculation in Africa." *Journal of African History* 16, no. 4 (1975): 539–59.

Higginson, Francis. "Higginson's Journal of his Voyage." Repr. in *Chronicles of the First Planters of the Colony of Massachusetts Bay, from 1623 to 1636*, ed. Alexander Young, 215–38. Boston, 1846.

———. *New Englands Plantation. Or, A Short and True Description of the Commodities and Discommodities of that Countrey*. London: Printed by T.C. and R.C. for Michael Sparke, 1630.

Hopkins, Donald R. *Princes and Peasants*. Chicago: University of Chicago Press, 1983.

Hubbard, William. *A General History of New England, from the Discovery to 1680 (ca. 1682)*. Repr. Collections of the Massachusetts Historical Society, 2nd ser., vol. 5. Boston, 1848.

Hulme, Peter. *Colonial Encounters: Europe and the Native Caribbean 1492–1797*. New York: Methuen, 1986.

Humins, John H. "Squanto and Massasoit: A Struggle for Power." *The New England Quarterly* 60, no. 1 (March 1987): 54–70.

Jenner, Edward. *An Inquiry into the Causes and Effects of the Variolae Vaccinae*. London: Printed by Sampson Low, 1798.

Jennings, Francis. *The Invasion of America: Indians, Colonialism and the Cant of Conquest*. New York: Norton, 1975.

Johnson, Charles. *Middle Passage*. New York: Atheneum, 1990.

Johnson, Edward. *A History of New-England [Wonder-Working Providence of Sions Saviour in New-England]*. London: Printed for Nath. Brooke, 1654.

Johnson, Steven. *The Ghost Map: The Story of London's Most Terrifying Epidemic—and How It Changed Science, Cities, and the Modern World*. New York: Penguin, 2006.

Jones, David S. *Rationalizing Epidemics: Meanings and Uses of American Indian Mortality since 1600*. Cambridge, MA: Harvard University Press, 2004.

———. "Virgin Soils Revisited." *William and Mary Quarterly* 60 (2003): 703–42.

Josselyn, John. *An Account of two Voyages to New-England*. 2nd ed. London: Printed for G. Widdowes, 1675.

Kamensky, Jane. *Governing the Tongue: The Politics of Speech in Early New England*. New York: Oxford University Press, 1997.

Kibbey, Ann. *The Interpretation of Material Shapes in Puritanism: A Study of Rhetoric, Prejudice, and Violence*. New York: Cambridge University Press, 1986.

Kittredge, George Lyman. "Cotton Mather's Election into the Royal Society." *Transactions of the Colonial Society of Massachusetts, 1911–1913*, 14. Boston, 1913: 81–114. Repr., Cohen, vol. 1.

———. "Cotton Mather's Scientific Communications with the Royal Society." *Proceedings of the American Antiquarian Society*. Worcester, 1916: 3–42. Repr., Cohen, vol. 1.

———. "Dr. Robert Child the Remonstrant." *Transactions of the Colonial Society of Massachusetts* 21. Boston, 1920: 1–146.

———. "Further Notes on Cotton Mather and the Royal Society." *Transactions of the Colonial Society of Massachusetts, 1911–1913*. Boston, 1913: 281–92. Repr., Cohen, vol. 1.

———. "Some Lost Works of Cotton Mather." *Proceedings of the Massachusetts Historical Society* 45. Boston, 1912: 418–79.

Klebs, Arnold C. "The Historic Evolution of Variolation." *Bulletin of the Johns Hopkins Hospital* 24, no. 265 (1913): 69–83, 70. Repr., Cohen, vol. 1.

Knight, Janice. *Orthodoxies in Massachusetts: Rereading American Puritanism.* Cambridge, MA: Harvard University Press, 1994.

Kupperman, Karen Ordahl. *Indians and English: Facing Off in Early America.* Ithaca, NY: Cornell University Press, 2000.

Lang, Amy Shrager. *Prophetic Woman: Anne Hutchinson and the Problem of Dissent in the Literature of New England.* Berkeley: University of California Press, 1987.

Lilienfeld, Abraham M., and David E. Lilienfeld. *Foundations of Epidemiology.* 2nd ed. New York: Oxford University Press, 1980.

Locke, John. *Two Treatises of Government* (1690). Ed. Peter Laslett. Cambridge, UK: Cambridge University Press, 2005.

Mackenthun, Gesa. *Metaphors of Dispossession: American Beginnings and the Translation of Empire 1492–1637.* Norman: University of Oklahoma Press, 1997.

Macpherson, C. B. *The Political Theory of Possessive Individualism: Hobbes to Locke.* New York: Oxford University Press, 1962.

Malan, Rian. "AIDS in Africa: In Search of the Truth." *Rolling Stone,* November 22, 2001: 70+.

———. "Megadeath and Megahype." *San Francisco Chronicle,* January 6, 2002: D1+.

Marten, Benjamin. *A New Theory of Consumptions: More Especially of a Phthisis, or Consumption of the Lungs.* London: Printed for R. Knaplock, A. Bell, J. Hooke, and C. King, 1720.

Massey, Edmund. *A Sermon against the Dangerous and sinful Practice of Inoculation.* 3rd ed. London 1722; repr. Boston: Printed for Benjamin Indicott, 1730.

[Mather, Cotton]. *An Account of the Method and Success of Inoculating the Small-Pox in Boston, in New-England.* London: Printed for J. Peele, 1722.

[———]. *Sentiments on the Small Pox Inoculated.* Boston: Printed by S. Kneeland for J. Edwards, 1721.

Mather, Cotton. *The Angel of Bethesda.* Ed. Gordon W. Jones. Barre, MA: American Antiquarian Society, 1972.

———. *Diary of Cotton Mather.* 2 vols. New York: Ungar, 1957.

———. *Magnalia Christi Americana* (1702). Repr. Ed. Kenneth B. Murdock. Cambridge, MA: Harvard University Press, 1977.

———. *Selected Letters of Cotton Mather.* Ed. Kenneth Silverman. Baton Rouge: Louisiana State University Press, 1971.

Mather, Increase. *Several Reasons Proving that Inoculating or Transplanting the Small Pox, is a Lawful Practice, and that it has been Blessed by GOD for the Saving of many a Life.* Boston: Printed by S. Kneeland for J. Edwards, 1721.

———. *Some further Account from London, of the Small-Pox Inoculated.* 2nd ed. Boston: Printed for J. Edwards, 1721.

Mausner, Judith S., and Anita K. Bahn. *Epidemiology: An Introductory Text.* Philadelphia: Saunders, 1974.

McNeill, William. *Plagues and Peoples.* New York: Anchor Books, 1998.

Middlekauff, Robert. *The Mathers: Three Generations of Puritan Intellectuals, 1596–1728.* New York: Oxford University Press, 1971.

Miller, Genevieve. *The Adoption of Inoculation for Smallpox in England and France.* Philadelphia: University of Pennsylvania Press, 1957.

Miller, Perry. *Errand into the Wilderness.* Cambridge, MA: Harvard University Press, 1956.

———. *The New England Mind: From Colony to Province.* Cambridge, MA: Harvard University Press, 1953.

———. *The New England Mind: The Seventeenth Century.* Cambridge, MA: Harvard University Press, 1939.

——. *Orthodoxy in Massachusetts 1630–1650: A Genetic Study.* Cambridge, MA: Harvard University Press, 1933.

Minardi, Margot. "The Inoculation Controversy of 1721–1722: An Incident in the History of Race." *The William and Mary Quarterly* 61, no. 1 (2004): 47–76.

Morgan, Edmund S. *Visible Saints: The History of a Puritan Idea.* New York: New York University Press, 1963.

Morrison, Toni. *Song of Solomon.* New York: Penguin, 1977.

Morton, Nathaniel. *New Englands Memoriall.* Cambridge: Printed by S.G. and M.J. for John Usher, 1669.

Morton, Thomas. *New English Canaan.* Amsterdam: Printed by Jacob Frederick Stam, 1637.

Mulford, Carla. "New Science and the Question of Identity in Eighteenth-Century British America." In *Finding Colonial Americas Essays Honoring J.A. Leo Lemay.* Eds. Mulford and David S. Shields, 79–103. Newark: University of Delaware Press, 2001.

——. "Pox and 'Hell-Fire': Boston's Smallpox Controversy, the New Science, and Early Modern Liberalism." In *Periodical Literature in Eighteenth-Century America.* Eds. Mark L. Kamrath and Sharon M. Harris, 7–27. Knoxville: University of Tennessee Press, 2005.

Murray, Iain H. *Jonathan Edwards: A New Biography.* Carlisle, PA: Banner of Truth Trust, 1987.

Newell, Margaret E. "Robert Child and the Entrepreneurial Vision: Economy and Ideology in Early New England." *The New England Quarterly* 68, no. 2 (1995): 223–56.

Norton, Mary Beth. *Founding Mothers & Fathers: Gendered Power and the Forming of American Society.* New York: Knopf, 1996.

Parrish, Susan Scott. *American Curiosity: Cultures of Natural History in the Colonial British Atlantic World.* Chapel Hill: University of North Carolina, 2006.

Patton, Cindy. *Globalizing AIDS.* Minneapolis: University of Minnesota Press, 2002.

——. "Performativity and Spatial Distinction: The End of AIDS Epidemiology." In *Performativity and Performance.* Eds. Andrew Parker and Eve Kosofsky Sedgwick, 173–96. New York: Routledge, 1995.

Pearce, Roy Harvey. *Savagism and Civilization.* Berkeley: University of California Press, 1988.

Pettit, Norman. *The Heart Prepared: Grace and Conversion in Puritan Spiritual Life.* 2nd ed. Middletown, CT: Wesleyan University Press, 1989.

Pope, Robert G. *The Half-Way Covenant: Church Membership in Puritan New England.* Princeton, NJ: Princeton University Press, 1969.

Pudaloff, Ross J. "Sign and Subject: Antinomianism in Massachusetts Bay." *Semiotica* 54 (1985): 147–63.

Reed, Ishmael. *Mumbo Jumbo.* New York: MacMillan, 1972.

Reiss, Oscar. *Medicine in Colonial America.* Lanham, MD: University Press of America, 2000.

Richardson, Margaret V., and Arthur T. Hertig. "New England's First Recorded Hydatidiform Mole." *New England Journal of Medicine* 207, no. 11 (March 1959): 544–45.

Rosenberg Charles E., and Janet Golden. *Framing Disease: Studies in Cultural History.* New Brunswick, NJ: Rutgers University Press, 1992.

Round, Phillip. *By Nature and by Custom Cursed: Transatlantic Civil Discourse and New England Cultural Production, 1620–1660.* Hanover, NH: University Press of New England, 1999.

Schutte, Anne Jacobson. "'Such Monstrous Births': A Neglected Aspect of the Antinomian Controversy." *Renaissance Quarterly* 38, no. 1 (1985): 85–106.

Shilts, Randy. *And the Band Played On: Politics, People, and the AIDS Epidemic.* New York: St. Martin's, 1987.

Shuffelton, Frank. "Indian Devils and Pilgrim Fathers: Squanto, Hobomok, and the English Conception of Indian Religion." *The New England Quarterly* 49, no. 1 (March 1976): 108–16.

Shurtleff, Nathaniel B., ed. *Records of the Governor and Company of the Massachusetts Bay in New England.* Vol. 1. Boston: W. White, 1853.

Smith, Henry Nash. *Virgin Land: The American West as Symbol and Myth.* Cambridge, MA: Harvard University Press, 1970.

Smith, John. *Advertisements for the Unexperienced Planters of New-England, or any where. Or, the Pathway to experience to erect a Plantation.* London: Printed by John Haviland, 1631.

———. *A Description of New England: Or The Observations, and discoveries, of Captain John Smith (Admirall of that Country) in the North of America, in the year of our Lord 1614.* London: Printed by Humfrey Lownes for Robert Clerke, 1616.

———. *The Generall Historie of Virginia, New-England, and the Summer Isles with the names of the Adventurers, Planters, and Governours from their first Beginning Anno 1584 to this present 1624.* London: Printed by I.D. and I.H. for Michael Sparkes, 1624.

———. *New Englands Trials.* 2nd ed. London: Printed by William Jones, 1622.

Snow Dean R., and Kim M. Lanphear. "European Contact and Indian Depopulation in the Northeast: The Timing of the First Epidemics." *Ethnohistory* 35 (Winter 1988): 15–33.

Snow, John. *On the Mode of Communication of Cholera* (1855). Repr. in *Snow on Cholera.* London: Oxford University Press, 1936.

Spiess, Arthur J., and Bruce D. Spiess. "The New England Pandemic of 1616–1622: Cause and Archaeological Implication." *Man in the Northeast* 34 (1987): 71–83.

Stearn, E. Wagner, and Allen E. Stearn. *The Effect of Small-Pox on the Destiny of the Amerindian.* Boston: Humphries, 1945.

Stearns, Raymond P. *Science in the British Colonies of America.* Urbana: University of Illinois Press, 1970.

Thornton, Russell. "Aboriginal North American Population and Rates of Decline, ca. A.D. 1500–1900." *Current Anthropology* 38, no. 2 (April 1997): 310–15.

Timmreck, Thomas C. *An Introduction to Epidemiology.* 3rd ed. Boston: Jones, 2002.

Tobin, Lad. "A Radically Different Voice: Gender and Language in the Trials of Anne Hutchinson." *Early American Literature* 25 (1990): 253–70.

Traister, Bryce. "Anne Hutchinson's 'Monstrous Birth' and the Feminization of Antinomianism." *Canadian Review of American Studies /Revue canadienne d'études américaines* 27, no. 2 (1997): 133–58.

Van De Wetering, Maxine. "A Reconsideration of the Inoculation Controversy." *The New England Quarterly* 58, no. 1 (1985): 46–67.

Wald, Priscilla. *Contagious: Cultures, Carriers, and the Outbreak Narrative.* Durham, NC: Duke University Press, 2008.

———. "Future Perfect: Grammar, Genes, and Geography." *New Literary History* 31 (2000): 681–708.

———. "Imagined Immunities." In *Cultural Studies and Political Theory.* Ed. Jodi Dean, 189–208. Ithaca, NY: Cornell University Press, 2000.

Walker, Williston. *The Creeds and Platforms of Congregationalism* (1893). Repr. Boston: Pilgrim, 1960.

———. *A History of the Congregational Churches in the United States.* New York: Christian Literature Co., 1894.

Warner, Margaret Humphreys. "Vindicating the Minister's Medical Role: Cotton Mather's Concept of the *Nishmath-Chajim* and the Spiritualization of Medicine." *Journal of the History of Medicine and Allied Sciences* 36, no. 3 (1981): 278–95.

Waters, John T. "Hingham, Massachusetts, 1631–1661: An East Anglican Oligarchy in the New World." *Journal of Social History* 1, no. 4 (1968): 351–70.

Watson, Patricia A. *The Angelical Conjunction: The Preacher-Physicians of Colonial New England.* Knoxville: University of Tennessee Press, 1991.

Watts, Sheldon. *Epidemics and History: Disease, Power and Imperialism.* New Haven, CT: Yale University Press, 1997.

Webster, Noah. *A Brief History of Epidemic and Pestilential Diseases.* 2 vols. Hartford: Printed by Hudson and Goodwin, 1799.

Wheelwright, John. "A Fast Day Sermon." Repr. in Hall, ed., *The Antinomian Controversy,* 152–72.

[White, John]. *The Planters Plea. Or The Grounds of Plantations Examined, and Usuall Objections Answered.* London: Printed by William Jones, 1630.

Wideman, John Edgar. *Fever.* New York: Penguin, 1989.

Wigglesworth, Michael. *The Diary of Michael Wigglesworth, 1653–1657.* Ed. Edmund S. Morgan. New York: Harper & Row, 1965.

———. "God's Controversy with New England." *Electronic Texts in American Studies.* Ed. Reiner Smolinski. Lincoln: University of Nebraska Press, 2007.

Williams, Roger. *The Correspondence of Roger Williams, 1629–1653,* vol. 1. Ed. Glenn W. LaFantasie. Providence, RI: Brown University Press, 1988.

Winship, Michael P. *Making Heretics: Militant Protestants and Free Grace in Massachusetts, 1636–1641.* Princeton, NJ: Princeton University Press, 2002.

Winslow, Edward. *Good Newes From New England. A True Relation of Things Very Remarkable at the Plantation of Plimoth in New England* (1624). Repr. Bedford, MA: Applewood Books, 1996.

———. *Hypocrisie Unmasked.* London: Printed by Rich. Cotes for John Bellamy, 1646.

———. *New-Englands Salamander.* London: Printed by Ric. Cotes, for John Bellamy, 1647.

Winslow, Ola Elizabeth. *A Destroying Angel: The Conquest of Smallpox in Colonial Boston.* Boston: Houghton Mifflin, 1974.

Winthrop, John. *Antinomians and Familists Condemned By the Synod of Elders in New England.* London: Printed for Ralph Smith, 1644.

———. *Generall Considerations for the Plantation in New England, with an Answer to Several Objections* (1629). Repr. in *The Winthrop Papers.* vol. 2. Ed. Stewart Mitchell. Boston: Massachusetts Historical Society, 1931.

———. *The Journal of John Winthrop 1630–1649.* Eds. Richard S. Dunn, James Savage, and Laetitia Yeandle. Cambridge, MA: Harvard University Press, 1996.

———. "A Model of Christian Charity." Repr. in *The Norton Anthology of American Literature.* 7th ed., Vol. A. Eds. Nina Baym, et al., 147–58. New York: Norton, 2007.

———. *A Short Story of the Rise, reign, and ruin of the Antinomians, Familists & Libertines, that infected the Churches of New-England* (1644). Repr. in Hall, ed., *The Antinomian Controversy,* 199–310.

———. *The Winthrop Papers,* Vol. 2, *1623–1630.* Ed. Stewart Mitchell. Boston: Massachusetts Historical Society, 1931.

———. *The Winthrop Papers,* Vol. 3, *1631–1637.* Ed. Allyn Bailey Forbes. Boston: Massachusetts Historical Society, 1943.

Wolf, Leonard A. "Squanto's Role in Pilgrim Diplomacy." *Ethnohistory* 11, no. 3 (Summer 1964): 247–61.

Wood, William. *New England's Prospect* (1634). Repr. Ed. Alden T. Vaughan. Amherst: University of Massachusetts Press, 1977.

Yarbrough, Slayden. "The Influence of Plymouth Colony Separatism on Salem: An Interpretation of John Cotton's Letter of 1630 to Samuel Skelton." *Church History* 51 (1982): 290–303.

Young, Alexander, ed. *Chronicles of the First Planters of the Colony of Massachusetts Bay, from 1623 to 1636.* Boston: Little and Brown, 1846.

———, ed. *Chronicles of the Pilgrim Fathers of the Colony of Plymouth from 1602 to 1625.* Boston: Little and Brown, 1844.

Ziff, Larzer. *Puritanism in America: New Culture in a New World.* New York: Viking Compass, 1973.

———. "The Salem Puritans in the 'Free Aire of a New World.'" *The Huntington Library Quarterly* 20 (1956): 373–84.

INDEX

Africa
  African knowledge appropriated, 169,
    173–74, 176, 178, 220n102
  African sailor infected with smallpox, 142,
    169
  Africans represented as untrustworthy
    narrators, 174–75, 182
  and Early American studies, 184–85
  and history of smallpox, 158
  HIV/AIDS in, 184–87, 189–91
  inoculation tested on Africans in Boston,
    169
  medical practices in, 151, 176
  representation of African speech, 171–76,
    182
  smallpox and slavery, 177–79
  source of inoculation in, 22, 169–73
  See also inoculation controversy; Onesimus
agricultural tropes, 28–29
Anabaptism. *See* Baptism
Anderson, Benedict, 8, 21, 165–66
Angel of Bethesda, 153–62, 173–74. *See also*
    Mather, Cotton
Anglo–American colonists
  defined immunologically, 14, 44, 106–8,
    111, 115, 138–39
  fear of traveling to Europe, 113
  shifting epidemiological patterns among,
    11, 19, 103–4, 117, 125, 132–33
  See also English colonists
Animalcula, 158–62
Anti-inoculators, 144–50. *See also* Douglass,
    William; Franklin, James; Grainger,
    Samuel
Antinomian controversy, 18–19
Antinomians defined, 80–81

assembly of women prohibited during, 99
civil prosecutions during, 83–86
charges of sedition in, 83–87
covenant of works and, 80–82
epidemiology and, 74–78, 85, 92–93,
    95–98
epistemology and, 91–92, 94, 99
fast-day sermon, 82–83
as figural epidemic, 74, 76–77, 97
gender and, 85–91, 96–97, 209n112
historiography of, 75–76, 85–87, 95–96
and justification, 81
as language controversy, 74, 81–83, 91–92,
    94, 98, 208n78
and orthodoxy, 76, 91–92
petition of remonstrance and, 84, 86,
    88–89
and sanctification, 80–81
trope of infection in, 74, 78–79
See also Hutchinson, Anne
Arneil, Barbara, 35–36, 44, 46–47

Backhouse, William, 68
Baillie, Robert, 68, 78, 122, 205n43
baptism, 69, 123–28, 130–32. *See also*
    Congregationalism; halfway covenant
Baudrillard, Jean, 75
Beall, Otho, 156
Bender, Thomas, 183
Bercovitch, Sacvan, 126, 129–30, 132–33
Biological determinism. *See* immunological
    determinism
Black, Francis, 48–50
Bonner, John, 107
Book of Common Prayer, 67–68